AF479234

PERIPHERAL VASCULAR INTERVENTIONS 1993

A Bibliographic Reference Manual

Gerald Dorros, M.D.
Clinical Professor in Medicine
University of Wisconsin-Madison
Madison, Wisconsin

Medical Director
The William Dorros-Isadore Feuer
Interventional Cardiovascular Disease Foundation, Ltd.
Milwaukee, Wisconsin

Cardiovascular Interventionist
Milwaukee Heart & Vascular Clinic, S.C.
Milwaukee, Wisconsin

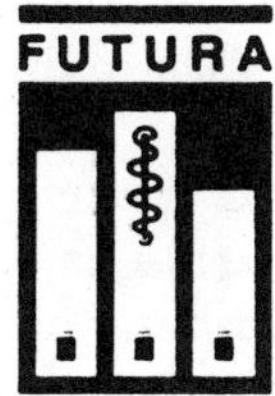

Futura Publishing Company
Mount Kisco, NY

Library of Congress Cataloging-in-Publication Data
is available.

Dorros, Gerald.
    Peripheral vascular interventions 1993 : a bibliographic reference
manual / Gerald Dorros.
        p.   cm.
    Includes bibliographical references and index.
    ISBN 0-87993-567-7 (alk. paper)
    1. Blood-vessels—Surgery—Bibliography. 2. Transluminal
angioplasty—Bibliography. 3. Thrombolytic therapy—Bibliography.
I. Title.
    [DNLM: 1. Angioplasty, Balloon—bibliography. 2. Fibrinolytic
Agents—therapeutic use—bibliography. 3. Vascular Diseases—
therapy—bibliography.   ZWG 500 D716p 1993]
Z6667.V35D674   1993
[RD598.5]
016.6174'13—dc20
DNLM/DLC
for Library of Congress   93-11900
                                                                         CIP

Copyright 1993
Futura Publishing Company, Inc.

Published by

Futura Publishing Company, Inc.
2 Bedford Ridge Road
Mount Kisco, New York 10549

L.C. No.: 93-11900
ISBN 0-87993-567-7

<u>Dedication</u>

This book is dedicated to the memory of my father,
William Dorros, and my grandfather, Isadore Feuer;
its purpose is to perpetuate their thoughts and
deeds which were to make the future better.

Acknowledgment

This book was made possible through a grant from

SANOFI WINTHROP PHARMACEUTICALS

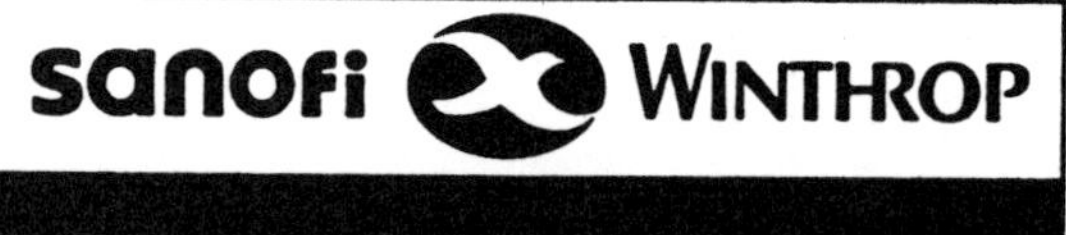

Foreword

Enhanced diagnostic techniques, improved balloon technology, atherectomy devices, percutaneous grafts, stents, and thrombolytic therapy have enabled and encouraged more and more radiologists, cardiologists, and vascular surgeons, each having their own unique perspective, to employ these percutaneous interventions.

Peripheral Vasular Interventions 1993: A Bibliographical Reference Manual becomes more important since it provides a rapid, concise, and easy method of accessing published data concerning percutaneous peripheral vascular interventions. Authors have been listed alphabetically and references have been arranged by topic [e.g., balloon angioplasty, atherectomy, laser applications, stents, intravascular ultrasound, and thrombolytic therapies (with the thrombolytic section including synopses of pertinent articles)].

Percutaneous interventions have become the standard of care for peripheral vascular disease and, as such, the cardiovascular interventionist should have a reference book that can assist in providing more effective interventional care.

Gerald Dorros, M.D., FACC, FESC (Eur.),
FSCAI, FACP, FACA, FCCP, SCVIR (Member)
Cardiovascular Interventionist

Contents

Section 4.

Thrombolytic Agents

Section 5.

Section 1

Angioplasty

I. Aorta or Mesenteric Vessels

Abad J, Hidalgo EG, Cantarero JM, Parga G, Fernandez R, Gomez M, Colina F, Moreno E (1989) Hepatic artery anastomotic stenosis after transplantation: treatment with percutaneous transluminal angioplasty. Radiology 171: 661–662.

Anonymous (1991) Balloon dilatation of native aortic coarctation [letter]. Int J Cardiol 31: 363–369.

Arai T, Mizuno K, Fujikawa A, Nakagawa M, Kikuchi M (1990) Infrared absorption spectra ranging from 2.5 to 10 microns at various layers of human normal abdominal aorta and fibrofatty atheroma in vitro. Lasers Surg Med 10: 357–362.

Archie JP Jr (1981) Balloon catheter for dilatation and thrombectomy for acute aortoiliac occlusion. Cardiovasc Dis Bull Texas Heart Inst 8: 546–549.

Attia IM, Lababidi ZA (1988) Early results of balloon angioplasty of native aortic coarctation in young adults. Am J Cardiol 61: 930–931.

Attia IM, Lababidi ZA (1988) Transumbilical balloon coarctation angioplasty. Am Heart J 116: 1623–1624.

Bahl VK, Das GS, Sharma S (1990) Percutaneous balloon angioplasty of congenital aortic stenosis and associated aortic coarctation in an adult. Am Heart J 120: 432–433.

Balaji S, Oommen R, Rees PG (1991) Fatal aortic rupture during balloon dilatation of recoarctation. Br Heart J 65: 100–101.

Belli AM, Hemingway AP, Cumberland DC, Welsh CL (1989) Percutaneous transluminal angioplasty of the distal abdominal aorta. Eur J Vasc Surg 3: 449–453.

Bongard O, Schneider PA, Krahenbuhl B, Bounameaux H (1992) Transluminal angioplasty of the aorta, renal and mesenteric arteries in Takayasu's arteritis: report of two cases. Eur J Vasc Surg 6(5): 567–571.

Brewster DC, Darling RC (1981) Optimum methods of aortoiliac reconstruction. Surgery 84: 739–748.

Brothers TE, Greenfield LJ (1990) Long-term results of aortoiliac reconstruction. J Vasc Intervent Radiol 1(1): 49–55.

Buchler JR, Braga SL, Fontes VF, Sousa JE (1987) Angioplasty for primary treatment of aortic coarctation: immediate results in two adult patients. Int J Cardiol 17: 7–14.

Bunt TJ (1986) Aortic reconstruction vs extra-anatomic bypass and angioplasty. Thoughts on evolving a protocol for selection. Arch Surg 121: 1166–1171.

Calderon M, Reul GJ, Gregoric ID, Jacobs MJ, Duncan JM, Ott DA, Livesay, JJ, et al. (1992) Long-term results of the surgical management of symptomatic chronic intestinal ischemia. J Cardiovasc Surg 33(6): 723–728.

Castaneda-Zuniga WR, Laerum F, Rysavy J, Rusnak B, Amplatz K (1982) Paralysis of arteries by intraluminal balloon dilatation. An experimental study. Radiology 144: 75–76.

Castaneda-Zuniga WR, Lock JE, Vlodaver Z, Rusnak B, Rysavy JP, Herrere M, Amplatz K (1982) Transluminal dilatation of coarctation of the abdominal aorta. An experimental study in dogs. Radiology 143: 693–697.

Charlebois N, Saint-Georges G, Hudon G (1986) Percutaneous transluminal angioplasty of the lower abdominal aorta. AJR 146: 369–371.

Chopra PS, Grassi CJ (1992) Superior mesenteric artery angioplasty with the TEGwire: usefulness and technical difficulties. J Vasc Intervent Radiol 3(3): 523–526.

Choy M, Rocchini AP, Beekman RH, Rosenthal A, Dick M, Crowley D, Behrendt D, Snider AR (1987) Paradoxical hypertension after repair of coarctation of the aorta in children: balloon angioplasty versus surgical repair. Circulation 75: 1186–1191.

Clugston RA, Eisenhauer AC, Matthews RV (1992) Atherectomy of the distal aorta using a "kissing-balloon" technique for the treatment of blue toe syndrome. AJR 159(1): 125–127.

Cooper JC, Welsh CL (1991) The role of percutaneous transluminal angioplasty in the treatment of critical ischaemia. Eur J Vasc Surg 5: 261–264.

Cooper RS, Ritter SB, Rothe WB, Chen CK, Griepp R, Golinko RJ (1987) Angioplasty for coarctation of the aorta: long-term results. Circulation 75: 600–604.

Cooper SG, Sullivan ID, Wren C (1989) Treatment of recoarctation: balloon dilation angioplasty. JACC 14: 413–419; discussion 420–421.

Da Costa AG, Iwahashi ER, Atik E, Rati MA, Ebaid M (1992) Persistence of hypoplastic and recoarcted fifth aortic arch associated with type A aortic arch interruption: surgical and balloon angioplasty results in an infant. Pediatr Cardiol 13(2): 104–106.

De Lezo JS, Sancho M, Pan M, Romero M, Olivera C, Luque M (1989) Angiographic follow-up after balloon angioplasty for coarctation of the aorta. JACC 13: 689–695.

Dev V, Kaul U, Jain P, Reddy S, Sharma S, Pandey G, Rajani M (1989) Percutaneous transluminal balloon angioplasty for obstruction of the suprahepatic inferior vena cava and cavo-atrial graft stenosis. Am J Cardiol 64: 397–399.

Dev V, Shrivastava S, Rajani M (1990) Percutaneous transluminal balloon angioplasty in Takayasu's aortitis: persistent benefit over two years. Am Heart J 120: 222–224.

Duckworth FP, Souch K, Roberts WN (1989) Takayasus' arteritis (clinical conference). VA Med Mon 116: 218–219, 222–223.

El Ashmaoui A, do DD, Triller J, Stirnemann P, Mahler F (1991) Angioplasty of the terminal aorta: follow-up of 20 patients treated by PTA or PTA with stents. Eur J Radiol 13: 113–117.

Erbel R, Bednarczyk I, Pop T, Todt M, Henrichs KJ, Brunier A, Thelen M, Meyer J (1990) Detection of dissection of the aortic intima and media after angioplasty of coarctation of the aorta. An angiographic, computer tomographic, and echocardiographic comparative study. Circulation 81: 805–814.

Fawzy ME, Dunn B, Galal O, Wilson N, Shaikh A, Sriram R, Duran CM (1992) Balloon coarctation angioplasty in adolescents and adults: early and intermediate results. Am Heart J 124(1): 167–171.

Feigin RD, Glickson M, Varstending A, Luria B, Gordon RL, Ring EJ, Tur-Kaspa R (1990) Familial Budd-Chiari syndrome due to membranous obstruction of the right hepatic vein treated with transluminal angio plasty. Am J Gastroenterol 85: 94–97.

Fontes VF, Esteves CA, Braga SL, da Silva MV, E Silva MA, Sousa JE, de Souza JA (1990) It is valid to dilate native aortic coarctation with a balloon catheter. Int J Cardiol 27: 311–316.

Frainas PL (1941) A new technique for arteriographic examination of the abdominal aorta and its branches. Am J Roentgenol 46: 641–645.

Furui S, Yamauchi T, Ohtomo K, Tsuchiya K, Makita K, Takenaka E (1988) Hepatic inferior vena cava obstructions: clinical results of treatment with percutaneous transluminal laser-assisted angioplasty. Radiology 166: 673–677.

Galal O, Qureshi SA, al Halees Z (1990) Reopening of the arterial duct after balloon dilatation of native coarctation. Int J Cardiol 27: 133–135.

Ginsburg R, Thorpe P, Bowles CR, Wright AM, Wexler L (1989) Pull-through approach to percutaneous angioplasty of totally occluded common iliac arteries. Radiology 172: 111–113.

Gu ZM, Lin G, Yi JR, Li JM, Zhou J, Pan WM (1988) Transluminal catheter angioplasty of abdominal aorta in Takayasu's arteritis. Acta Radiol 29: 509–513.

Haiart DC, Callam MJ, Muri JA, Ruckley CV, Jenkins AM (1991) Reoperations for late complications following abdominal aortic operation. Br J Surg 78: 204–206.

Harrison JK, Sheikh KH, Davidson CJ, Kisslo KB, Leithe ME, Himmelstein SI, Kanter RJ, Bashore TM (1990) Balloon angioplasty of coarctation of the aorta evaluated with intravascular ultrasound imaging. J Am Coll Cardiol 15: 906–909.

Henriksen LO, Jorgensen B, Holstein PE, Tonnesen KH, Karle A, Sager P

(1988) Percutaneous transluminal angioplasty of infrarenal arteries in intermittent claudication. Acta Chir Scand 154(10): 573–576.

Hess J, Mooyaart EL, Busch HJ, Bergstra A, Landsman ML (1986) Percutaneous transluminal balloon angioplasty in restenosis of coarctation of the aorta. Br Heart J 55: 459–461.

Hijazi ZM, Fahey JT, Kleinman CS, Hellenbrand WE (1991) Balloon angioplasty for recurrent coarctation of aorta. Immediate and long-term results. Circulation. 84: 1150–1156.

Ho SY, Somerville J, Yip WC, Anderson RH (1988) Transluminal balloon dilation of resected coarcted segments of thoracic aorta: histological study and clinical implications. Int J Cardiol 19: 99–105.

Hosie KB, Bolia A, Watkin DF (1988) Treatment of Budd-Chiari syndrome by percutaneous transluminal angioplasty [letter]. Lancet 2: 158–159.

Howd A, Loose H, Chamberlain J (1987) Transluminal angioplasty in the treatment of mesenteric vein graft stenosis. Cardiovasc Intervent Radiol 10: 43–45.

Hunter DW, So SK, Castaneda-Zuniga WR, Coleman CE, Sutherland DE, Amplatz K (1983) Failing or thrombosed Brescia-Cimino arteriovenous dialysis fistulas. Angiographic evaluation and percutaneous transluminal angioplasty. Radiology 149: 105–109.

Insall RL, Loose HW, Chamberlain J (1993) Long-term results of double-balloon percutaneous transluminal angioplasty of the aorta and iliac arteries. Eur J Vasc Surg 7(1): 31–36.

Isner JM, Donaldson RF, Fulton D, Bhan I, Payne DD, Cleveland RJ (1987) Cystic medial necrosis in coarctation of the aorta: a potential factor contributing to adverse consequences observed after percutaneous balloon angioplasty of coarctation sites. Circulation 75: 689–695.

Iyer SS, Hall P, Dorros G (1991) Brachial approach to management of an abdominal aortic occlusion with prolonged lysis and subsequent angioplasty. Cath Cardiovas Diagnosis. 23: 290–293.

Jenkins RD, Sinclair IN, Anand RK, James LM, Spears JR (1988) Laser balloon angioplasty: effect of exposure duration on shear strength of welded layers of postmortem human aorta. Lasers Surg Med 8: 392–396.

Johnston KW (1991) Aortoiliac disease treatment. A surgical comment [comment]. Circulation 83 (Suppl 2): I61–62.

Joyce DH, McGrath LB (1990) Pseudo-aneurysm formation following balloon angioplasty for recurrent coarctation of the aorta. Cathet Cardiovasc Diagn 20(2): 133–135.

Khalilullah M, Tyagi S (1992) Percutaneous transluminal angioplasty in Takayasu's arteritis. Heart Vessels 7(Suppl): 146–153.

Khalilullah M, Tyagi S, Lochan R, Yadav BS, Nair M, Gambhir DS, Khanna SK (1987) Percutaneous transluminal balloon angioplasty of the aorta in patients with aortitis. Circulation 76: 597–600.

Krotovsky GS, Turpitko SA, Gerasimov VB, Zabelskaya TF, Mamedov DM, Klokov KI, Uchkin IG, Papandopulos E (1991) Surgical treatment and prevention of vasculopathic impotence in conjunction with revascularisation of the lower extremities in Leriche's syndrome. J Cardiovasc Surg 32: 340–343.

Kumar S, Mandalam KR, Rao VR, Subramanyan R, Gupta AK, Joseph S, Unni M, Rao AS (1989) Percutaneous transluminal angioplasty in nonspecific aortoarteritis (Takayasu's disease): experience of 16 cases. Cardiovasc Intervent Radiol 12: 321–325.

Kumpe DA (1981) Percutaneous dilatation of an abdominal aortic stenosis: Three-balloon catheter technique. Radiology 141: 536–538.

Laissy JP, Thiebot J, Peillon C, Watelet J, Testart J, Benozio M (1987) Axillo-femoral bypass failure secondary to axillary stenosis: ultrasound-guided percutaneous transluminal angioplasty. Bildgebung 56: 185–186.

Laufer G, Wollenek G, Hohla K, Horvat R, Henke KH, Buchelt M, Wutzl G, Wolner E (1988) Excimer laser-induced simultaneous ablation and spectral identification of normal and atherosclerotic arterial tissue layers. Circulation 78: 1031–1039.

Lee BI, Becker GJ, Waller BF, Barry KJ, Connolly RJ, Kaplan J, Shapiro AR, Nardella PC (1989) Thermal compression and molding of atherosclerotic vascular tissue with use of radiofrequency energy: implications for radiofrequency balloon angioplasty. J Am Coll Cardiol 13: 1167–1175.

Levy PJ, Haskell L, Gordon RL (1987) Percutaneous transluminal angioplasty of splanchnic arteries: an alternative method to elective revascularisation in chronic visceral ischaemia. Eur J Radiol 7: 239–242.

Lewis AB, Takahashi M (1988) Plasma catecholamine responses to balloon angioplasty in children with coarctation of the aorta. Am J Cardiol 62: 649–650.

Lewis VD, 3d, Meranze SG, McLean GK, O'Neill JA, Jr, Berkowitz HD, Burke DR (1988) The midaortic syndrome: diagnosis and treatment [see comments]. Comment in: Radiology 1989 Feb;170(2): 571–2. Radiology 167: 111–113.

Lo RN, Leung MP, Yau KK, Cheung DL (1989) Transvenous antegrade balloon angioplasty for recoarctation of the aorta in an infant. Am Heart J 117: 1157–1159.

Lock JE, Casteneda-Zuniga WR, Bass JL, Foker JE, Amplatz K, Anderson RW (1982) Balloon dilatation of excised aortic coarctations. Radiology 143: 689–691.

Lois JF, Hartzman S, McGlade CT, Gomes AS, Grant EC, Berquist W, Perrella RR, Busuttil RW (1989) Budd-Chiari syndrome: treatment with percutaneous transhepatic recanalization and dilation. Radiology 170: 791–793.

Loya YS, Sharma S, Amrapurkar DN, Desai HG (1989) Complete membranous obstruction of inferior vena cava: case treated by balloon dilatation. Cathet Cardiovasc Diagn 17(3): 164–167.

Mandalam KR, Rao VR, Neelakandhan KS, Kumar S, Unnikrishnan M, Mukhopadhyay S (1992) Hyperperfusion syndrome following balloon angioplasty and bypass surgery of aortic arch vessels: a report of 3 cases. Cardiovasc Intervent Radiol 15(2): 108–112.

Mantoni MY, Holstein P (1990) Aorto-femoral digital subtraction angiography in old patients with symptoms of peripheral arterial disease. Findings, efficacy, and consequences. Dan Med Bull 37: 192–193.

Martin RP, Qureshi SA, Arnold R (1989) Percutaneous balloon aortoplasty of recoarctation: an alternative approach using the axillary artery. Int J Cardiol 22: 119–121.

McShane MD, Proctor A, Spencer P, Cumberland DC, Welsh CL (1992) Mesenteric angioplasty for chronic intestinal ischaemia. Eur J Vasc Surg 6(3): 333–336.

Mee C (1989) Treatment of chronic mesenteric ischaemia by percutaneous transluminal angioplasty. Radiogr Today 55: 19–21.

Millward SF, Jaward MA, Henderson DR (1989) Percutaneous transluminal angioplasty of stenosis at the common iliac artery origin using a single-balloon technique. Can Assoc Radiol J 40: 38–39.

Minich LL, Beekman RH 3d, Rocchini AP, Heidelberger K, Bove EL (1992) Surgical repair is safe and effective after unsuccessful balloon angioplasty of native coarctation of the aorta. J Coll Cardiol 19(2): 389–393.

Mitchell SE, Kadir S, Kaufman SL, Chang R, Williams GM, Kan JS, White RI Jr (1983) Percutaneous transluminal angioplasty of aortic graft stenoses. Radiology 149: 439–444.

Moneta GL, Schneider E, Jager K, Brulisauer M, Thuring-Vollenweider U, Bollinger A (1988) Laser Doppler flux and vasomotion in patients before and after transluminal angioplasty for limb salvage. Vasa 17: 26–31.

Morag B, Garniek A, Bass A, Schneiderman J, Walden R, Rubinstein ZJ (1993) Percutaneous transluminal aortic angioplasty: early and late results. Cardiovasc Intervent Radiol 16(1): 37–42.

Morag B, Rubinstein Z, Kessler A, Schneiderman J, Levinkopf M, Bass A (1987) Percutaneous transluminal angioplasty of the distal abdominal aorta and its bifurcation. Cardiovasc Intervent Radiol 10: 129–133.

Morris GC. DeBakey ME (1961) Abdominal angina: diagnosis and treatment. JAMA 176: 89–92.

Morrow WR, Vick GW 3rd, Nihill MR, Rokey R, Johnston DL, Hedrick TD, Mullins CE (1988) Balloon dilation of unoperated coarctation of the aorta: short- and intermediate-term results. JACC 11: 133–138.

Motarjeme A, Keifer JW, Zuska AJ (1981) Percutaneous transluminal angioplasty as a complement to surgery. Radiology 141: 341–346.

Nawa S, Nakayama Y, Teramoto S, Mori K, Dohi T (1989) Coarctation restenosis after isthmosubclavioplasty. A consideration on operative procedure and intraluminal balloon angioplasty. Chest 95: 247–250.

Nevelsteen A, Beyens G, Duchateau J, Suy R (1990) Aorto-femoral reconstruction and sexual function: a prospective study. Eur J Vasc Surg 4: 247–251.

Norstein J, Brekke IB, Holdaas H, Vatne K (1990) Arterial stenoses in duct occluded segmental pancreatic grafts treated with percutaneous transluminal angioplasty. Transplant Proc 22: 599–601.

Odurny A, Colapinto RF, Sniderman KW, Johnston KW (1989) Percutaneous transluminal angioplasty of abdominal aortic stenoses. Cardiovasc Intervent Radiol 12: 1–6.

Odurny A, Sniderman KW, Colapinto RF (1988) Intestinal angina: percutaneous transluminal angioplasty of the celiac and superior mesenteric arteries. Radiology 167: 59–62.

Palmaz JC, Encarnacion CE, Garcia OJ, Schatz RA, Rivera FJ, Laborde JC, Dougherty SP (1991) Aortic bifurcation stenosis: treatment with intravascular stents. J Vasc Intervent Radiol 2(3): 319–323.

Park JH, Han MC, Kim SH, Oh BH, Park YB, Seo JD (1989) Takayasu's arteritis: angiographic findings and results of angioplasty. AJR AM J Roentgenol 153: 1069–1074.

Pavlovic D, Suarez de Lezo J, Medina A, Romero M, Hernandez E, Pan M, Tejero I, Melian F (1992) Sequential transcatheter treatment of combined coarctation of aorta and persistent ductus arteriosus. Am Heart J 123(1): 249–250.

Pelikan P, French WJ, Ruiz C, Laks H, Criley JM (1988) Percutaneous double-balloon angioplasty of a stenotic modified Fontan aortic homograft conduit. Cathet Cardiovasc Diagn 15: 47–51.

Raby N, Karani J, Thomas S, O'Grady J, Williams R (1991) Stenoses of vascular anastomoses after hepatic transplantation: treatment with balloon angioplasty. AJR 157: 167–171.

Radner S (1948) Thoracal aortography by catheterization from the radial artery. Arch Radiol (Diagn) (Stockh) 29: 178–180.

Rao PS (1991) Fatal aortic rupture during balloon dilatation of recoarctation [letter]. Br Heart J 66: 406–407.

Rao PS (1991) Pseudoaneurysm following balloon angioplasty? [letter] Cathet Cardiovasc Diag 23: 150–152.

Rao PS (1989) Balloon angioplasty and valvuloplasty in infants, children, and adolescents. REVIEW ARTICLE: 225 REFS. Curr Probl Cardiol 14: 417–497.

Rao PS (1989) Balloon angioplasty of aortic coarctation: a review. REVIEW ARTICLE: 80 REFS. Clin Cardiol 12: 618–628.

Rao PS (1989) Balloon valvuloplasty and angioplasty in infants and children. REVIEW ARTICLE: 77 REFS. J Pediatr 114: 907–914.

Rao PS (1989) Which aortic coarctations should we balloon-dilate (editorial) Am Heart J 117: 987–989.

Rao PS (1987) Balloon angioplasty for coarctation of the aorta in infancy. J Pediatr 110: 713–718.

Rao PS, Carey P (1989) Remodeling of the aorta after successful balloon coarctation angioplasty. J Am Coll Cardiol 14: 1312–1317.

Rao PS, Chopra PS (1991) Role of balloon angioplasty in the treatment of aortic coarctation. Ann Thorac Surg 52: 621–631.

Rao PS, Najjar HN, Mardini MK, Solymar L, Thapar MK (1988) Balloon angioplasty for coarctation of the aorta: immediate and long-term results. REVIEW ARTICLE: 56 REFS. Am Heart J 115: 657–665.

Rao PS, Solymar L (1988) Transductal balloon angioplasty for coarctation of the aorta in the neonate: preliminary observations. Am Heart J 116: 1558–1562.

Rao PS, Thapar MK, Kutayli F, Carey P (1989) Causes of recoarctation after balloon angioplasty of unoperated aortic coarctation. JACC 13: 109–115.

Ravimandalam K, Rao VR, Kumar S, Gupta AK, Joseph S, Unni M, Rao AS (1991) Obstruction of the infrarenal portion of the abdominal aorta: results of treatment with balloon angioplasty. AJR 156: 1257–1260.

Ritter SB (1989) Coarctation and balloons: inflated or realistic? J Am Coll Cardiol 13: 696–699.

Salahuddin N, Wilson AD, Rao PS (1991) An unusual presentation of coarctation of the aorta in infancy: role of balloon angioplasty in the critically ill infant. Am Heart J 122: 1772–1775.

Sanyal SK, Wilson N, Twum-Danso K, Abomelha A, Sohel S (1990) Moraxella endocarditis following balloon angioplasty of aortic coarctation. Am Heart J 119: 1421–1423.

Selby JB Jr, Matsumoto AH, Tegtmeyer CJ, Hartwell GD, Tribble CG, Daniel TM, Kron IL et al. (1993) Balloon angioplasty above the aortic arch: immediate and long-term results. AJR 160(3): 631–635.

Sharma S, Bhagwat AR, Loya YS (1991) Percutaneous balloon angioplasty for native coarctation of the aorta. Early and intermediate term results. J Assoc Physicians India 39(8): 610–613.

Sharma S, Loya YS, Daxini BV (1991) Coarctation of aorta with unusual association of diverticulum of the left ventricle and double orifice mitral valve. Int J Cardiol 30: 113–115.

Sharma S, Rajani M, Kaul U, Talwar KK, Dev V, Shrivastava S (1990) Initial experience with percutaneous transluminal angioplasty in the management of Takayasu's arteritis. Br J Radiol 63: 517–522.

Sharma S, Rajani M, Shrivastava S, Kaul U, Kamalakar T, Talwar KK, Saxena A (1991) Non-specific aorto-arteritis (Takayasu's disease) in children. Br J Radiol 64: 690–698.

Shimshak TM, Giorgi LV, Hartzler GO (1988) Successful percutaneous transluminal angioplasty of an obstructed abdominal aorta secondary to a chronic dissection. Am J Cardiol 61: 486–487.

Sise MJ, Counihan CM, Shackford SR, Rowley WR (1988) The clinical spectrum of Takayasu's arteritis. Surgery 104: 905–910.

Soulen RL, Kan J, Mitchell S, White RI Jr (1987) Evaluation of balloon angioplasty of coarctation restenosis by magnetic resonance imaging. Am J Cardiol 60: 343–345.

Stoney RJ, Ehrenfeld WK, Wylie EJ (1977) Revascularization methods in chronic visceral ischemia caused by atherosclerosis. Ann Surg 186: 468–476.

Tadavarthy AK, Sullivan WA Jr, Nicoloff D, Castaneda-Zuniga WR, Hunter DW, Amplatz K (1989) Aorta balloon angioplasty: 9-year follow-up. Radiology 170: 1039–1041.

Tegtmeyer CJ, Hartwell GD, Selby JB, Robertson R Jr, Kron IL, Tribble CG (1991) Results and complications of angioplasty in aortoiliac disease [comments]. Circulation 83 (Suppl 2): I53–60.

Tegtmeyer CJ, Wellons HA, Thompson RN (1980) Balloon dilatation of the abdominal aorta. JAMA 244: 2636–2637.

Tyagi S, Arora R, Kaul UA, Sethi KK, Gambhir DS, Khalilullah M (1992) Balloon angioplasty of native coarctation of the aorta in adolescents and young adults. Am Heart J 123(3): 674–680.

Tyagi S, Kaul UA, Nair M, Sethi KK, Arora R, Khalilullah M (1992) Balloon angioplasty of the aorta in Takayasu's arteritis: initial and long-term results. Am Heart J 124(4): 876–882.

Van Beers B, Roche A, Cauquil P (1988) Transluminal angioplasty of a stenotic surgical splenorenal shunt. Acta Radiol 29: 327–329.

VanDeinse WH, Zawacki JK, Phillips D (1986) Treatment of acute mesenteric ischemia by percutaneous transluminal angioplasty. Gastroenterology 91: 475–478.

Velasquez G, Castaneda-Zuniga W, Formanek A, Zollikofer C, Barreto A, Nicoloff D, Amplatz K, Sullivan A (1980) Nonsurgical aortoplasty in Leriche syndrome. Radiology 143: 359–360.

Volodos NL, Karpovich IP, Troyan VI, Kalashnikova YuV, Shekhanin VE, Ternyuk NE, Neoneta AS, Ustinov NI, Yakovenko LF (1991) Clinical experience of the use of self-fixing synthetic prostheses for remote endoprosthetics of the thoracic and the abdominal aorta and iliac arteries through the femoral artery and as intraoperative endoprosthesis for aorta reconstruction. Vasa Suppl 33: 93–95.

Vorwerk D, Gunther RW, Bohndorf K, Keulers P (1991) Stent placement for failed angioplasty of aortic stenoses: report of two cases. Cardiovasc Intervent Radiol 14: 316–319.

Waldman JD (1991) Make balloon dilatation an approved procedure for recurrent coarctation in children [editorial; comment] Circulation 84: 1440–1441.

Walker PJ, Harris JP, May J (1991) Combined percutaneous transluminal angioplasty and extraanatomic bypass for symptomatic unilateral iliac artery occlusion with contralateral iliac artery stenosis. Ann Vasc Surg 5: 209–216.

Walstra BR, Janevski BK (1987) Sequential PTA of abdominal aorta. Haemodynamic evaluation and IV-DSA follow-up. ROFO 146: 446–449.

Williams DM, Andrews JC, Marx MV, Abrams GD (1993) Creation of reentry tears in aortic dissection by means of percutaneous balloon fenestration: gross anatomic and histologic considerations. J Vasc Intervent Radiol 4(1): 75–83.

Williams DM, Brothers TE, Messina LM (1990) Relief of mesenteric ischemia in type III aortic dissection with percutaneous fenestration of the aortic septum. Radiology 174: 450–452.

Williams DM, Simon HJ, Marx MV, Starkey TD (1992) Acute traumatic aortic rupture: intravascular US findings. Radiology 182: 247–249.

Wilms G, Baert AL (1986) Transluminal angioplasty of superior mesenteric artery and celiac trunk. Ann Radiol (Paris) 29: 535–538.

Yakes WF, Kumpe DA, Brown SB, Parker SH, Lattes RG, Cook PS, Haas DK, Gibson MD, Hopper KD, Reed MD, et al (1989) Percutaneous transluminal aortic angioplasty: techniques and results. Radiology 172: 965–970.

Zheng D, Fan D, Liu L (1992) Takayasu's arteritis in China: a report of 530 cases. Heart Vessels 7(Suppl): 32–36.

II. Brachiocephalic

Allen HD, Marx GR, Ovitt TW, Goldberg SJ (1986) Balloon dilation angioplasty for coarctation of the aorta. Am J Cardiol 57: 828–832.

Angelini P, Bush HS (1988) Brachial artery injury as a complication of cardiac catheterization: percutaneous transluminal angioplasty and streptokinase as a treatment alternative. Cathet Cardiovasc Diagn 15: 243–246.

Appleberg M (1977) Graduated internal dilatation in the treatment of fibromuscular dysplasia of the internal carotid artery. SA Med J 51: 244–246.

Bachman DM, Kim RM (1980) Transluminal dilatation for subclavian steal syndrome. AJR 135: 995–996.

Baker RN, Carroll-Ramseyer J, Schauartz WS (1968) Prognosis in patients with transient ischemic attacks. Neurology 18: 1157–1165.

Barnwell SL, Higashida RT, Halbach VV, Dowd CF, Wilson CB, Hieshima GB (1989) Transluminal angioplasty of intracerebral vessels for cerebral arterial spasm: reversal of neurological deficits after delayed treatment. Neurosurgery 25: 424–429.

Barth KH (1983) A modified catheter for transluminal angioplasty of the femoropopliteal artery. Radiology 149: 598–599.

Basche S, Ritter H, Gaerisch F, Grossman K, Heerklotz I, Schumann E (1983) Percutaneous transluminal angioplasty of the subclavian artery. Zentralbl Chir 108: 142–149.

Bean WJ, Rodan BA, Franqui DA (1984) Subclavian steal: treatment with percutaneous transluminal angioplasty. South Med J 77: 1044–1046.

Beekman RH, Rocchini AP, Behrendt DM, Bove EL, Dick M 2d, Crowley DC, Snider AR, Rosenthal A (1986) Long-term outcome after repair of coarctation in infancy: subclavian angioplasty does not reduce the need for reoperation. JACC 8: 1406–1411.

Beekman RH, Rocchine AP, Dick M 2nd, Snider AR, Crowley DC, Serwer GA, Spicer RL, Rosenthal A (1987) Percutaneous balloon angioplasty for native coarctation of the aorta. JACC 10: 1078–1084.

Belan A, Vesela M, Vanek I, Weiss K, Peregrin JH (1982) Percutaneous transluminal angioplasty of fibromuscular dysplasia of the internal carotid artery. Cardiovasc Intervent Radiol 5: 79–81.

Belz M, Marshall JJ, Cowley MJ, Vetrovec GW (1992) Subclavian balloon angioplasty in the management of the coronary-subclavian steal syndrome. Cathet Cardiovas Diag 25(2): 161–163.

Bird CR, Hasso AN (1983) Transluminal angioplaslty of the carotid artery, in Castaneda-Zuniga WR (ed) New Applications of Transluminal Angio-plasty. New York, Thieme-Stratton, Inc., pp 154–161.

Bockenheimer SA, Mathias K (1983) Percutaneous transluminal angio-plasty in arteriosclerotic internal carotid artery stenosis. AJNR 4: 791–792.

Bockenheimer SAM, Mathias K (1983) Percutaneous transluminal angio-plasty in supra-aortic artery disease. Medicamundi 28: 87–89.

Brady HR, Fitzcharles B, Goldberg H, Huraib S, Richardson T, Simons M, Uldall PR (1989) Diagnosis and management of subclavian vein throm-bosis occurring in association with subclavian cannulation for hemodi-alysis. Blood Purif 7: 210–217.

Brandt C, Sandhu A (1988) Subclavian steal syndrome and its management by angioplasty. Radiography 54: 83–85.

Braun IF, Battey PM, Fulenwider JT, Per-Lee JH (1986) Transcatheter carotid occlusion: an alternative to the surgical treatment of cervical carotid aneurysms. J Vasc Surg 4: 299–302.

Bret J (1981) Neuroradiology; Recanalization of Sylvian aqueduct. Eur J Radiol 1: 67–70.

Brosnahan D, McFadzean RM, Teasdale E (1992) Neuro-ophthalmic fea-tures of carotid cavernous fistulas and their treatment by endoarterial balloon embolisation. J Neurol Neurosurg Psychiatry 55(7): 553–556.

Brothers MF, Holgate RC (1990) Intracranial angioplasty for treatment of vasospasm after subarachnoid hemorrhage: technique and modifica-tions to improve branch access. AJNR 11: 239–247.

Brown MM, Butler P, Gibbs J, Swash M, Waterston J (1990) Feasibility of percutaneous transluminal angioplasty for carotid artery stenosis. J Neurol Neurosurg Psychiatry 53: 238–243.

Bruckmann H (1988) Vertebral percutaneous transluminal angioplasty (let-ter). AJNR 9: 607–608.

Bruckmann H, Ringelstein EB, Buchner H, Zeumer H (1986) Percutaneous transluminal angioplasty of the vertebral artery. A therapeutic alterna-tive to operative reconstruction of proximal vertebral artery stenoses. J Neurol 233: 336–339.

Burke DR, Gordon RL, Mishkin JD, McLean GK, Meranze SG (1987) Percu-taneous transluminal angioplasty of subclavian arteries. Radiology 164: 699–704.

Campbell DB, Bartholomew M, Waldhausen JA (1986) The case for subcla-vian flap repair (editorial). JACC 8: 1412.

Cartlidge NEF, Whisnant JJP, Elveback LR (1977) Carotid and vertebral basilar transient cerebral ischemic attacks. Mayo Clin Proc 52: 117–120.

Cook AM, Dyet JF (1989) Six cases of subclavian stenosis treated by percutaneous angioplasty. Clin Radiol 40: 352–354.

Courtheoux P, Theron J, Maiza D, Derlon JM, Pelouze GA, Henriet JP, Evrard C, Commeau P (1984) Endoluminal angioplasty for atheromatous stenoses of supra-aortic trunks. The brachiocephalic arterial trunk, subclavian arteries. J Radiol 65: 845–851.

Courtheoux P, Tournade A, Theron J, Henriet JP, Maiza D, Derlon JM, Pelouze G, Evrard C (1985) Transcutaneous angioplasty of vertebral artery atheromatous ostial structure. Neuroradiology 27: 259–264.

Culicchia F, Spetzler RF, Flom RA (1991) Failure of transluminal angioplasty in the treatment of myointimal hyperplasia of the internal carotid artery: case report. Neurosurgery 28: 148–151.

Damuth HD Jr, Diamond AB, Rappoport AS, Renner JW (1983) Angioplasty of subclavian artery stenosis proximal to the vertebral origin. AJNR 4: 1239–1242.

Daniell SJ, Dacie JE (1988) Percutaneous transluminal angioplasty of brachiocephalic vein stenoses in patients with dialysis shunts [letter]. Radiology 169: 280–281.

DeBakey ME, Crawford ES, Cooley DA, Morris GC Jr, Garrett E, Fields WS (1965) Cerebral arterial insufficiency. One to 11 years result following arterial reconstructive operation. Am J Surg 161: 921–945.

Deligonul U, Gabliani G, Kern MJ, Vandormael M (1988) Percutaneous brachial catheterization: the hidden hazard of high brachial artery bifurcation. Cathet Cardiovasc Diagn 14: 44–45.

Delos Reyes RA, Ausman JI, Diaz FG, Pak H, Pearce JE, Dujouny M (1983) The surgical management of vertebrobasilar insufficiency. Acta Neurochir 68: 203–216.

DeMonte F, Peerless SJ, Rankin RN (1989) Carotid transluminal angioplasty with evidence of distal embolization. Case report [see comments]. Comment in: J Neurosurg 71: 301. J Neurosurg 70: 138–141.

Derauf BJ, Erickson DL, Castaneda-Zuniga WR, Cardella JF, Amplatz K (1986) Washout: technique for brachiocephalic angioplasty. AJR 146: 849–851.

Donald JJ, Raphael MJ (1991) Pulsatile tinnitus relieved by angioplasty. Clin Radiol 43: 132–134.

Dorros G (1984) The brachial artery method to peripheral transluminal angioplasty. Cathet Cardiovasc Diagn 10: 115–127.

Dorros G, Lewin RF (1987) Percutaneous transluminal angioplasty of a brachial artery occlusion after cardiac catheterization. Am J Cardiol 59: 163.

Dorros G, Lewin RF, Jamnadas P, Mathiak LM (1990) Peripheral transluminal angioplasty of the subclavian and innominate arteries utilizing the brachial aproach: acute outcome and follow-up. REVIEW ARTICLE: 17 REFS. Cathet Cardiovasc Diagn 19: 71–76.

Duber C, Klose KJ, Kopp H, Schmiedt W (1992) Percutaneous transluminal angioplasty for occlusion of the subclavian artery: short- and long-term results. Cardiovasc Intervent Radiol 15(4): 205–210.

Dublin AB, Baltaxe HA, Cobb CA 3rd (1983) Percutaneous transluminal carotid angioplasty in fibromuscular dysplasia. Case report. J Neurosurg 59: 162–165.

Dublin AB, Baltaxe HA, Cobb CA 3rd (1984) Percutaneous transluminal carotid angioplasty and detachable balloon embolization in fibromuscular dysplasia. AJNR 5: 646–648.

Effeney DJ, Ehrenfeld WK, Stoney RJ, Wylie EJ (1980) Why operate on carotid fibromuscular dysplasia? Arch Surg 115: 1261–1265.

Erbstein RA, Wholey MH, Smoot S (1988) Subclavian artery steal syndrome: treatment by percutaneous transluminal angioplasty. AJR 151: 291–294.

Eskridge JM, Newell DW, Pendleton GA (1990) Transluminal angioplasty for treatment of vasospasm. Neurosurg Clin N Am 1(2): 387–399.

Farina C, Mingoli A, Schultz RD, Castrucci M, Feldhaus RJ, Rossi P, Cavallaro A (1989) Percutaneous transluminal angioplasty versus surgery for subclavian artery occlusive disease. Am J Surg 158: 511–514.

Feld H, Nathan P, Raninga D, Shani J (1992) Symptomatic angina secondary to coronary-subclavian steal syndrome treated successfully by percutaneous transluminal angioplasty of the subclavian artery. Cathet Cardiovasc Diagn 26(1): 12–14.

Ferris EJ (1981) Why operate on carotid fibromuscular dysplasia? Radiology 139: 534.

Freitag G, et al (1986) Percutaneous angioplasty of carotid artery stenoses. Neuroradiology 28: 126–127.

Freitag G, Freitag J, Koch RD, Heinrich P, Wagemann W, Hennig HP, Deike R (1987) Transluminal angioplasty for the treatment of carotid artery stenoses. Vasa 16: 67–71.

Gale SS (1989) Residual lesions and early recurrent stenosis after carotid endarterectomy [letter; comment]. Comment on: J Vasc Surg 1987 May; 5(5): 731–737. J Vasc Surg 10: 705–707.

Galichia JP, Bajaj AK, Vine DL, Roberts RW (1983) Subclavian artery stenosis treated by transluminal angioplasty: six cases. Cardiovasc Intervent Radiol 6: 78–81.

Garrido E, Garofola JH (1983) Intraluminal dilatation of the innominate artery before extracranial-intracranial bypass: case report. Neurosurgery 13: 581–583.

Garrido E, Montoya J (1981) Transluminal dilatation of internal carotid artery in fibromuscular dysplasia: a preliminary report. Surg Neurol 16: 469–471.

George SM Jr, Noon GP, Hausknecht MJ (1991) Coronary-subclavian steal: correction of recurrent angina and cerebrovascular symptoms. J Cardiovasc Surg 32: 523–526.

Giller CA, Mathews D, Purdy P, Kopitnik TA, Batjer HH, Samson DS (1992) The transcranial Doppler appearance of acute carotid artery occlusion. Ann Neurol 31(1): 101–103.

Gordon RL, Haskell L, Hirsch M, Shifrin E, Weinman E, Romanoff H (1985) Transluminal dilatation of the subclavian artery. Cardiovasc Intervent Radiol 8: 14–19.

Grantzig A, Hopff H (1974) Perkutane rekanalisation chronischer arterieller verschluse mit rinem neuren dilatations-catheter. Dtsch Med Wochenschr 99: 2502–2505.

Grimes CM (1991) Cerebral balloon angioplasty for treatment of vasospasm after subarachnoid hemorrhage. Heart & Lung 20(5Pt 1): 431:435.

Grote R, Freyschmidt J, Walterbusch G (1983) Percutaneous transluminal angioplasty in proximal subclavian stenoses. ROFO 138: 660–664.

Hanakita J, Suwa H, Nishihara K, Iihara K, Sakaida H (1991) Giant pseudoaneurysm of the extracranial vertebral artery successfully treated using intraoperative balloon catheters. Neurosurgery 28: 738–741.

Hasso AN, et al (1981) Fibromuscular dysplasia of the internal carotid artery: percutaneous transluminal angioplasty. AJR 136: 955–960.

Hasso AN, Bird CR, Zinke DE, Thompson JR (1981) Fibromuscular dysplasia of the internal carotid artery: percutaneous transluminal angioplasty. AJNR 2: 175–180.

Hebrang A, Maskovic J, Tomac B (1991) Percutaneous transluminal angioplasty of the subclavian arteries: long-term results in 52 patients. AJR 156: 1091–1094.

Herring M (1977) The subclavian steal syndrome: a review. Surgery 43: 222–228.

Hieshima GS, Higashida RT, Halbach VV (1990) Intravascular treatment of aneurysms. Clin Neurosurg 36: 338–343.

Higashida RT, Halbach VV, Cahan LD, Brant-Zawadzki M, Barnwell S, Dowd C, Hieshima GB (1989) Transluminal angioplasty for treatment of intracranial arterial vasospasm. J Neurosurg 71: 648–653.

Higashida RT, Halbach VV, Dormandy B, Bell J, Brant-Zawadzki M, Hieshima GB (1990) New microballoon device for transluminal angioplasty of intracranial arterial vasospasm. AJNR 11: 233–238.

Higashida RT, Hieshima GB, Halbach VV (1991) Advances in the treatment of complex cerebrovascular disorders by interventional neurovascular techniques. Circulation 83: 1196–206.

Higashida RT, Hieshmia GB, Tsai FY, Bentson JR, Halbach VV (1986) Percutaneous transluminal angioplasty of the subclavian and vertebral arteries. Acta Radiol Suppl (Stockh) 369: 124–126.

Higashida RT, Hieshima GB, Tsai FY, Halbach VV, Norman D, Newton TH (1987) Transluminal angioplasty of the vertebral and basilar artery. AJNR 8: 745–749.

Hilal, SK (1967) New techniques in cerebral angiography with particular emphasis on the study of cerebrovascular disease. Angiology 18: 316–322.

Hodgins GW, Dutton JW (1982) Subclavian and carotid angioplasties for Takayasu's arteritis. J Can Assoc Radiol 33: 205–207.

Ingram TL, Reid SH, Tisnado J, Cho SR, Posner MP (1988) Percutaneous transluminal angioplasty of brachiocephalic vein stenoses in patients with dialysis shunts. Radiology 166: 45–47.

Ishii K, Hirota Y, Kita Y, Kawamura K, Suma H, Takeuchi A (1991) Coronary-subclavian steal corrected with percutaneous transluminal angioplasty. J Cardiovasc Surg 32: 275–277.

Jacobs MJ, Gregoric ID, Reul GJ (1992) Profunda femoral artery pseudoaneurysm after percutaneous transluminal procedures manifested by neuropathy. J Cardiovasc Surg 33(6): 729–731.

Jaschke W, Menges HW, Ockert D, Huck K, Georgi M (1989) PTA of the subclavian and innominate artery: short- and long-term results. Ann Radiol (Paris) 32: 29–33.

Kachel R, Basche S, Heerklotz I, Grossmann K, Endler S (1991) Percutaneous transluminal angioplasty (PTA) of supra-aortic arteries especially the internal carotid artery. Neuroradiology 33: 191–194.

Kachel R, Endert G, Basche S, Grossmann K, Glaser FH (1987) Percutaneous transluminal angioplasty (dilatation) of carotid, vertebral, and innominate artery stenoses. Cardiovasc Intervent Radiol 10 (3): 142–146.

Kamada RO, Fergusson DJ, Itagaki RK (1988) Percutaneous entry of the brachial artery for transluminal coronary angioplasty. Cathet Cardiovasc Diagn 15: 132–133.

Kerber CW, Cromwell LD, Loehden OL (1980) Catheter dilatation of proximal carotid stenosis during distal bifurcation endarterectomy. AJNR 1: 348–349.

Khalilullah M, Tyagi S (1992) Percutaneous transluminal angioplasty in Takayasu's arteritis. Heart Vessels 7(Suppl): 146–153.

Khayata M, Aymard A, Guichard JP, Merland JJ (1992) Interventional neuroradiology. Curr Opinion Radiol 4(1): 71–78.

Kichikawa K, Nakagawa H, Yoshiya K, Ide K, Ohishi H, Uchida H, Iida N, Kyoi K, Utsumi S (1985) Percutaneous transluminal angioplasty in a case of left subclavian and brachiocephalic artery stenosis due to aortitis syndrome. Rinsho Hoshasen 1: 121–124.

Kobina GS, Bergmann H Jr (1983) Angioplasty in stenosis of the innominate artery. Cardiovasc Intervent Radiol 6: 82–85.

Koike T, Minakawa T, Abe H, Takeuchi S, Sasaki O, Nishimaki K, Tanaka R (1992) PTA of supra-aortic arteries with temporary balloon occlusion to avoid distal embolism. Neurol Med Chir (Toyko) 32(3): 140–147.

Laissy JP, Thiebot J, Peillon C, Watelet J, Testart J, Benozio M (1987) Axillo-femoral bypass failure secondary to axillary stenosis: ultrasound-guided percutaneous transluminal angioplasty. Bildgebung 56: 185–186.

Lang EV, Bookstein JJ (1989) Accelerated thrombolysis and angioplasty for hand ischemia in Buerger's disease. Cardiovasc Intervent Radiol 12: 95–97.

Laub GW, Muralidharan S, Naidech H, Fernandez J, Adkins M, McGrath LB (1991) Percutaneous transluminal subclavian angioplasty in a patient with postoperative angina. Ann Thorac Surg 52: 850–851.

Lazar L, Pasztor E, Czirjak S' Lanyi F, Deak G (1982) Experiences in the endovascular treatment of cerebral arteriovenous angiomas. Neurol Res 4: 235–252.

Leipzig TJ, Mullan SF (1983) Deflation of metrizamide-filled balloon used to occlude a carotid-cavernous fistula. Case report. J Neurosurg 59: 524–528.

Levien LJ, Fritz VU (1985) Intra-operative transluminal angioplasty in the management of symptomatic aortic arch vessel stenosis. S Afr J Surg 23: 49–52.

Levitt RG, Jarmolowski CR, Wholey MH (1991) Myocardial ischemia caused by postoperative malfunction of a patent internal mammary coronary arterial graft [letter; comment]. J Vasc Surg 13: 177–178.

Levitt RG, Wholey MH, Jarmolowski CR (1992) Subclavian artery angioplasty for treatment of coronary artery steal syndrome. J Vasc Intervent Radiol 3(1): 73–76.

Liang GC, Nemickas R, Madayag M (1989) Multiple percutaneous transluminal angioplasties and low dose pulse methotrexate for Takayasu's arteritis. J Rheumatol 16: 1370–1373.

Linskey ME, Horton JA, Rao GR, Yonas H (1991) Fatal rupture of the intracranial carotid artery during transluminal angioplasty for vasospasm induced by subarachnoid hemorrhage. Case report. J Neurosurg 74: 985–990.

Loftus CM, Quest DO (1983) Current status of carotid endarterectomy for atheromatous disease. Neurosurgery 12: 718–723.

Lowman BG, Queral LA, Holbrook WA, Estes JT, Bayly B (1981) The treatment of innominate artery stenosis by intraoperative transluminal angioplasty. Surgery 89: 565–568.

Lowman BG, Queral LA, Holbrook WA, Estes JT, Bayly B, Dagher FY

(1983) The correction of cerebrovascular insufficiency by transluminal dilatation: a preliminary report. Am Surg 11: 621–624.

Luessernhop A, Spence W (1960) Artificial embolization of cerebral arteries: report of use in a case of arteriovenous malformation. JAMA 172: 1153.

Mandalam KR, Rao VR, Neelakandhan KS, Kumar S, Unnikrishnan M, Mukhopadhyay S (1992) Hyperperfusion syndrome following balloon angioplasty and bypass surgery of aortic arch vessels: a report of 3 cases. Cardiovasc Intervent Radiol 15(2): 108–112.

Maouad J, Guermonprez JL (1988) Percutaneous femoral transluminal angioplasty of a right brachial artery occluded after Sones coronary angiography. Cathet Cardiovasc Diagn 14: 165–168.

Marks LA, Mehta AV, Marangi D (1991) Percutaneous transluminal balloon angioplasty of stenotic standard Blalock-Taussig shunts: effect on choice of initial palliation in cyanotic congenital heart disease. J Am Coll Cardiol 18: 546–551.

Mathias K (1977) Ein neuartiges Kathetersystem zur perkutanen transluminalen Angioplastie von Karotisstenosen. Fortschr Med 95 (15): 1007–1011.

Mathias K, Mitlermeyer C, Ensinger H, Neff W (1980) Percutane Katheterdilatation von karotiseteuosen. Fortscr Roetgenstr 133: 348–361.

Mathias K, Mitterman C, Eninger H, Neff W (1980) (GE) Percutaneous catheter dilatation of carotid stenoses: animal experiments. ROFO 133: 258–261.

Mathias K, Rau WS, Rohrbach R, Neff W (1977) Percutaneous transluminal angioplasty of carotid artery stenosis: experimental studies and possible application in patients. XIV Congress of radiologie, Rio de Janeiro, 23–29 October 1977. Excerpta Medica, Amsterdam, pp 45.

Mathias K, Rohrbach R, Neff W, Ensinger H (1978) Percutaneous transluminal dilatation (PTD) of carotid artery stenosis In: E Zeitler, et al (eds) Percutaneous Vascular Recanalization. Berlin, Heidelberg, New York, Springer, chap 10, pp 66–72.

Mathias K, Staiger J, Thron A, Spillner G, Heiss HW, Konrad-Graf S (1980) Perkutane Katheterangioplastik der Arteria Subclavia. Dtsch Med Wochenschr 105: 16–18.

Mathias VK, Schlosser V, Reinke M (1980) Katheterrekanalisation eines Subklaviaverschlusses. ROFO 132: 346–347.

McLean L, Jeans WD, Horrocks M, Baird RN (1987) The place of percutaneous transluminal angioplasty in the treatment of patients having angiography for ischaemic disease of the lower limb. Clin Radiol 38: 157–160.

Merland JJ, Reizine D, Riche MC, George B, Guimaraens L, Laurent A, Melki JP (1986) Endovascular treatment of vertebral arteriovenous fistulas in twenty-two patients. Ann Vasc Surg 1: 73–78.

Mizuno K, Arai T, Satomura K, Shibuya T, Arakawa K, Okamoto Y, Miyamoto A, Kurita A, Kikuchi M, Nakamura H, et al (1989) New percutaneous transluminal coronary angioscope. J Am Coll Cardiol 13: 363–368.

Moore T, Russell W, Parent A, Parket L, Smith R (1981) Nonsurgical treatment of "subclavian steal syndrome" with percutaneous transluminal angioplasty. Neurosurgery 9: 466.

Morris GC, Lechter A, DeBakey ME (1968) Surgical treatment of fibromuscular disease of the carotid arteries. Arch Surgery 96: 636–643.

Morrow WR, Vick GW, 3d Nihill MR, Rokey R, Johnston DL, Hedrick TD, Mullins CE (1988) Balloon dilation of unoperated coarctation of the aorta: short- and intermediate-term results. J Am Coll Cardiol 11: 133–138.

Motarjeme A, Keifer JW, Zuska AJ (1982) Percutaneous transluminal angioplasty of the brachiocephalic arteries. AJNR 3: 169–174.

Motarjeme A, Keifer JW, Zuska AJ (1982) Percutaneous transluminal angioplasty of the brachiocephalic arteries. AJR 138: 457–462.

Motarjeme A, Keifer JW, Zuska AJ (1981) Percutaneous transluminal angioplasty of the vertebral arteries. Radiology 139: 715–717.

Motarjeme A, Keifer JW, Zuska AJ, Nabawi P (1985) Percutaneous transluminal angioplasty for treatment of subclavian steal. Radiology 155: 611–613.

Mullan S, Duda EE, Patronas NJ (1980) Some examples of balloon technology in neurosurgery. J Neurosurg 52: 321–329.

Nawa S, Nakayama Y, Teramoto S, Mori K, Dohi T (1989) Coarctation restenosis after isthmosubclavioplasty. A consideration on operative procedure and intraluminal balloon angioplasty. Chest 95: 247–250.

Newell DW, Eskridge JM, Mayberg MR, Grady MS, Winn HR (1989) Angioplasty for the treatment of symptomatic vasospasm following subarachnoid hemorrhage. J Neurosurg 71: 654–660.

Nicholson AA, Kenan NM, Sheridan WG, Ruttley MS (1991) Percutaneous transluminal angioplasty of the subclavian artery. Ann R Coll Surg Eng 73: 46–52.

Numaguchi Y, Puyau FA, Provenza LJ, Richardson DE (1984) Percutaneous transluminal angioplasty of the carotid artery. Its application to post surgical stenosis. Neuroradiology 26: 527–530.

O'Leary DH, Clouse ME (1984) Percutaneous transluminal angioplasty of the cavernous carotid artery for recurrent ischemia. AJNR 5: 644–645.

Olbert F, Mendel H, Muzika N, Schlegl A (1983) Percutaneous transluminal vasodilatation. Long-term results and report on experiences with a new system of catheters: transaxillary technic. Wien Klin Wochenschr 95: 528–536.

Perler BA, Mitchell SE (1986) Percutaneous transluminal angioplasty and transaxillary first rib resection. A multidisciplinary approach to the thoracic outlet syndrome. Am Surg 52: 485–488.

Pernes JM, Brenot P, Seurot M, Angel C, Ferrer J, Renaudin JM, Fabiani JN, D'Allaines C, Gaux JC (1984) Percutaneous endoluminal angioplasty of the supra-aortic arterial trunks. Immediate and remote results. Presse Med 12: 1075–1078.

Pilla TJ, Tantana S, Smith KR (1988) Percutaneous transluminal angioplasty prior to carotid cavernous fistula embolization. AJNR 9: 789–790.

Portsman W (1973) Ein Never Korsett Balloon Katheter Zur Transluminalen Rehanalisation nach Dotter Unter besonderer Berucksickt, gung Von Obliterationen on den Beckenarterien. Radiol Diagn 14: 239–241.

Pritz MB, Smolin MF (1984) Treatment of tandem lesions of the extracranial carotid artery. Neurosurgery 15: 233–236.

Rabkin IKH, Matevosov AL, Shekhter IUI (1984) X-ray endovascular dilatation of the subclavian artery. Grudn Khir 2: 76–78.

Reid TL (1986) Balloon therapy for cranial aneurysm (letter). Arch Neurol 43: 756.

Riles TS, Imparato AM, Mintzer R, Baumann EG (1982) Comparison of results of bilateral and unilateral carotid endarterectomy five years after surgery. Surgery 91: 258–262.

Ringelstein EB, Zeumer H (1984) Delayed reversal of vertebral artery blood flow following percutaneous transluminal angioplasty for subclavian steal syndrome. Neuroradiology 26: 189–198.

Romanowski CA, Fairlie NC, Procter AE, Cumberland DC (1992) Percutaneous transluminal angioplasty of the subclavian and axillary arteries: initial results and long term follow-up. Clin Radiol 46(2): 104–107.

Rosenblum J, Stertzer SH, Schechtmann NS, Hidalgo B, Baciewicz PA, Myler RK (1991) Brachial rotational atherectomy. J Cathet Cardiovas Diagn 24: 32–36.

Rossi P, Sciacca V, Castrucci M, Farina C, Mingoli A, Di Marzo L, Pavone P, Cavallaro A (1988) Percutaneous transluminal angioplasty of subclavian artery. Comparative study with axillo-contralateral bypass. Ann Radiol (Paris) 31: 87–91.

Rubenstein RB, Tatkon-Coker J (1984) Nonsurgical treatment of subclavian steal syndrome by percutaneous transluminal angioplasty. Iowa Med 74: 109–111.

Sanders RJ, Haug C (1990) Subclavian vein obstruction and thoracic outlet syndrome: a review of etiology and management. REVIEW ARTICLE: 66 REFS. Ann Vasc Surg 4: 397–410.

Scheel JN, Gardner TJ, Kan JS (1991) Balloon dilatation of a stenotic Waterston shunt with long-term follow-up. Am J Cardiol 68: 821–822.

Schlosser V (1984) Subclavian steal syndrome: correction by transthoracic orextraanatomic repair. Vasc Surg 289–293.

Schulz H, et al (1981) Dilatation of vertebral artery stenosis. N Engl J Med 732.

Selby JB Jr, Matsumoto AH, Tegtmeyer CJ, Hartwell GD, Tribble CG, Daniel TM, Kron IL (1993) Balloon angioplasty above the aortic arch: immediate and long-term results. AJR 160(3): 631–635.

Shapira S, Braun SD, Puram B, Patel G, Rotman H (1991) Percutaneous transluminal angioplasty of proximal subclavian artery stenosis after left internal mammary to left anterior descending artery bypass surgery. J Am Coll Cardiol 18: 1120–1123.

Sharma S, Kaul U, Misra N, Rajani M (1990) Percutaneous supra-aortic angioplasty in a high risk coronary patient. Clin Radiol 42: 57–59.

Sharma S, Kaul U, Rajani M (1991) Identifying high-risk patients for percutaneous transluminal angioplasty of subclavian and innominate arteries. Acta Radiologica 32: 381–385.

Sharma S, Rajani M, Kaul U, Talwar KK, Dev V, Shrivastava S (1990) Initial experience with percutaneous transluminal angioplasty in the management of Takayasu's arteritis. Br J Radiol 63: 517–522.

Sharma S, Rajani M, Shrivastava S, Kaul U, Kamalakar T, Talwar KK, Saxena A (1991) Nonspecific aorto-arteritis (Takayasu's disease) in children. Br J Radiol 64: 690–698.

Slutzker DM, Capeless MA, Brown KA (1990) Subclavian stenosis presenting as progressive exertional angina pectoris. Clin Cardiol 13: 221–223.

Smith LL, Smith DC, Killeen JD, Hasso AN (1987) Operative balloon angioplasty in the treatment of internal carotid artery fibromuscular dysplasia. J Vasc Surg 6: 482–487.

Soulen MC, Sullivan KL (1991) Subclavian artery angioplasty proximal to a left internal mammary-coronary artery bypass graft: case report. Cardiovasc Intervent Radiol 14(6): 355–357.

Staller BJ, Maleki M (1989) Percutaneous transluminal angioplasty for innominate artery stenosis and total occlusion of subclavian artery in Takayasu's-type arteritis. Cathet Cardiovasc Diagn 16: 91–94.

Stanley JC, Fry WJ, Seeger JF, Hoffman GL, Gabrielsen TO (1974) Extracranial internal carotid and vertebral artery fibrodysplasia. Arch Surg 109: 215–221.

Sundt TM Jr, Smith HC, Campbell JK, Vlietstra RE, Cucchiara RF, Stanson AW (1980) Transluminal angioplasty for basilar artery stenosis. Mayo Clin Proc 55: 673–680.

Sundt TM Jr, Smith HC, Piepgras DG, Campbell LJK (1982) Bypass and transluminal dilatation procedures for advanced occlusive disease of the posterior circulation. Neurosurg Rev 5: 65–72.

Takahashi M, Miyawaki M, Bussaka H, Saito R (1985) Use of short-tapered catheters in combination with a balloon catheter for markedly stenotic renal and brachiocephalic arteries. Br J Radiol 58: 751–753.

Theron J (1989) Carotid angioplasty techniques (letter). J Neurosurg 71: 301.

Theron J, Courtheoux P, Henriet JP, Pelouze G, Derlon JM, Maiza D (1984) Angioplasty of supraaortic arteries. J Neuroradiol 11: 187–200.

Theron J, Melancon D, Ethier R (1985) Pre: subclavian steal syndromes and their treatment by angioplasty. Hemodynamic classification of subclavian artery stenoses. Neuroradiology 27: 265–270.

Theron J, Olivier A, Melancon D, Ethier R (1985) Left carotido-cavernous fistula with right exophthalmos: treatment by detachable balloon. Case report and literature review. Neuroradiology 27 (4): 349–353.

Theron J, Raymond J, Casasco A, Courtheoux F (1987) Percutaneous angioplasty of atherosclerotic and postsurgical stenosis of carotid arteries. AJNR 8: 495–500.

Theron J, Tyler JL (1987) Takayasu's arteritis of the aortic arch: endovascular treatment and correlation with positron emission tomography. AJNR 8: 621–626.

Thomas ES, Williams DO (1988) Simultaneous double balloon coronary angioplasty through a single guiding catheter for bifurcation lesions. Cathet Cardiovasc Diagn 15: 260–264.

Thompson MM, Sayers RD, Budd JS, London NJ, Bell PR (1992) Therapeutic options in subclavian artery disease. JR Coll Surg Edinb 37(6): 377–380.

Tievsky AL, Druy EM, Mardiat JG (1983) Transluminal angioplasty in postsurgical stenosis of the extracranial carotid artery. AJNR 4: 800–802.

Tournade A, Zenglein JP, Braun JP, Courtheoux P, Tajahmady T (1986) Percutaneous transluminal angioplasty of the vertebral and subclavian arteries. An angiographic-velocimetry comparison. J Neuroradiol 13: 95–110.

Tsai FY, Hieshima G, Mehringer CM, Gallacher DJ, Lewis G, Pribram HFW (1984) Arterial digital subtractionangiography with particulate intravascular embolization and angioplasty. Surg Neurol 22: 204–212.

Tsai FY, Matovich V, Hieshima G, Shah DC, Mehringer CM, Tiu G, Higashida R, Pribram HF (1986) Percutaneous transluminal angioplasty of the carotid artery. AJNR 7: 349–358.

Turnbull IW, Bannister CM (1992) Can laser angioplasty replace carotid endarterectomy in the management of nonstenotic atheromatous disease of the carotid bifurcation? Surg Neurol 38(1): 73–76.

Van den Hoven RW, Mali WP, Theodorides T (1988) Transluminal dilatation of the internal carotid artery in fibromuscular dysplasia: a case history. Angiology 39: 272–275.

Vinuela F, Dion J, Lylyk P, Duckwiler G (1989) Update on interventional neuroradiology. REVIEW ARTICLE: 73 REFS. AJR Am J Roentgenol 153: 23–33.

Vitek JJ (1983) Percutaneous transluminal angioplasty of the external carotid artery. AJNR 4: 796–799.

Vitek JJ (1986) Percutaneous transluminal angioplasty of the carotid artery (letter). AJNR 7: 1103–1104.

Vitek JJ (1989) Subclavian artery angioplasty and the origin of the vertebral artery. Radiology 170: 407–409.

Vitek JJ, Keller FS, Duvall ER, Gupta KL, Chandra-Sekar B (1986) Brachiocephalic artery dilation by percutaneous transluminal angioplasty. Radiology 158: 779–785.

Vitek JJ, Morawetz RB (1982) Percutaneous transluminal angioplasty of the external carotid artery: preliminary report. AJNR 3: 451–546.

Vitek JJ, Raymon BC, Oh SJ (1984) Innominate artery angioplasty. AJNR 5: 113–114.

Von KaChel R, Ritter H, Gobmann K, Glasa FH (1986) Frgebmisse der perkutanen tranluminalen dilatation (PTD) von hirngefabstenosen. Fortschr Rontgenstr 144: 338–342.

Weil SM, van Loveren HR, Tomsick TA, Quallen BL, Tew JM, Jr (1987) Management of inoperable cerebral aneurysms by the navigational balloon technique. REVIEW ARTICLE: 55 REFS. Neurosurgery 21: 296–302.

Whitaker SC, Gregson RH (1991) Case report: occlusion of subclavian artery treated by percutaneous angioplasty. Clin Radiol 44: 199–200.

Wiggle U, Gratzl O (1983) Transluminal angioplasty of stenotic carotid arteries: case reports and protocol. AJNR 4: 793–795.

Williams SJ 2nd (1986) Chronic upper extremity ischemia: current concepts in management. Surg Clin North Am 66: 355–375.

Wilms G, Baert A, Dewaele D, Vermylen J, Nevelsteen A, Suy R (1987) Percutaneous transluminal angioplasty of the subclavian artery: early and late results. Cardiovasc Intervent Radiol 10: 123–128.

Wilms G, Nevelsteen A, Baert A, Suy R (1987) Intraoperative angioplasty. Cardiovasc Intervent Radiol 10: 8–12.

Yamanashi WS, Patil AA, Hill DL, Lepage JR, Yassa NA, Valentine JL, Lester PD (1988) Precision surgery with an electromagnetically induced current convergence probe application in aneurysm treatment, angioplasty, and brain tumor resection in in vivo and in vitro models. Med Instrum 22: 205–216.

Yamanashi WS, Yassa NA, Hill DL, Lewis JE, Patil AA, Lester PD (1988)

Electromagnetic field focusing probe (EFFP)—a new angioplasty tool. Angiology 39: 1014–1021.

Zeitler E, Berger G, Schmitt-Ruth R (1983) Percutaneous transluminal angioplasty of the supra-aortic arteries. In CT Dotter, A Gruentzig, et al (eds) Berlin, Heidelberg, Springer-Verlag, pp 245–261.

Zubkov YN, Nikiforov BM, Shustin VA (1984) Balloon catheter technique for dilatation of constricted cerebral arteries after aneurysmal SAH. Acta Neurochir (Wien) 70: 65–79.

III. Femoro-Popliteal

Adar R, Critchfield GC, Eddy DM (1989) A confidence profile analysis of the results of femoropopliteal percutaneous transluminal angioplasty in the treatment of lower-extremity ischemia. J Vasc Surg 10: 57–67.

Ahn S, Rutherford RB (1992) A multicenter prospective randomized trial to determine the optimal treatment of patients with claudication and isolated superficial femoral artery occlusive disease: conservative versus endovascular versus surgical therapy. J Vasc Surg 15(5): 889–891.

Armstrong MW, Torrie EP, Galland RB (1992) Consequences of immediate failure of percutaneous transluminal angioplasty. Ann R Coll Surg Engl 74(4): 265–268.

Barnes RW (1982) Initial results after percutaneous transluminal angioplasty in femoral and iliac obstruction. Vasa 11: 301–304.

Bauriedel G, DeMaio SJ Jr, Hofling B (1992) Sheath introducer technique for recanalizing total occlusions of the superficial femoral artery. Cathet Cardiovasc Diagn 25(1): 66–70.

Baxi RK (1982) A case report of percutaneous transluminal angioplasty following failure of femoro-popliteal venous bypass graft. Cardiovasc Interventional Radiol 5: 30–33.

Belli AM, Cumberland DC, Procter AE, Welsh CL (1991) Follow-up of conventional angioplasty versus laser thermal angioplasty for total femoropopliteal artery occlusions: results of a randomized trial. J Vasc Intervent Radiol 2(4): 485–488.

Belli AM, Cumberland DC, Procter AE, Welsh CL (1991) Total peripheral artery occlusions: conventional versus laser thermal recanalization with a hybrid probe in percutaneous angioplasty—results of a randomized trial [comments]. Radiology 181: 57–60.

Bendick PJ, Price JL, Glover JL (1992) Limb perfusion. An objective measure of hemodynamic improvement after angioplasty. Arch Surg 127(7): 806–811.

Berkowitz HD, Fox AD, Deaton DH (1992) Reversed vein graft stenosis: early diagnosis and management. J Vasc Surg 15(1): 130–141; discussion 141–142.

Boyd AM (1960) The natural course of atherosclerosis of the lower extremities. Angiology 11: 10–14.

Brown KT, Moore ED, Getrajdman GI, Saddekni S (1993) Infrapopliteal angioplasty: long-term follow-up. J Vasc Intervent Radiol 4(1): 139–144.

Capek P, McLean GK, Berkowitz HD (1991) Femoropopliteal angioplasty. Factors influencing long-term success. Circulation 83: I70–80.

Colapinto RF, Harries-Jones EP, Johnston KW (1980) Percutaneous transluminal angioplasty of peripheral vascular disease: a two-year experience. Cardiovasc Interventional Radiol 3: 213–218.

Colapinto RF, Harries-Jones EP, Johnston KW (1980) Percutaneous transluminal dilatation and recanalization in the treatment of peripheral vascular disease. Radiology 135: 583–587.

Cole SE, Baird RN, Horrocks M, Jeans WD (1987) The role of balloon angioplasty in the management of lower limb ischaemia. Eur J Vasc Surg 1: 61–65.

Cooper JC, Welsh CL (1991) The role of percutaneous transluminal angioplasty in the treatment of critical ischaemia. Eur J Vasc Surg 5: 261–264.

Creasy TS, Tonnesen KH (1992) Retrograde femoral angioplasty: a new technique (letter). Br J Surg 79(7): 710.

Dacie JE, Daniell SJ (1991) The value of percutaneous transluminal angioplasty of the profunda femoris artery in threatened limb loss and intermittent claudication. Clin Radiol 44(5): 311–316.

Dacie JE, Tennant D (1990) A new approach to percutaneous transluminal angioplasty of profunda femoris origin stenosis. Cardiovasc Intervent Radiol 13: 67–70.

Dalman RL, Taylor LM Jr, Moneta GL, Yeager RA, Porter JM (1991) Simultaneous operative repair of multilevel lower extremity occlusive disease. J Vasc Surg 13: 211–219.

Dalsing MC, Cockerill E, Deupree R, Wolf G, Wilson S (1991) Outcome predictors in selection of balloon angioplasty or surgery for peripheral arterial occlusive disease. Veterans Administration Cooperative Study No. 199. Surgery 110: 636–643; discussion 643–664.

Darcy MD (1992) Reanalyzing the reanalysis of femoropopliteal angioplasty (editorial; comment). Radiology 183(3): 621–622.

Do-dai-Do, Triller J, Walpoth BH, Stirnemann P, Mahler F (1992) A comparison study of self-expandable stents vs balloon angioplasty alone in femoropopliteal artery occlusions. Cardiovasc Intervent Radiol 15(5): 306–312.

Dorros G, Iyer S, Zaitoun R, Lewin R, Cooley R, Olson K (1991) Acute angiographic and clinical outcome of high-speed percutaneous rotational atherectomy (Rotablator). Cathet Cardiovas Diagn 22: 157–166.

Dotter CT (1971) Clinical indications for transluminal dilatation in the management of atheromatous leg ischema. Cardiovasc Clin 3: 104–111.

Dotter CT (1974) Catheter technics in diagnosing and treating femoral artery atherosclerosis. Geriatrics 29: 93–102.

Dotter CT, Judkins MP (1964) Transluminal treatment of arteriosclerotic obstruction: description of a new technique and preliminary report of its application. Circulation 30: 654–670.

Dotter CT, Judkins MP (1968) Transluminal recanalization in occlusive disease of the leg arteries. GP 37: 98–106.

Dotter CT, Judkins MP (1969) Transluminal dilatation for atherosclerotic ischemia of the lower extremity. Geriatrics 24: 108–111.

Dotter CT, Krippaehne WW, Judkins MP (1965) Transluminal recanalization and dilatation in atherosclerotic obstruction of the femoral popliteal system. Am Surg 31: 453–459.

Douek PC, Leon MB, Geschwind H, Cook PS, Selzer P, Miller DL, Bonner RF (1991) Occlusive peripheral vascular disease: a multicenter trial of fluorescence-guided, pulsed dye laser-assisted balloon angioplasty. Radiology 180: 127–133.

Fletcher JP, Little JM, Fermanis GG, Simmons K (1986) Percutaneous transluminal angioplasty for severe lower extremity ischaemia. Aust N Z J Surg 56: 121–125.

Flueckiger F, Lammer J, Klein GE, Hausegger K, Pilger E, Waltner F, Aschauer M (1992) Percutaneous transluminal angioplasty of crural arteries. Acta Radiol 33(2): 152–155.

Freiman DB, Ring EJ, Oleaga JA, Berkowitz H, Roberts B (1979) Transluminal angioplasty of the iliac, femoral, and popliteal arteries. Radiology 132: 285–288.

Freiman DB, Spence R, Gatenby R, Gertner M, Roberts B, Berkowitz HD, Ring EJ, Oleaga JA (1981) Transluminal angioplasty of the iliac and femoral arteries: follow-up results without anticoagulation. Radiology 141: 347–350.

Glover JL, Bendick PJ, Dilley RS, Becker GJ, Richmond BC, Yune HY, Holden RW (1983) Balloon catheter for limb salvage. Arch Surg 118: 557–560.

Glover JL, Bendick PJ, Dilley RS, Holden RW, Yune HY, Richmond BD, Klatte EC (1982) Efficacy of balloon catheter dilatation for lower extremity atherosclerosis. Surgery 91: 560–565.

Graor RA, Young JR, McCandless M, Swift C, Smith JA, Ruschaupt WF, Risius B, Zelch MG (1984) Percutaneous transluminal angioplasty: review of iliac and femoral dilatations at the Cleveland Clinic. Clev Clin Q 51: 149–154.

Graziani L (1987) Percutaneous recanalization of total iliac and femoro-popliteal artery occlusions. Eur J Radiol 7: 91–93.

Greenfield AJ (1980) Femoral, popliteal, and tibial arteries: percutaneous transluminal angioplasty. AJR 135: 927–935.

Gunther RW, Vorwerk D, Bohndorf K, Peters I, el-Din A, Messmer B (1989) Iliac and femoral artery stenoses and occlusions: treatment with intravascular stents. Radiology 172: 725–730.

Gupta SK, Veith FJ, Kram HB, Wengerter KA (1990) Significance and management of inflow gradients unexpectedly generated after femoro-femoral, femoropopliteal, and femoroinfrapopliteal bypass grafting. J Vasc Surg 12: 278–283.

Haapanen A, Keski-Nisula L, Ala-Ketola L (1984) Percutaneous dilatation of lower leg arteries. Ann Clin Res 16 Suppl 40: 7–9.

Harris RW, Dulawa LB, Andros G, Oblath RW, Salles-Cunha SX, Apyan RL (1991) Percutaneous transluminal angioplasty of the lower extremities by the vascular surgeon. Ann Vasc Surg 5: 345–353.

Henriksen LO, Jorgensen B, Holstein PE, Tonnesen KH, Karle A, Sager P (1988) Percutaneous transluminal angioplasty of infrarenal arteries in intermittent claudication. Acta Chir Scand 154: 573–576.

Hewes RC, White RI Jr, Murray RR, Kaufman SL, Chang R, Kadir S, Kinnison ML, Mitchell SE, Auster M (1986) Long-term results of superficial femoral artery angioplasty. AJR 146: 1025–1029.

Hoffmann U, Schneider E, Bollinger A (1992) Percutaneous transluminal angioplasty (PTA) of the deep femoral artery. Vasa 21(1): 69–75.

Hunink MG, Donaldson MC, Meyerovitz MF, Polak JF, Whittemore AD, Kandarpa K, Grassi CJ, et al. (1993) Risks and benefits of femoropopliteal percutaneous balloon angioplasty. J Vasc Surg 17(1): 183–192; discussion 192–194.

Ingrisch H, Schatzl M, Hess H, Mietaschk A, Frey KW (1980) Microdensitometric controls for quantification of the results in percutaneous transluminal recanalization of the femoral artery. Ann Radiol 23: 283–285.

Jester HG, Sinapius D (1978) Morphologic alterations after percutaneous transluminal recanalization of chronic femoral atherosclerosis. In: Zeitler E, et al (eds) Percutaneous Vascular Recanalization. Springer, Berlin Heidelberg New York, chap. 8, pp 51–56.

Johnston KW (1992) Factors that influence the outcome of aortoiliac and femoropopliteal percutaneous transluminal angioplasty. Surg Clin North Am 72(4): 843–850.

Johnston KW (1992) Femoral and popliteal arteries: reanalysis of results of balloon angioplasty (see comments). Radiology 183(3): 767–771.

Johnston KW, Colapinto RF, Harries-Jones EP, DeMorais D, Kalman PG, Baird RJ, Goldman BS, Key JA, Weisel RD (1980) Transluminal dilatation in the treatment of peripheral arterial occlusive disease. Can J Surg 23: 547–548.

Johnston KW, Rae M, Hogg-Johnston SA, Colapinto RF, Walker PM, Baird RJ, Sniderman KW, Kalman P (1987) 5-year results of a prospective study of percutaneous transluminal angioplasty. Ann Surg 206: 403–413.

Jorgensen B, Henriksen LO, Karle A, Sager P, Holstein PE, Tonnesen KH (1988) Percutaneous transluminal angioplasty of iliac and femoral arteries in severe lower-limb ischaemia. Acta Chir Scand 154: 647–652.

Jorgensen B, Meisner S, Holstein P, Tonnesen KH (1990) Early rethrombosis in femoropopliteal occlusions treated with percutaneous transluminal angioplasty. Eur J Vasc Surg 4: 149–152.

Jorgensen B, Tonnesen KH, Bulow J, Nielsen JD, Jorgensen M, Holstein P, Andersen E (1989) Femoral artery recanalization with percutaneous angioplasty and segmentally enclosed plasminogen activator [see comments]. Comment in: Lancet 1989 Aug 12;2(8659): 390–391. Lancet 1: 1106–1108.

Jorgensen B, Tonnesen KH, Holstein P (1991) Late hemodynamic failure following percutaneous transluminal angioplasty fopr long and multifocal femoropopliteal stenoses. Cardiovas Intervent Radiol 14: 290–292.

Jorgensen B, Tonnesen KH, Nielsen JD, Holstein P, Bulow J, Jorgensen M, Andersen E (1991) Segmentally enclosed thrombolysis in percutaneous transluminal angioplasty for femoropopliteal occlusions: a report from a pilot study. Cardiovasc Intervent Radiol 14: 293–298.

Kalman PG, Sniderman KW (1988) Salvage of in situ femoropopliteal and femorotibial saphenous vein bypass with interventional radiology. J Vasc Surg 7: 429–432.

Kalman PG, Colapinto RF, Harries-Jones EP, Silver MD, Johnston KW (1980) Preliminary results of transluminal dilatation in the treatment of peripheral arterial occlusive disease. Surg Gynecol Obstet 150: 865–868.

Kashdan BJ, Trost DW, Jagust MB, Rackson ME, Sos TA (1992) Retrograde approach for contralateral iliac and infrainguinal percutaneous transluminal angioplasty: experience in 100 patients. J Vasc Intervent Radiol 3(3): 515–521.

Katzen BT (1984) Percutaneous transluminal angioplasty for arterial disease of the lower extremities. AJR 142: 23–25.

Khangure MS, Chow KC, Christensen MA (1982) Accurate and safe puncture of a pulseless femoral artery: an aid in performing iliac artery percutaneous transluminal angioplasty. Radiology 144: 927–928.

Kinnison ML, Kadir S (1984) Superficial femoral artery occlusion: observations that influence patient selection criteria for angioplasty. Cardiovasc Interventional Radiol 7: 102–103.

Korogi Y, Takahashi M, Bussaka H, Miyawaki M, Yamashita Y (1987) Percutaneous transluminal angioplasty of the ilio-femoro-popliteal arteries: initial and long-term results. Radiat Med 5: 68–74.

Krayenbuhl B (1980) Treatment of arterial occlusive diseases of the lower limbs (in French). Ther Umsch 37: 132, 136.

Krepel VM, Van Andel GJ, Van Erp WF, Breslau, PJ (1985) Percutaneous transluminal angioplasty of the femoropopliteal artery: initial and long-term results. Radiology 156: 325–328.

Kumpe DA, Kempczinski RF (1980) Percutaneous transluminal angioplasty in the selected management of proximal arterial occlusive disease of the lower extremities: a preliminary report. Surgery 87: 488–493.

Lai ST, Cheng KJ (1991) Results of angioscopy-assisted intraoperative transluminal angioplasty of the iliac and femoral artery. Chung Hua I Hsueh Tsa Chih 48: 25–30.

Lammer J, Pilger E, Decrinis M, Quehenberger F, Klein GE, Stark G (1992) Pulsed excimer laser versus continuous-wave Nd:YAG laser versus conventional angioplasty of peripheral arterial occlusions: prospective, controlled, randomised trial. Lancet 340(8829): 1183–1188.

Lammer J, Pilger E, Karnel F, Schurawitzki H, Horvath W, Riedl M, Umek H, Klein GE, Schreyer H, Kretschmer G, et al. (1991) Laser angioplasty: results of a prospective, multicenter study at 3-year follow-up. Radiology 178: 335–337.

Lancashire MJ, Torrie EP, Galland RB (1992) Percutaneous angioplasty in a district general hospital: impact and implications. J R Coll Surg Edinb 37(3): 183–186.

Leachman DR, Avedissian MG, Krajcer Z, Angelini P (1989) Transluminal laser angioplasty of the femoropopliteal circulation by use of a percutaneous popliteal approach. Am J Cardiol 64: 106–108.

Lee TC, Hartzler GO, Rutherford BD, McConahay DR (1990) Removal of an occlusive coronary dissection flap by using an atherectomy catheter. Cathet Cardiovasc Diagn 20: 185–188.

Liang GC, Nemickas R, Madayag M (1989) Multiple percutaneous transluminal angioplasties and low dose pulse methotrexate for Takayasu's arteritis. J Rheumatol 16: 1370–1373.

London NJ, Bolia A, Bell PR (1993) Subintimal angioplasty for femoropopliteal artery occlusion [letter]. Lancet 341(8839): 238.

Lu C, Zarins CK, Yang C, Sottiurai V (1982) Long-segment arterial occlusion: percutaneous transluminal angioplasty. AJR 138: 119–122.

Martin EC, Fankuchen EI, Karlson KB, Dolgin C, Collins RH, Voorhees AB Jr, Casarella WJ (1981) Angioplasty for femoral artery occlusion: comparison with surgery. AJR 137: 915–919.

Mathias K (1991) Local thrombolysis for salvage of occluded bypass grafts. Semin Thromb Hemost 17: 14–20.

Maynar M, Garcia-Pumarino JL, Salvador G, Rodriguez JE, Estevan MA, Diez-Valencia O, Gomez Martinez JLG, Seco YMA (1981) Angioplastia transluminal percutanea en extremidades inferiores. Radiologia 23: 73–82.

McLean L, Jeans WD, Horrocks M, Baird RN (1987) The place of percutaneous transluminal angioplasty in the treatment of patients having angiography for ischaemic disease of the lower limb. Clin Radiol 38: 157–160.

Milford MA, Weaver FA, Lundell CJ, Yellin AE (1988) Femoropopliteal percutaneous transluminal angioplasty for limb salvage. J Vasc Surg 8: 292–299.

Minar E, Ahmadi R, Ehringer H (1986) Excessive ectasia of the femoral artery: an unknown late sequel of percutaneous transluminal angioplasty (case report). Vasa 15: 88–90.

Minar E, Ehringer H, Ahmadi R, Dudczak R, Leitha T, Koppensteiner R, Jung M, Stumpflen A (1989) Platelet deposition at angioplasty sites and its relation to restenosis in human iliac and femoropopliteal arteries. Radiology 170: 767–772.

Moody P, Gould DA, Harris PL (1990) Vein graft surveillance improves patency in femoropopliteal bypass. Eur J Vasc Surg 4: 117–121.

Moore WS (1991) Therapeutic options for femoropopliteal occlusive disease. Circulation 83: I91–93.

Morgenstern BR, Getrajdman GI, Laffey KJ, Bixon R, Martin EC (1989) Total occlusions of the femoropopliteal artery: high technical success rate of conventional balloon angioplasty. Radiology 172: 937–940.

Morin JF, Johnston KW, Rae M (1986) Improvement after successful percutaneous transluminal dilation treatment of occlusive peripheral arterial disease. Surg Gynecol Obstet 163: 453–457.

Morin JF, Johnston KW, Wasserman L, Andrews D (1986) Factors that determine the long-term results of percutaneous transluminal dilatation for peripheral arterial occlusive disease. J Vasc Surg 4: 68–72.

Motarjeme A, Keifer JW, Zuska AJ (1980) Percutaneous transluminal angioplasty of the deep femoral artery. Radiology 135: 613–617.

Murray RR Jr, Hewes RC, White RI Jr, Mitchell SE, Auster M, Chang R, Kadir S, Kinnison ML, Kaufman SL (1987) Long-segment femoropopliteal stenoses: is angioplasty a boon or a bust? Radiology 162: 473–476.

Neiman HL, Bergan JJ, Yao JST, Brandt TD, Greenberg M, O'Mara CS (1982) Hemodynamic assessment of transluminal angioplasty for lower extremity ischemia. Radiology 143: 639–643.

Odink HF, de Valois HC, Eikelboom BC (1991) Femoropopliteal arterial occlusions: laser-assisted versus conventional percutaneous transluminal angioplasty. Radiology 181: 61–66.

Olbert F, Weidinger P, Schlegl A, Teiner G, Hagmuller GW, Denck H (1981) Combined transluminal percutaneous dilation and surgical reconstruction of the iliac, femoral and popliteal arteries. Ann Radiol (Paris) 24: 369–374.

O'Mara CS, Neiman HL, Flinn WR, Herman RJ, Yao JST, Bergan JJ (1981) Hemodynamic assessment of transluminal angioplasty for lower extremity ischemia. Surgery 89: 106–117.

Page JE, Buckenham TM, Taylor RS (1992) Accelerated thrombolysis facilitated by direct puncture of occluded prosthetic femoral grafts. Australas Radiol 36(3): 230–233.

Peterkin GA, Belkin M, Cantelmo NL, Guben J, Greenfield AJ, Johnson WC, Menzoian JO (1990) Combined transluminal angioplasty and infra-inguinal reconstruction in multilevel atherosclerotic disease. Am J Surg 160: 277–279.

Podlas H, Snychess FD (1980) Successful transluminal recanalization in legs. S Afr Med J 57: 15–17.

Probst P, Cerny P, Owens A, Mahler F (1983) Patency after femoral angioplasty: correlation of angiographic appearance with clinical findings. AJR 140: 1227–1232.

Rao PS (1991) Pseudoaneurysm following balloon angioplasty? [letter]. Cathet Cardiovasc Diagn 23: 150–152.

Ratner SW, Reilly CH, Gudas CJ (1983) Percutaneous transluminal angioplasty in the treatment of ischemic disease of the lower extremity. J Foot Surg 22: 86–91.

Reilly DT, Packer SG, Morrison N, van Rij AM (1988) Percutaneous transluminal angioplasty for the ischaemic lower limb: the early Dunedin experience. N Z Med J 101: 129–132.

Saab MH, Smith DC, Aka PK, Brownlee RW, Killeen JD (1992) Percutaneous transluminal angioplasty of tibial arteries for limb salvage. Cardiovasc Intervent Radiol 15(4): 211–216.

Sclafani SJ, Shaftan GW (1982) Transcatheter treatment of injuries to the profunda femoris artery. AJR 138: 463–466.

Shanahan D, Grieve NW, Bennett CE, Thomas MH (1991) Retrograde femoral angioplasty: a new technique. Br J Surg 78: 1134–1135.

Sinning MA, Dixon GD, Pinkerton JA Jr (1983) Percutaneous transluminal angioplasty. Therapy for vascular occlusive disease of the lower extremities. J Kans Med Soc 84: 331–334, 355.

Spence RK, Freiman DB, Gatenby R, Hobbs CL, Barker CF, Berkowitz HD, Robert B, McClean G, Oleaga J, Ring EJ (1981) Long-term results of transluminal angioplasty of the iliac and femoral arteries. Arch Surg 116: 1377–1386.

Spies JB, LeQuire MH, Brantley SD, Williams JE, Beckett WC, Mills JL (1990) Comparison of balloon angioplasty and laser thermal angioplasty in the treatment of femoropopliteal atherosclerotic disease: initial results of a prospective randomized trial. Work in progress (see comments). J Vasc Intervent Radiol 1(1): 39–42.

Stokes KR, Strunk HM, Campbell DR, Gibbons GW, Wheeler HG, Clouse ME (1990) Five-year results of iliac and femoropopliteal angioplasty in diabetic patients. Radiology 174: 977–982.

Strauss AL, Schaberle W, Rieger H, Roth FJ (1991) Use of duplex scanning in the diagnosis of arteria profunda femoris stenosis. J Vasc Surg 13: 698–704.

Sugrue ME, Lee M, Hederman WP, Legge D (1988) Percutaneous transluminal angioplasty in the treatment of lower limb ischaemia. Ir J Med Sci 157: 104–106.

Tamura S, Sniderman KW, Beinart C, Thomas A (1982) Percutaneous transluminal angioplasty of the popliteal artery and its branches. Radiology 143: 645–648.

The SH, Gussenhoven EJ, Zhong Y, Li W, Van Egmond F, Pieterman H, Van Urk H, Gerritsen GP, Borst C, Wilson RA, et al (1992) Effect of balloon angioplasty on femoral artery evaluated with intravascular ultrasound imaging. Circulation 86(2): 483–493.

Thorvinger B, Norgrn L, Albrechtsson U (1992) Patency after iliac and femoro-popliteal angioplasty. Difference between angiographic and clinical results. Acta Radiol 33(1): 29–30.

Tonnesen KH, Holstein P, Andersen E (1991) Femoro-popliteal artery occlusions treated by percutaneous transluminal angioplasty and enclosed thrombolysis: results in 55 patients. Eur J Vasc Surg 5: 429–434.

Tonnesen KH, Sager P, Karle A, Henriksen L, Jorgensen B (1988) Percutaneous transluminal angioplasty of the superficial femoral artery by retrograde catheterization via the popliteal artery. Cardiovasc Intervent Radiol 11: 127–131.

Van Andel GJ (1981) Long-term results of iliac and femoral angioplasty. Ann Radiol 24: 365–368.

Van der Vliet JA, Mulling FJ, Heijstraten FM, Reinaerts HH, Buskens FG (1992) Femoropopliteal arterial reconstruction with intraoperative iliac transluminal angioplasty for disabling claudication: results of a combined approach. Eur J Vasc Surg 6(6): 607–609.

Van Urk H (1990) The optimal approach to the treatment of acute femoro-popliteal occlusion. REVIEW ARTICLE: 29 REFS. Acta Chir Scand 555 Suppl: 59–62.

Villavicencio R, Meier B (1991) Left axillary approach for balloon recanalization of an occlusion of the right common femoral artery. Vasa 20: 186–187.

Vroegindeweij D, Kemper FJ, Tielbeek AV, Buth J, Landman G (1992) Recurrence of stenoses following balloon angioplasty and Simpson atherectomy of the femoro-popliteal segment. A randomised comparative 1-year follow-up study using colour flow duplex. Eur J Vasc Surg 6(2): 164–171.

Waltman AC (1980) Percutaneous transluminal angioplasty of iliac and deep femoral arteries. AJR 135: 921–925.

Waltman AC, Greenfield AJ, Novelline RA, Abbott WM, Brewster DC, Darling RC, Moncure AC, Ottinger LW, Athanasoulis CA (1982) Transluminal angioplasty of the iliac and femoropopliteal arteries. Arch Surg 117: 1218–1221.

Weibull H, Bergqvist D, Jonsson K, Karlsson S, Takolander R (1987) Complications after percutaneous transluminal angioplasty in the iliac, femoral, and popliteal arteries. J Vasc Surg 5: 681–686.

Welsh CL, Cumberland DC (1986) The role of percutaneous transluminal angioplasty for atherosclerotic disease of the lower extremities (letter). Ann R Coll Surg Engl 68: 54–55.

Whyman MR, Ruckley CV, Fowkes FG (1991) Angioplasty for mild intermittent claudication [editorial]. Br J Surg 78: 643–645.

Wilson SE, White GH, Wolf G, Cross AP (1990) Proximal percutaneous balloon angioplasty and distal bypass for multilevel arterial occlusion. Veterans Administration Cooperative Study No. 199. Ann Vasc Surg 4: 351–355.

Wollenweber J, Henne W, Kiefer H, Meves M, Schmarsow R (1986) Early and late results after percutaneous transluminal angioplasty in peripheral arterial occlusive disease. Vasa 15: 67–70.

Zajko AB, McLean GK, Freiman DB, Oleaga JA, Ring EJ (1981) Percutaneous puncture of venous bypass grafts for transluminal angioplasty. AJR 137: 799–802.

Zarins CK, Lu CT, McDonnel AE, Whitehouse WM (1980) Limb salvage by percutaneous transluminal recanalization of the occluded superficial femoral artery. Surgery 87: 701–708.

Zeitler E (1980) Percutaneous dilatation and recanalization of iliac and femoral arteries. Cardiovasc Interventional Radiol 3: 207–212.

Zeitler E (1985) Primary and late results of percutaneous transluminal angioplasty (PTA) in iliac and femoro-popliteal obliterations. Int Angiol 4: 81–85.

IV. Iliac

Ahmadi R, Dudczak R, Ehringer H, Minar E (1989) Platelet disposition at angioplasty sites and platelet survival time after PTA in iliac and femoral arteries (letter). Vasa 18: 79.

Alpert JR, Ring EJ, Freiman DB, Oleaga JA, Gordon R, Berkowitz HD, Roberts B (1980) Treatment of stenosis of the iliac artery by balloon catheter dilation. Surg Gynecol Obstet 150: 481–485.

Alpert JR, Ring EJ, Freiman DB, Oleaga JA, Gordon R, Berkowitz HD, Roberts O (1980) Balloon dilation of iliac stenosis with distal arterial surgery. Arch Surg 115: 715–717.

Angelini P, Fighali S (1987) Early experience with balloon angioplasty of internal iliac arteries for vasculogenic impotence. Catheterization Cardiovasc Diagn 13: 107–110.

Arfvidsson B, Davidsen JP, Persson B, Spansen L (1983) Percutaneous transluminal angioplasty (PTA) for lower extremity arterial insufficiency. Acta Chir Scand 149: 43–47.

Armstrong MW, Torrie EP, Galland RB (1992) Consequences of immediate failure of percutaneous transluminal angioplasty. Ann R Coll Surg Engl 74(4): 265–268.

Auster M, Kadir S, Mitchell SE, Williams GM, Perler BA, Chang R, White RI Jr (1984) Iliac artery occlusion: management with intrathrombus streptokinase infusion and angioplasty. Radiology 153: 385–388.

Bachman DM, Casarella WJ, Sos TA (1979) Percutaneous illiofemoral angioplasty via the contralateral femoral artery. Radiology 130: 617–621.

Barnes RW (1982) Initial results after percutaneous transluminal angioplasty in femoral and iliac obstruction. Vasa 11: 301–304.

Bendick PJ, Price JL, Glover JL (1992) Limb perfusion. An objective measure of hemodynamic improvement after angioplasty. Arch Surg 127(7): 806–811.

Bergqvist D, Takolander R, Jonsson K, Karlsson S, Hellekant C (1984) Percutaneous transluminal angioplasty of artheriosclerotic lesions in the pelvis and lower extremities. Acta Chir Scand 150: 445–449.

Bjork L (1991) Arterial phlebography of the leg. Acta Radiol 32: 141–142.

Blankensteijn JD, van Vroonhoven TJ, Lampmann L (1986) Role of percutaneous transluminal angioplasty in aorto-iliac reconstruction. J Cardiovasc Surg (Torino) 27: 466–468.

Blattler W, Cappius G, Haeberli A, Foullon N, Roth FJ (1986) Thrombinemia during percutaneous transluminal angioplasty of chronic femoral artery occlusions. Vasa 15: 379–386.

Bolia A, Brennan J, Bell PR (1989) Recanalisation of femoro-popliteal occlusions: improving success rate by subintimal recanalisation (letter). Clin Radiol 40: 325.

Bookstein JJ, Wexler L (1987) Angioplastic treatment of impotence. A hard look at soft data (letter). Cathet Cardiovasc Diagn 13: 425–426.

Borozan PG, Schuler JJ, Spigos DG, Flanigan DP (1985) Long-term hemodynamic evaluation of lower extremity percutaneous transluminal angioplasty. J Vasc Surg 2: 785–793.

Brahme F, Swedenborg J, Tibel B (1969) Evaluation of transluminal recanalisation of the femoral artery. Acta Chir Scand 135:679–684.

Breslau PJ, van Soest M, Janevski B, Jorning PJ (1985) Hemodynamic evaluation of transluminal iliac artery balloon dilatation. Neth J Surg 37: 145–147.

Brewer ML, Kinnison ML, Perler BA, White RI Jr (1988) Blue toe syndrome: treatment with anticoagulants and delayed percutaneous transluminal angioplasty. Radiology 166: 31–36.

Brewster DC, Cambria RP, Darling RC, Athanasoulis CA, Waltman AC, Geller SC, Moncure AC, Lamuraglia GM, Freehan M, Abbott WM (1989) Long-term results of combined iliac balloon angioplasty and distal surgical revascularization. Ann Surg 210: 324–330; discussion 331.

Brothers TE, Greenfield LJ (1990) Long-term results of aortoiliac reconstruction. J Vasc Intervent Radiol 1(1): 49–55.

Brunner U, Gruentzig A (1978) Vascular surgery and transluminal dilatation/recanalization: complementary procedures for the reconstruction of peripheral occlusive diseases. In: Zeitler E, et al (eds) Percutaneous Vascular Recanalization. Springer, Berlin Heidelberg New York, pp 160–166.

Castaneda-Zuniga WR, Amplatz Ka (1983) Transluminal angioplasty of pelvic arteries in the management of vasculogenic erectile impotence. In: Castaneda-Zuniga WR, (ed) Transluminal Angioplasty, Thieme-Stratton Inc, New York, pp 192–195.

Castaneda-Zuniga WR, Smith A, Kaye K, Rusnak, Herrera M, Miller R, Amplatz, Weens C, Ketchum D (1982) Transluminal angioplasty for treatment of vasculogenic impotence. AJR 139: 371–373.

Chong WK, Cross FW, Raphael MJ (1990) Iliac artery rupture during percutaneous angioplasty. REVIEW ARTICLE: 10 REFS. Clin Radiol 41: 358–359.

Cikrit DF, Helikson MA, Nichols WK, Silver D (1991) Complete external iliac artery disruption after percutaneous aortic valvuloplasty in two young children: successful repair with hypogastric artery transposition. Surgery 109: 623–626.

Cikrit DF, O'Donnell DM, Dalsing MC, Sawchuk AP, Lalka SG (1991) Clinical implications of combined hypogastric and profunda femoral artery occlusion. Am J Surg 162: 137–140.

Cluley SR, Brener BJ, Hollier L, Schoenfeld R, Novick A, Vilkomerson D, Ferrara-Ryan M, et al. (1993) Transcutaneous ultrasonography can be used to guide and monitor balloon angioplasty. J Vasc Surg 17(1): 23–30; discussion 30–31.

Colapinto RF, Harries-Jones EP, Johnston KW (1981) Percutaneous transluminal recanalization of complete iliac artery occlusions. Arch Surg 116: 277–281.

Colapinto RF, Stronell RD, Johnston WK (1986) Transluminal angioplasty of complete iliac obstructions. AJR 146: 859–862.

Cook AM, Dyet JF (1990) Percutaneous angioplasty of the superior gluteal artery in the treatment of buttock claudication. Clin Radiol 41: 63–65.

Cooper JC, Woods DA, Spencer P, Procter AE (1991) The development of an infected false aneurysm following iliac angioplasty. Br J Radiol 64: 759–760.

Coy KM, Park JC, Fishbein MC, Laas T, Diamond GA, Adler L, Maurer G, et al. (1992) In vitro validation of three-dimensional intravascular ultrasound for the evaluation of arterial injury after balloon angioplasty [see comments]. J Am Coll Cardiol 20(3): 692–700.

Cumberland DC (1982) Percutaneous angioplasty in complete iliac occlusions. Vasa 11(4): 297–300.

Daskalakis MK (1978) Fibromuscular hyperplasia of external iliac arteries. West J Med 128: 345–346.

Davidson CJ, Sheikh, Harrison JK, Himmelstein SI, Leithe ME, Kisslo KB, Bashore TM (1990) Intravascular ultrasonography versus digital subtraction angiography: a human in vivo comparison of vessel size and morphology. J Am Coll Cardiol 16: 633–636.

Demer LL, Ariani M, Siegel RJ (1991) High intensity ultrasound increases distensibility of calcific atherosclerotic arteries. JACC 18: 1259–1262.

DeSouza NM, King DH, Pilgrim P, Bates P, Reidy JF, Gosling RG (1991) Quickscan: Doppler ultrasound emulation of angiography—its value prior to arteriography in peripheral vascular disease. Br J Radiol 64: 479–484.

Dewar ML, Blundell PE, Lidstone D, Herba MJ, Chiu RC (1985) Effects of abdominal aneurysmectomy, aortoiliac bypass grafting and angioplasty on male sexual potency: a prospective study. Can J Surg 28: 154–156, 159.

Do-dai-Do, Triller J, Walpoth BH, Stirnemann P, Mahler F (1992) A comparison study of self-expandable stents vs balloon angioplasty alone in femoropopliteal artery occlusions. Cardiovasc Intervent Radiol 15(5): 306–312

Dorros G, Mathiak L (1993) Direct deployment of the iliofemoral balloon expandable (Palmaz) stent utilizing a small (7.5 French) arterial puncture. Cathet Cardiovasc Diagn 28(1): 80–82.

Dotter CT, Judkins MP, Frische LH, Mueller R (1966) The "non-surgical" treatment of ilio-femoral arteriosclerotic obstruction. Radiology 86: 871–875.

Dotter CT, Judkins MP, Frische LH, Rosch J (1968) Tratamiento transluminal de la obstruccion arteriosclerotica. Rev Argent Angiol II: 27–36.

Dotter CT, Rosch J, Anderson JM, Antonovic R, Robinson M (1974) Transluminal iliac artery dilatation—nonsurgical catheter treatment of atheromatous narrowing. JAMA 230: 117–124.

Eidemiller ER, Porter JM, Rosch J, Dotter CT, Krippaehne WW (1974) Surgical treatment of bilateral iliac artery occlusive disease in high-risk patients. Am Surg 40: 511–517.

el-Bayar H, Roberts A, Hye R, Davis G, Freischlag J (1992) Determinants of failure in superficial femoral artery angioplasty. Angiology 43(11): 877–885.

Engel A, Adler OB, Rosenberger A (1982) Percutaneous transluminal angioplasty of the iliac and lower limb vessesl: one year's experience. Isr J Med Sci 18: 921–927.

Fradet G. Lidstone D, Herba M, Chiu RC, Blundell PE (1984) Percutaneous transluminal angioplasty of iliac arteries: the importance of functional studies. Can J Surg 27: 359–361.

Francois F, Picard E, Nicaud P, Albat B, Thevenet A (1991) Femoro-femoral crossover bypass for noninfective complications of aortoiliac surgery. Ann Vasc Surg 5: 46–49.

Freiman DB, Ring EJ, Oleaga JA, Berkowitz H, Roberts B (1979) Transluminal angioplasty of the iliac, femoral, and popliteal arteries. Radiology 132: 285–288.

Freiman DB, Spence R, Gatenby R, Gertner M, Roberts B, Berkowitz HD, Ring EJ, Oleaga JA (1981) Transluminal angioplasty of the iliac and femoral arteries: follow-up results without anticoagulation. Radiology 141: 347–350.

Galichia JP, Duick GF, Bajaj AK, Roberts RW (1982) Percutaneous transluminal angioplasty. The treatment of stenotic or occluded iliac arteries. J Kans Med Soc 83: 553–557.

Gibson PH (1992) Balloon angioplasty versus surgery [letter; comment]. Radiology 185(3): 908–909.

Ginsburg R, Thorpe P, Bowles CR, Wright AM, Wexler (1989) Pull-through approach to percutaneous angioplasty of totally occluded common iliac arteries. Radiology 172: 111–113.

Goldwasser B, Carson CC 3d, Braun SD, McCann RL (1985) Impotence due to the pelvic steal syndrome: treatment by iliac transluminal angioplasty. J Urol 133: 860–861.

Graor RA, Young JR, McCandless M, Swift C, Smith JA, Ruschaupt WF, Risius B, Zelch MG (1984) Percutaneous transluminal angioplasty: review of iliac and femoral dilatations at the Cleveland Clinic. Clev Clin Q 51: 149–154.

Graziani L (1987) Percutaneous recanalization of total iliac and femoropopliteal artery occlusions. Eur J Radiol 7: 91–93.

Greenfield AJ (1980) Femoral, popliteal, and tibial arteries: percutaneous transluminal angioplasty. AJR 135: 927–935.

Griffith CD, Harrison JD, Gregson RH, Makin GS, Hopkinson BR (1989) Transluminal iliac and angioplasty with distal bypass surgery in patients with critical limb ischaemia. J R Coll Surg Edinb 34: 253–255.

Gunn IG, Cowie TN, Forrest H, Quin RO, Sheldon C, Vallance R (1981) Haemodynamic assessment following iliac artery dilatation. Br J Surg 68: 858–860.

Gunther RW, Vorwerk D, Antonucci F, Beyssen B, Essinger A, Gaux JC, Joffre F, Raynaud A, Rousseau H, Zollikofer CL (1991) Iliac artery stenosis or obstruction after unsuccessful balloon angioplasty: treatment with a self-expandable stent. AJR 156: 389–393.

Gunther RW, Vorwerk D, Bohndorf K, Peters I, el-Din A, Messmer B (1989) Iliac and femoral artery stenoses and occlusions: treatment with intravascular stents. Radiology 172: 725–730.

Henriksen LO, Jorgensen B, Holstein PE, Tonnesen KH, Karle A, Sager P (1988) Percutaneous transluminal angioplasty of infrarenal arteries in intermittent claudication. Acta Chir Scand 154: 573–576.

Hodgson KJ, Sumner DS (1988) Buttock claudication from isolated bilateral internal iliac arterial stenoses. J Vasc Surg 7: 446–448.

Howd A, Spencer H. Loose H, Chamberlain J, Proud G (1986) The widening indications for transluminal angioplasty in peripheral vascular disease. Int Angiol 5: 275–279.

Howell HS, Ingram CH, Parham AR, Miller IB, Harriss WF, Wood JL, Tester DR (1983) Transluminal angioplasty of the iliac artery combined with femorofemoral bypass. South Med J 76: 49–51.

Hunink MG, Donaldson MC, Meyerovitz MF, Polak JF, Whittemore AD, Kandarpa K, Grassi CJ, et al. (1993) Risks and benefits of femoropopliteal percutaneous balloon angioplasty. J Vasc Surg 17(1): 183–192; discussion 192–194.

Insall RL, Loose HW, Chamberlain J (1993) Long-term results of double-balloon percutaneous transluminal angioplasty of the aorta and iliac arteries. Eur J Vasc Surg 7(1): 31–36.

Johnston KW (1991) Aortoiliac disease treatment. A surgical comment [comment]. Circulation 83 (2 Suppl): I61–62.

Johnston KW (1992) Factors that influence the outcome of aortoiliac and femoropopliteal percutaneous transluminal angioplasty. Surg Clin North Am 72(4): 843–850.

Johnston KW (1992) Femoral and popliteal arteries: reanalysis of results of balloon angioplasty (see comments). Radiology 183(3): 767–771.

Johnston KW (1993) Iliac arteries: reanalysis of results of balloon angioplasty. Radiology 186(1): 207–212.

Jorgensen B, Henriksen LO, Karle A, Sager P, Holstein PE, Tonnesen KH (1988) Percutaneous transluminal angioplasty of iliac and femoral arteries in severe lower-limb ischaemia. Acta Chir Scand 154: 647–652.

Joseph N, Levy E, Lipman S (1987) Angioplasty-related iliac artery rupture: treatment by temporary balloon occlusion. Cardiovasc Interventional Radiol 10: 276–279.

Kadir S, White RI Jr, Kaufman SL, Barth KH, Williams GM, Burdick JF, O'Mara CS, Smith GW, Stonesifter GL Jr, Ernst CB, Minken SL (1983) Long-term results of aortoiliac angioplasty. Surgery 94: 10–14.

Kashdan BJ, Trost DW, Jagust MB, Rackson ME, Sos TA (1992) Retrograde approach for contralateral iliac and infrainguinal percutaneous transluminal angioplasty: experience in 100 patients. J Vasc Intervent Radiol 3(3): 515–521.

Kaufman SL, Barth KH, Kadir S, Williams GM, Smith GW, Stonesifer GL Jr, Leand PM, Adams PE, Wenham F, White RI Jr (1982) Hemodynamic measurements in the evaluation and follow-up of transluminal angioplasty of the iliac and femoral arteries. Radiology 142: 329–336.

Khangure MS, Chow KC, Christensen MA (1982) Accurate and safe puncture of a pulseless femoral artery: an aid in performing iliac artery percutaneous transluminal angioplasty. Radiology 144: 927–928.

Khoury M, Batra S, Berg R, Rama K, Kozul V (1992) Influence of arterial access sites and interventional procedures on vascular complications after cardiac catheterizations. Am J Surg 164(3): 205–209.

Korogi Y, Takahashi M (1986) Percutaneous transluminal angioplasty of totally occluded iliac arteries in high-risk patients. Br J Radiol 59: 1167–1170.

Korogi Y, Takahashi M, Bussaka H, Miyawaki M, Yamashita Y (1987) Percutaneous transluminal angioplasty of the ilio-femoro-popliteal arteries: initial and long-term results. Radiat Med 5: 68–74.

Kwasnik EM, Siouffi SY, Jay ME, Khuri SF (1987) Comparative results of angioplasty and aortofemoral bypass in patients with symptomatic iliac disease. Arch Surg 122: 288–291.

Lai ST, Cheng KJ (1991) Results of angioscopy-assisted intraoperative transluminal angioplasty of the iliac and femoral artery. Chung Hua I Hsueh Tsa Chih 48: 25–30.

Laissy JP, Peillon C, Clavier E, Pernes JM, Gaux JC, Watelet J, Testart J, Benozio M (1990) Transluminal angioplasty of failing infrainguinal arterial by-pass grafts: initial and long-term results in 13 patients. Cardiovasc Intervent Radiol 13: 14–17.

Lalka SG, Lash JM, Unthank JL, Lalka VK, Cikrit DF, Sawchuk AP, Dalsing MC (1991) Inadequacy of saphenous vein grafts for cross-femoral venous bypass. Vasc Surg 13: 622–630.

Lammer J, Pilger E, Decrinis M, Quehenberger F, Klein GE, Stark G (1992) Pulsed excimer laser versus continuous-wave Nd:YAG laser versus conventional angioplasty of peripheral arterial occlusions: prospective, controlled, randomised trial. Lancet 340(8829): 1183–1188.

Levade M, Joffre F, Railhac JJ, Sabatier JC, Putois (1981) Notre experience du traitement des stenoses des arteres iliaques angioplastie transluminale percutanee. J de Radiol 62: 134.

Liddicoat AJ, Ruttley MS (1992) Deflating an angioplasty balloon [letter]. Clin Radiol 46(2): 148–149.

Lomas DJ, Britton PD (1991) CT demonstration of acute and chronic iliofemoral thrombosis. J Comput Assist Tomogr 15: 861–862.

London NJ, Bolia A, Bell PR (1993) Subintimal angioplasty for femoropopliteal artery occlusion [letter]. Lancet 341(8839): 238.

Loose HW, Ryall CJ (1988) Common iliac artery occlusion: treatment with pull-through angioplasty. Radiology 168: 273–274.

Lorentzen JE, Jorgensen L, Johansen JJ (1990) The ideal operation for unilateral iliac occlusion. Should the asymptomatic iliac artery also be reconstructed? Acta Chir Scand Suppl 555: 69–71.

Lu C, Zarins CK, Yang C, Sottiurai V (1982) Approach to transluminal angioplasty in patients with groin scarring or vascular grafts. Radiology 143: 395–398.

Miller BV, Sharp WJ, Shamma AR, Kresowik TF, Petrone S, Corson JD (1991) Surveillance for recurrent stenosis after endovascular procedures, a prospective study. Arch Surg 126: 867–871.

Millward SF, Jaward MA, Henderson DR (1989) Percutaneous transluminal angioplasty of stenosis at the common iliac artery origin using a single-balloon technique. Can Assoc Radiol J 40: 38–39.

Mittal V, Karl EM, Atkinson JB, Virmani R (1986) Early and late morphologic changes after transluminal balloon angioplasty of the iliac arteries. Am J Cardiol 58: 182–184.

Molpus WM, McCowan TC, Eidt JF (1991) External iliac artery rupture during angioplasty: control by balloon tamponade. So Med J 84: 1138: 1139.

Monaghan D, Gaines PA (1992) Case report: perforation of angioplasty balloon by Palmaz stent. Clin Radiol 46(2): 133–134.

Morse SS, Cambria R, Strauss EB, Kim B, Sniderman KW (1986) Transluminal angioplasty of the hypogastric artery for treatment of buttock claudication. Cardiovasc Intervent Radiol 9: 136–138.

Nevelsteen A, Beyens G, Duchateau J, Suy R (1990) Aorto-femoral reconstruction and sexual function: a prospective study. Eur J Vasc Surg 4: 247–251.

Olbert F, Weidinger P, Schlegl A, Teiner G, Hagmuller GW, Denck H (1981) Combined transluminal percutaneous dilation and surgical reconstruction of the iliac, femoral and popliteal arteries. Ann Radiol (Paris) 24: 369–374.

Page JE, Buckenham TM, Taylor RS (1992) Accelerated thrombolysis facilitated by direct puncture of occluded prosthetic femoral grafts. Australas Radiol 36(3): 230–233.

Palmaz JC, Richter GM, Noeldge G, Schatz RA, Robinson PD, Gardiner GA Jr, Becker GJ, McLean GK, Denny DF Jr, Lammer J, et al (1988) Intraluminal stents in atherosclerotic iliac artery stenosis: preliminary report of a multicenter study. Radiology 168: 727–731.

Parnell AP, Loose HW, Chamberlain J (1988) Fibromuscular dysplasia of the external iliac artery: treatment by percutaneous transluminal angioplasty. Br J Radiol 61: 1080–1082.

Postmann W. Wierny L (1967) Intravasale rekanalisation inoperabler arterieller obliterationen. Zentralbl Chir 92: 1586–1591.

Poulias GE, Doundoulakis N, Prombonas E, Haddad H, Papaioannou K, Lymberiades D, Savopoulos G (1992) Aorto-femoral bypass and determinants of early success and late favourable outcome. Experience with 1000 consecutive cases. J Cardiovasc Surg 33(6): 664–678.

Rees CR, Palmaz JC, Garcia O, Roeren T, Richter GM, Gardiner G Jr, Schwarten D, Schatz RA, Root HD, Rogers W (1989) Angioplasty and stenting of completely occluded iliac arteries. Radiology 172: 953–959.

Reilly DT, Packer SG, Morrison N, van Rij AM (1988) Percutaneous transluminal angioplasty for the ischaemic lower limb: the early Dunedin experience. N Z Med J 101: 129–132.

Ring EJ, Freiman DB, McLean GK, Schwarz W (1982) Percutaneous recanalization of common iliac artery occlusions: an unacceptable complication rate? AJR 139: 587–589.

Rubinstein ZJ, Morag B, Peer A, Bass A, Schneiderman J (1987) Percutaneous transluminal recanalization of common iliac artery occlusions. Cardiovasc Interventional Radiol 10: 16–20.

Saab MH, Smith DC, Aka PK, Brownlee RW, Killeen JD (1992) Percutaneous transluminal angioplasty of tibial arteries for limb salvage. Cardiovasc Intervent Radiol 15(4): 211–216.

Saddekni S, Srur M, Cohn DJ, Rozenblit G, Wetter EB, Sos TA (1985) Antegrade catheterization of the superficial femoral artery. Radiology 157: 531–532.

Saibil EA, Maggisano R (1988) Combined antegrade-retrograde catheterization of the occluded common iliac artery prior to angioplasty. Can Assoc Radiol J 39: 228–229.

Sawchuk AP, Flanigan DP, Tober JC, Eton D, Schwarcz TH, Eldrup-Jorgensen J, Meyer JP, Durham JR, Schuler JJ (1990) A rapid, accurate, noninvasive technique for diagnosing critical and subcritical stenoses in aortoiliac arteries. J Vasc Surg 12: 158–167.

Schmidtke I, Zeitler E, Schoop W (1975) Langzeitergebnisse der perkutanen katheterbehandlung (Dotter-technik) bei femoro-poplitealen arterienverschlussen im stadium II. Vasa 4: 210–226.

Schmidtke L, Zeitler E, Schoop W (1978) Late results of percutaneous catheter treatment (Dotter's technique) in occlusion of the femoropopliteal arteries, State II. In: Zeitler E, et al (eds) Percutaneous Vascular Recanalization. Springer, Berlin Heidelberg New York, chap. 15, pp 96–110.

Schmidtke L, Zeitler E, Schoop W (1978) Spatergebnisse (5–8Jahre) der perkutanen katheterbehandlung (Dotter-technik) bei femoro-poplitealen arterienverschlussen im stadium II. Vasa 7: 4–15.

Schoop W (1981) Dilatation of pelvic artery stenoses. Ann Radiol 24: 375–376.

Schoop W, Levy H, Cappius G, Mansjoer H, Zeitler E (1978) Early and late results of PTR in iliac stenosis. In: Zeitler E, et al (eds) Percutaneous Vascular Recanalization. Springer, Berlin Heidelberg New York, chap. 16, pp 111–117.

Schwarten DE (1984) Percutaneous transluminal angioplasty of the iliac arteries: intravenous digital subtraction angiography for follow-up. Radiology 150: 363–367.

Shanahan D, Grieve NW, Bennett CE, Thomas MH (1991) Retrograde femoral angioplasty: a new technique. Br J Surg 78: 1134–1135.

Simonetti G, Bonomo L, Falappa PG, Feltrin GP, Fugazzola C, Lupatelli L, Montesi A, Petrillo G (1985) Percutaneous transluminal angioplasty of iliac arteries. Ann Radiol (Paris) 28: 159–162.

Simonetti G, Rossi G, Passariello R, Caboni M, Caratelli M (1981) PTA in external iliac artery occlusion. Eur J Radiol 1: 184–186.

Simonetti G, Rossi P, Passariello R, Caboni M, Gastrucci M, Pesce B (1984) PTA in peripheral arteries. Ann Radiol (Paris) 27: 55–64.

Simonetti G, Urigo F, Guazzaroni M, Biglioli P, Dettori G, Bacciu PP (1986) Iliac artery lesions: a comparison between percutaneous transluminal angioplasty and surgery. Ann Radiol (Paris) 29: 127–129.

Strauss AL, Roth FJ, Rieger H (1993) Noninvasive assessment of pressure gradients across iliac artery stenoses: duplex and catheter correlative study. J Ultrasound Med 12(1): 17–22.

Tabbara MR, Mehringer CM, Cavaye DM, Schwartz M, Kopchok GE, Maselly M, White RA (1992) Sequential intraluminal ultrasound evaluation of balloon angioplasty of an iliac artery lesion. Ann Vasc Surg 6(2): 179–184.

Tamura S, Sniderman KW, Beinart C, Thomas A (1982) Percutaneous transluminal angioplasty of the popliteal artery and its branches. Radiology 143: 645–648.

Tegtmeyer CJ, Hartwell GD, Selby JB, Robertson R Jr, Kron IL, Tribble CG (1991) Results and complications of angioplasty in aortoiliac disease [comments]. Circulation 83 (2 Suppl): I53–60.

Tegtmeyer CJ, Moore TS, Chandler JG, Wellons HA, Rudolf LE (1979) Percutaneous transluminal dilatation of a complete block in the right iliac artery. AJR 133: 532–535.

Thorvinger B, Norgren L, Albrechtsson U (1992) Patency after iliac and femoro-popliteal angioplasty. Difference between angiographic and clinical results. Acta Radiol 33(1): 29–30.

Tonnesen KH, Holstein P, Andersen E (1991) Femoro-popliteal artery occlusions treated by percutaneous transluminal angioplasty and enclosed thrombolysis: results in 55 patients. Eur J Vasc Surg 5: 429–434.

Train JS, Dan SJ, Mitty HA, Dikman SH, Harrington EB, Miller CM, Jacobson JH, 2d (1988) Occlusion during iliac angioplasty: a salvageable complication. Radiology 168: 131–135.

Udoff EJ, Barth KL, Harrington DP, Kaufman SL, White RI (1979) Hemodynamic significance of iliac artery stenosis: Pressure measurements during angiography. Radiology 132: 289–293.

Valji K, Bookstein JJ (1988) Transluminal angioplasty in the treatment of arteriogenic impotence. REVIEW ARTICLE: 36 REFS. Cardiovasc Intervent Radiol 11: 245–252.

Van Andel GJ (1976) Percutaneous Transluminal Angioplasty. The Dotter Procedure. New York, American Elsevier Publishing Company.

Van Andel GJ (1980) Transluminal iliac angioplasty: long-term results. Radiology 135: 607–611.

Van Andel GJ (1981) Long-term results of iliac and femoral angioplasty. Ann Radiol 24: 365–368.

Van Andel GJ (1981) Transluminal iliac artery dilatation: technique of the Dotter procedure. Diagn Imaging 50: 32–42.

Van Andel GJ, Krepel VM (1979) De behandeling van stenosen in de arteriae iliacae met dilatatiecatheters (Dotter-methode). Ned Tijdschr Geneeskd 123: 873–878.

Van Andel GJ, Van Erp WF, Krepel VM, Breslau PJ (1985) Percutaneous transluminal dilatation of the iliac artery: long-term results. Radiology 156: 321–323.

Van Asten WN, Beijneveld WJ, Pieters BR, van Lier HJ, Wijn PF, Skotnicki SH (1991) Assesment of aortoiliac obstructive disease by Doppler spectrum analysis of blood flow velocities in the common femoral artery at rest and during reactive hyperemia. Surgery 109: 633–639.

Van der Vliet JA, Mulling FJ, Heijstraten FM, Reinaerts HH, Buskens FG (1992) Femoropopliteal arterial reconstruction with intraoperative iliac transluminal angioplasty for disabling claudication: results of a combined approach. Eur J Vasc Surg 6(6): 607–609.

Vanmaele RG, D'Archambeau OC, Van Schil PE, Van Landuyt KA, De Schepper AM (1993) Ruptured balloon separation during percutaneous transluminal renal artery angioplasty. Eur J Vasc Surg 7(1): 104–106.

Vawter M (1981) Percutaneous transluminal angioplasty of iliofemmoral arteries. Ariz Med 38: 687–689.

Veldhuyzen van Zanten GO, de Korte PJ, Visser R (1987) Pull-out method in percutaneous transluminal angioplasty of iliofemoral artery stenoses (letter). AJR 149: 1290.

Von Sommoggy S, Fraunhofer S, Wahba A, Blumel G, Maurer PC (1991) Coagulation in aortofemoral bifurcation bypass grafting. Eur J Vasc Surg 5: 247–253.

Von StoBlein F, Burger K, Wierny L, Widera R, (1981) Die kombinationstherapie arteriosklerotischer durchblutungsstorungen der unteren extremitat—perkutane transluminale angioplastik und chirurgische revaskularisation. Zentralbl Chir 106: 1521–1528.

Vorwerk D, Guenther RW (1990) Mechanical revascularization of occluded iliac arteries with use of self-expandable endoprostheses. Radiology 175: 411–415.

Vorwerk D, Gunther RW (1992) Stent placement in iliac arterial lesions: three years of clinical experience with the Wallstent. Cardiovasc Intervent Radiol 15(5): 285–290.

Walden R, Siegel Y, Rubinstein ZJ, Morag B, Bass A, Adar R (1986) Percutaneous transluminal angioplasty. A suggested method for analysis of clinical, arteriographic, and hemodynamic factors affecting the results of treatment. J Vasc Surg 3: 583–590.

Walker PJ, Harris JP, May J (1991) Combined percutaneous transluminal angioplasty and extra-anatomic bypass for symptomatic unilateral iliac artery occlusion with contralateral iliac artery stenosis. Ann Vasc Surg 5: 209–216.

Waltman AC (1980) Percutaneous transluminal angioplasty of iliac and deep femoral arteries. AJR 135: 921–925.

Waltman AC (1982) Catheter Systems Used in therapeutic angiography and methods of superselective vessel catheterization. In: Athanasoulis CA, Greene RE, Pfister RC, Roberson GH, Interventional Radiology, Philadelphia, W.B. Saunders Company, pp 14–21.

Waltman AC, Greenfield AJ, Novelline RA, Abbott WM, Brewster DC, Darling RC, Moncure AC, Ottinger LW, Athanasoulis CA (1982) Transluminal angioplasty of the iliac and femoropopliteal arteries. Arch Surg 117: 1218–1221.

Weber G, Kiss T (1989) Intraoperative balloon angioplasty. Eur J Vasc Surg 3: 153–157.

Weibull H, Bergqvist D, Jonsson K, Karlsson S, Takolander R (1987) Complications after percutaneous transluminal angioplasty in the iliac, femoral, and popliteal arteries. J Vasc Surg 5: 681–686.

Wellons HA Jr, Tegtmeyer CJ Jr, Crosby IK (1981) Balloon catheterization of the iliac artery: results in 34 patients. Va Med 108: 598–602.

Wexler L (1989) Percutaneous transluminal angioplasty of peripheral vascular occlusions: a clinical perspective [editorial]. J Am Coll Cardiol 13: 1555–1557.

Wheatley MJ, Hennein HA, Greenfield LJ (1991) Lower extremity arterial disease in systemic lupus erythematosus. Arch Surg 126: 109–110.

Wilson SE, Wolf GL, Cross AP (1989) Percutaneous transluminal angioplasty versus operation for peripheral arteriosclerosis. Report of a prospective randomized trial in a selected group of patients. J Vasc Surg 9: 1–9.

Youkey JR, Clagett GP, Cohen AJ, Huggins M, Olson DW, Nodalo L, Salander JM, Rich NM, Hutton JE (1983) Percutaneous transluminal balloon angioplasty of the iliac artery for contralateral ischemia. Surgery 94: 100–103.

Zeitler E (1978) Dilatation technique of iliac artery stenoses with balloon catheters. In: Zeitler E, et al (eds) Percutaneous Vascular Recanalization. Springer, Berlin Heidelberg New York, pp 24–32.

Zeitler E (1980) Percutaneous dilatation and recanalization of iliac and femoral arteries. Cardiovasc Interventional Radiol 3: 207–212.

Zeitler E (1985) Primary and late results of percutaneous transluminal angioplasty (PTA) in iliac and femoro-popliteal obliterations. Int Angiol 4: 81–85.

Zeitler E, Maresta A (1970) Ricanalizzazione transluminale percutanea delle occlusioni e delle stenosi arteriose nella arteriopatia aterosclerotica obliterative. G Clin Med 51: 381.

Zeitler E, Raithel D, Gailer H, Nippold AV, Kasprcak P (1987) PTA combined with surgical vascular operations in iliac and femoral obstruction. Ann Radiol (Paris) 30: 142–144.

Zorn-Bopp VE, Ingrisch H, Mietaschk A, Frey KW (1981) Transluminale GefaBdilatation der distalen Bauchaorta, der Arteria iliaca communis und externa. ROFO 134: 471–500.

V. Renal

Aaberg RA, Flaherty R, Smith RB (1991) Renal artery occlusive disease. Crit Care Nurs Clinics North Am 3: 507–514.

Abernethy LJ, Hendry GM, Reid JH (1989) Fibromuscular dysplasia of the renal artery in a child: detection by Doppler ultrasound and correction by percutaneous transluminal angioplasty. Pediatr Radiol 19: 539–540.

Abrass CK, Davidson WD, Guziel L, Grinnell V (1984) Therapeutic percutaneous renal artery occlusion with a detachable balloon. Am J Nephrol 4: 317–321.

Adam A, Winearls CG, Allison DJ (1983) Hypertension due to fibromuscular disease in a solitary kidney: treatment by percutaneous transluminal angioplasty. Br J Radiol 56: 494–496.

Adams CW, Reidy J (1987) Renal arterial pathology after percutaneous transluminal angioplasty. Atherosclerosis 63: 153–157.

Adler J, Ibrahim IM, Goldman M, Thomashow DF (1983) Combined thrombolysis with low-dose streptokinase and angioplasty in the treatment of renal artery occlusion. Urol Radiol 5: 113–116.

Alcaraz A, Talbot-Wright R, Alvarez-Vijande R, Cugat E, Bielsa O, Carretero P (1989) Prolonged anuria after failed percutaneous transluminal angioplasty in a kidney transplant patient solved by surgery. Eur Urol 16: 317–319.

Alfonzo JP, Caravia I, Nuviola B, Ugarte C, Banasco J, Martinez A, Alonso L, Coro R, Reyes R, Sotolongo Y, et al (1989) Renal autotransplant and percutaneous transluminal angioplast. Combined treatment in the management of renovascular hypertension—first report of two successful cases [letter]. Nephron 51: 143.

Aliabadi H, McLorie GA, Churchill BM, McMullin N (1990) Percutaneous transluminal angioplasty for transplant renal artery stenosis in children. J Urol 143: 569–572, discussion 572–573.

Archibald GR, Beckmann CF, Libertino JA (1988) Focal renal artery stenosis caused by fibromuscular dysplasia: treatment by percutaneous transluminal angioplasty. AJR 151: 593–596.

Ashenburg RJ, Blair RJ, Rivera FJ, Weigele JB (1990) Renal arterial rupture complicating transluminal angioplasty: successful conservative management. Radiology 174: 983–985.

Baert AL, Wilms G, Amery A, Vermylen J, Suy R (1990) Percutaneous transluminal renal angioplasty: initial results and long-term follow-up in 202 patients. Cardiovasc Intervent Radiol 13: 22–28.

Bailey RR, Lewis GR, Maling TM (1981) Percutaneous transluminal angioplasty: successful cure of malignant hypertension. NZ Med J 94: 256–257.

Baker KS, Sawyer RW Tisnado J, Cho SR (1986) Percutaneous transluminal angioplasty of the renal arteries: double-catheter technique. Radiology 159: 554–555.

Barbaric ZL (1982) Percutaneous transluminal angioplasty of the renal artery. Urol Clin North Am 9: 169–175.

Barth KH, Brusilow SW, Kaufman SL, Ferry FT (1981) Percutaneous transluminal angioplasty of homograft renal artery stenosis in a 10 year old girl. Pediatrics 67: 675–677.

Barth MO, Gagnadoux MF, Mareschal JL, Garel L, Mamou-Mani T, Brunelle FO (1989) Angioplasty of renal transplant artery stenosis in children. Pediatr Radiol 19: 383–387.

Bartlett ST, Dugoni WE, Jr, Ward RE (1990) Improved results with surgical treatment of renovascular hypertension: an individualized approach. J Cardiovasc Surg (Torino) 31: 351–355.

Barzi FM, Lupattelli L, Fiumicelli A (1987) Percutaneous transluminal angioplasty of radiation induced renal artery stenosis. Rays 12: 25–27, 99–100.

Baxi R, Epstein HY, Abitbol C (1981) Percutaneous transluminal renal artery angioplasty in hypertension associated with neurofibromatosis. Radiology 139: 583–584.

Beebe HG, Chesebro K, Merchant F, Bush W (1988) Results of renal artery balloon angioplasty limit its indications. REVIEW ARTICLE: 29 REFS. J Vasc Surg 8: 300–306.

Beinart C, Sos TA, Saddekni S, Weiner MA, Sniderman KW (1983) Arterial spasm during renal angioplasty. Radiology 149: 97–100.

Bell GM, Reid J, Buist TA (1987) Percutaneous transluminal angioplasty improves blood pressure and renal function in renovascular hypertension. Q J Med 63: 393–403.

Bennicke K, Ladefoged SD, Ulrich I, Sorensen K (1989) Results and complications of balloon dilatation of renal artery stenosis in patients with renovascular hypertension. Ugeskr Laeger 151: 557–560.

Benoit G, Hiesse C, Icard P, Bensadoun H, Bellamy J, Charpentier B, Jardin A, Fries D (1987) Treatment of renal artery stenosis after renal transplantation. Transplant Proc 19: 3600–3601.

Beraud JJ, Calvet B, Durand A, Mimran A (1989) Reversal of acute renal failure following percutaneous transluminal recanalization of an atherosclerotic renal artery occlusion. J Hypertens 7: 909–911.

Bergqvist D, Jonsson K, Weibull H (1987) Complications after percutaneous transluminal angioplasty of peripheral and renal arteries. Acta Radiol 28: 3–12.

Boijsen E, Kohler R (1963) Renal Artery Aneurysms. Acta Radiol (Diagn) (Stockh.) 1: 1077.

Bongard O, Schneider PA, Krahenbuhl B, Bounameaux H (1992) Transluminal angioplasty of the aorta, renal and mesenteric arteries in Takayasu arteritis: report of two cases. Eur J Vasc Surg 6(5): 567–571.

Boomsma H (1982) Percutaneous Transluminal Dilatation of Stenotic Renal Arteries in Hypertension. Groningen.

Born ML, Gerlock AJ Jr, Goncharenko V, Hollifield JW, MacDonell RC Jr (1981) Radionuclide evaluation of renal artery dilatation. Cardiovasc Intervent Radiology 4: 177–182.

Boruvka V; Stribrna J, Oppelt A, Belan A (1989) Recanalization and dilatation in chronic occlusion of the renal artery: 2 case reports. Cesk Radiol 43: 91–97.

Bover J, Montana J, Castelao AM, Seron D, Riera L, Camps I, Gil-Vernet S, Andres E, Franco E, Serrallach N, et al (1992) Percutaneous transluminal angioplasty for treatment of allograft renal artery stenosis. Transplant Proc 24(1): 94–95.

Brawn LA, Ramsay LE (1987) Is "improvement" real with percutaneous transluminal angioplasty in the management of renovascular hypertension? Lancet 2: 1313–1316.

Bredenberg CE, Sampson LN, Ray FS, Cormier RA, Heintz S, Eldrup-Jorgensen J (1992) Changing patterns in surgery for chronic renal artery occlusive diseases. J Vasc Surg 15(6): 1018–1023; discussion 1023–1024.

Bush WH, Burnett LL (1984) Balloon catheter angioplasty. Which patients with renovascular hypertension are candidates? Postgrad Med 76: 131–133, 136–139.

Cada E, Karnel F, Mayer G, Langle F, Schurawitzki H, Graf H (1989) Percutaneous transluminal angioplasty of failing arteriovenous dialysis fistulae. Nephrol Dial Transplant 4: 57–61.

Campieri C, Mignani R, Feletti C, Vangelista A, Bonomini V (1983) Percutaneous transluminal dilatation of posttransplant renal artery stenosis: beneficial effects in two cases at high surgical risk. Clin Exp Hypertens (A) 5: 803–813.

Canzanello VJ, Millan VG, Spiegel JE, Ponce PS, Kopelman RI, Madias NE (1989) Percutaneous transluminal renal angioplasty in management of atherosclerotic renovascular hypertension: results in 100 patients. Hypertension 13: 163–172.

Carmichael DJ, Mathias CJ, Snell ME, Peart S (1986) Detection and investigation of renal artery stenosis. Lancet 1: 667–670.

Carr D, Quin RO, Hamilton DN, Briggs JD, Junor BJR, Semple PF (1980)

Transluminal dilatation of transplant renal artery stenosis (technical note). Br Med J 281: 196–197.

Casarella WJ, Martin LG (1988) Failed percutaneous transluminal renal angioplasty: experience with lesions requiring operative intervention [letter]. J Vasc Surg 7: 821–822.

Cecile JP, Fournier A, Sorez JP, Louchart JC (1981) Diagnostik et traitement simple anodin et economique de l'hypertension arterielle renovasculaire (Angioplastie renale). Ann Radiol (Paris) 24: 508–514.

Chandrasoma P, Aberle AM (1986) Anastomotic line renal artery stenosis after transplantation. J Urol 135: 1159–1162.

Cianci M, Saccheri S, Giussani M, Sala C, Turolo L, et al (1991) Initial versus long-term results of percutaneous transluminal renal angioplasty in patients with renovascular hypertension. J Hypertens Suppl 9(6): S238–239.

Cicuto KP, McLean GK, Oleaga JA, Freiman DB, Grossman RA, Ring EJ (1981) Renal artery stenosis: anatomic classification for percutaneous transluminal angioplasty. AJR 137: 599–601.

Clements R, Evans C, Salaman JR (1987) Percutaneous transluminal angioplasty of renal transplant artery stenosis. Clin Radiol 38: 235–237.

Colapinto RF (1980) Inadvertent percutaneous transluminal dilatation of a renal artery with a four year follow-up. Radiology 135: 605–606.

Colapinto RF, Stronell RD, Harries-Jones EP, Gildiner M, Hobbs BB, Farrow GA, Wilson DR, Morrow JD, Logan AG, Birch SJ (1982) Percutaneous transluminal dilatation of the renal artery: follow-up studies on renovascular hypertension. AJR 139: 727–732.

Cook PG, Wells IP, Marshall AJ (1986) Case report: renovascular hypertension in Takayasu's disease treated by percutaneous transluminal angioplasty. Clin Radiol 37: 583–584.

Courtheoux P, Mani J, Mercier V, Alachkar F, Theron J (1988) Percutaneous intraluminal angioplasty in renal artery stenoses in a kidney considered to be solitary (solitary kidney, remaining kidney, before contralateral nephrectomy). Ann Radiol (Paris) 31: 177–180.

Cumberland DC (1982) Percutaneous transluminal angioplasty—experience in balloon dilatation of peripheral, coronary and renal arteries. Br J Radiol 55: 330–337.

Dal Canton A, Russo D, Iaccarino V, Caputo A, D'Anna F Andreucci VE (1983) Percutaneous angioplasty for treatment of renovascular hypertension. Proc Eur Dial Transplant Assoc 20: 582–586.

Davidson CJ, Newman GE, Sheikh KH, Kisslo K, Stack RS, Schwab SJ (1991) Mechanisms angioplasty in hemodialysis fistula stenoses evaluated by intravascular ultrasound. Kidney Inter 40: 91–95.

De Jong PE, De Zeeuw D, Smit AJ, Hoorntje SJ, Schuur KH, Donker AJ,

Van der Hem GK (1983) The effect of transluminal dilation of stenosed renal arteries on kidney function. Neth J Med 26: 266–270.

De Meyer M, Pirson Y, Dautrebande J, Squifflet JP, Alexandre GP, Van Ypersele de Strihou C (1989) Treatment of renal graft artery stenosis. Comparison between surgical bypass and percutaneous transluminal angioplasty. Transplantation 47: 784–788.

De Plaen JF, Maiter D (1987) The selection of hypertensive atherosclerotic patients for surgery or percutaneous transluminal angioplasty (PTA). Acta Clin Belg 42: 58–65.

Dean RH, Callis JT, Smith BM, Meacham PW (1987) Failed percutaneous transluminal renal angioplasty: experience with lesions requiring operative intervention. J Vasc Surg 6: 301–307.

Dell'Aria JC, Petrilli R, Schwartz E (1988) Acute occlusion of the left renal artery manifested by hypertensive crisis. J Emerg Med 6: 23–27.

Denny DF, Perlmutt LM, Bettmann MA (1984) Percutaneous recanalization of an occluded renal artery and delayed ethanol ablation of the kidney resulting in control of hypertension. Radiology 151: 381–382.

Diamond NG, Casarella WJ, Hardy MA, Appel GB (1979) Dilatation of critical transplant renal artery stenosis by percutaneous transluminal angioplasty. AJR 133: 1167–1169.

Dixon GD, Anderson S, Crouch TT (1986) Renal arterial rupture secondary to percutaneous transluminal angioplasty treated without surgical intervention. Cardiovasc Intervent Radiol 9: 83–85.

Dong ZJ, Li SH, Lu XC (1987) Percutaneous transluminal angioplasty for renovascular hypertension in arteritis: experience in China. Radiology 162: 477–479.

Doyle JE, Sequeira JC (1982) Treating renovascular hypertension: renal artery dilation. Am J Nurs; 82: 1563–1564.

Dunn FG, Husserl FE, Miller KD Jr, Tutton RH, Messerli FH, Dreslinski GR, Batson HM, Figueroa JE, Frohlich ED (1982) Transluminal angioplasty in the treatment of renovascular hypertension. J La State Med Soc 134: 24–27.

Dunnick NR, Sfakianakis GN (1991) Screening for renovascular hypertension. Radiol Clin North Am 29: 497–510.

Easterling TR, Brateng D, Goldman ML, Strandness DE, Zaccardi MJ (1991) Renal vascular hypertension during pregnancy. Obstet Gynecol 78:(5 Pt 2): 921–925.

Eckstein MR, Waltman AC, Athanasoulis CA (1984) Interventional angiography of the renal fossa. Radiol Clin North Am 22: 381–392.

Edwards JM, Zaccardi MJ, Strandness DE Jr (1992) A preliminary study of the role of duplex scanning in defining the adequacy of treatment of patients with renal artery fibromuscular dysplasia. J Vasc Surg 15(4): 604–609; discussion 609–611.

Ekelund L (1984) Increased kidney size following renal angioplasty. A 'new' observation. Acta Radiol (Diagn) (Stockh) 25: 401–405.

Ekelund L, Gerlock J Jr, Goncharenko V, Foster J (1978) Angiographic findings following surgical treatment for renovascular hypertension. Radiology 126: 345–359.

Ekelund L, Johnsson N, Lindstedt E, Stridbeck H, Lundquist SB (1981) Dilatation of experimental renal artery stenosis by balloon catheter. Acta Radiol Diagn 5: 561–569.

Elishu EH, Haire HM, Tew FT, Newton LW (1980) Control of malignant renovascular hypertension by percutaneous transluminal angioplasty and therapeutic renal embolization. AJR 134: 815–817.

England WL, Roberts SD, Grim CE (1987) Surgery or angioplasty for cost-effective renal revascularization? Med Decis Making 7: 84–91.

Englund R, Brown MA (1991) Renal angioplasty for renovascular disease: a reappraisal. J Cardiovasc Surg 32: 76–80.

Etheredge SB, Mahony JF, Savdie E, Waugh RC, Sheil AG (1982) Treatment of renal transplant artery stenosis by percutaneous transluminal dilatation. Clin Nephrol 17: 217–221.

Eurvilaichit C (1989) Percutaneous transluminal renal angioplasty (PTRA) in patients with renal artery stenosis. J Med Assoc Thai 72: 223–239.

Eyler WR, Clark MD, Garman JE, et al (1962) Angiography of the renal arterial stenoses in patients with and without hypertension. Radiology 78: 879–892.

Fallo F, Oberfield SE, Levine LS, Stoner E, Greig F, Sniderman K, Saddekni S, Sos T, New MI (1986) Percutaneous transluminal renal angioplasty in the treatment of renovascular hypertension in children. Clin Exp Hypertens (A) 8: 887–891.

Fauchald P, Vatne K, Paulsen D, Brodahl U, Sodal G, Holdaas H, Berg KJ, Flatmark A (1992) Long-term clinical results of percutaneous transluminal angioplasty in transplant renal artery stenosis. Nephrol Dial Transplan 7(3): 256–259.

Fava C, Grosso M, Sandrone M, Malfi B, Segoloni GP, Colla L (1988) Percutaneous transluminal angioplasty after renal transplantation. Radiol Med (Torino) 76: 1–7.

Flechner S, Novick AC, Vidt D, Buonocore E, Meaney T (1982) The use of percutaneous transluminal angioplasty for renal artery stenosis in patients with generalized atherosclerosis. J Urol 127: 1072–1075.

Flechner SM (1984) Percutaneous transluminal dilatation. A realistic appraisal in patients with stenosing lesions of the renal artery. Urol Clin North Am 11: 515–527.

Freiman DB (1985) Transluminal angioplasty of the renal arteries. Urol Clin North Am 12: 737–742.

Freiman DB, Helinek TG (1989) Angioplasty of bilateral renal artery occlusion—a case report. Angiology 40: 59–62.

Gardiner GA, Jr, Freedman AM, Shlansky-Goldberg R (1988) Percutaneous transluminal angioplasty: delayed response in neurofibromatosis. Radiology 169: 79–80.

Garfinkel HB, Rohr RE, Rottenberg RW (1984) Angioplasty of a stenotic aorto-renal artery saphenous vein bypass graft to a single kidney. Am J Kidney Dis 4: 171–174.

Gaux JC, Borquelot P, Raynaud A, Seurot M, Cattan S (1983) Percutaneous transluminal angioplasty of stenotic lesions in dialysis vascular accesses. Eur J Radiol 3: 189–193.

Gedroyc WM, Reidy JF, Saxton HM (1987) Arteriography of renal transplantation. Clin Radiol 38: 239–43.

Gemma K, Ohya T, Kumazaki T, Nishikawa H (1988) A Clinical experience with percutaneous transluminal angioplasty of bilateral stenotic renal arteries due to fibromuscular dysplasia. Rinsho Hoshasen 33: 523–526.

Gerard DF, Devin JB, Halasz NA, Collins GM (1982) Transplant renal artery thrombosis revascularization after 5 ½ hours of ischemia. Arch Surg 117: 361.

Gerlock AJ Jr, MacDonell RC Jr, Smith CW, Muhletaler CA, Parris WC, Johnson HK, Tallent MB, Richie RE, Kendall RI (1983) Renal transplant arterial stenosis: percutaneous transluminal angioplasty. AJR 140: 325–331.

Geyskes GG (1988) Treatment of renovascular hypertension with percutaneous transluminal renal angioplasty. REVIEW ARTICLE: 73 REFS. Am J Kidney Dis 12: 253–265.

Geyskes GG, de Bruyn AJ (1991) Captopril renography and the effect of percutaneous transluminal angioplasty on blood pressure in 94 patients with renal artery stenosis. Am J Hypertens 4(12 Pt 2): 685S–689S.

Geyskes GG, Oei HY, Faber JA (1986) Renography: prediction of blood pressure after dilatation of renal artery stenosis. Nephron 44 (Suppl 1): 54–59.

Geyskes GG, Oei HY, Klinge J, Kooiker CJ, Puylaert CB, Dorhout Mees EJ (1988) Renovascular hypertension: the small kidney updated. Q J Med 66: 203–217.

Geyskes GG, Puylaert CBAT, Oei HY, Boomsma JHB (1979) Intraluminal dilatation of renal artery stenosis. Clin Sci 57: 441–443.

Geyskes GG, Puylaert CB, Oei HY, Mees EJ (1983) Follow up study of 70 patients with renal artery stenosis treated by percutaneous transluminal dilatation. Br Med J 287: 333–336.

Ghisla R, Mahler F, Haertel M, Krneta A, Oetliker O, Rossi E (1983) Lasting antihypertensive effect of percutaneous transluminal angioplasty of renal artery stenoses in a child. Am J Dis Child 137: 600–601.

Giorgetti PL, Lovaria A, Saccheri S, Arpesani A, Rignano A, Bortolani EM, Galimberti M (1991) Locoregional fibrinolysis using tissue plasminogen activator in 2 cases of acute thrombosis of the renal artery. Panminerva Med 33(4): 180–184.

Glanz S, Gordon D, Butt KM, Hong J, Adamson R, Sclafani SJ (1984) Dialysis access fistulas: treatment of stenoses by transluminal angioplasty. Radiology 152: 637–642.

Glorioso N, Dessi' Fulgheri P, Madeddu P, Rappelli A (1982) Persistence of unilateral secretion and contralateral renin suppression after successful percutaneous transluminal dilatation in a normotensive patient. Acta Cardiol (Brux) 37: 451–454.

Gmelin E, Winterhoff R, Rinast E (1989) Insufficient hemodialysis access fistulas: late results of treatment with percutaneous balloon angioplasty. Radiology 171: 657–660.

Goertz KK, Linshaw MA, Lee KR, Hermreck A, Mattioli L, Bailie MD (1982) Transluminal arterial dilation of a postsurgical stenosis of renal artery implant in a child with recurrent hypertension. Pediatrics 69: 489–491.

Gordon DH, Glanz S, Butt KM, Adamsons RJ, Koenig MA (1982) Treatment of stenotic lesions in dialysis access fistulas and shunts by transluminal angioplasty. Radiology 143: 53–58.

Gosse P, Choussat A, Dallocchio M (1988) The role of transluminal angioplasty in the treatment of renovascular arterial hypertension. Presse Med 17: 187–188.

Gosse P, Choussat A, Tap R, Baudet E, Fontan F, Dallocchio M (1988) Treatment of renovascular arterial hypertension: angioplasty versus surgery. Arch Mal Coeur 81 Spec No: 213–216.

Greenstein SM, Verstandig A, McLean GK, DaFoe DC, Burke DR, Meranze SG, Naji A, Brayman KL, Grossman RA, Perloff LJ, et al (1987) Percutaneous transluminal angioplasty: the procedure of choice for renal allograft artery stenosis. Transplant Proc 19: 2194–2196.

Greenstein SM, Verstandig A, McLean GK, DaFoe DC, Burke DR, Meranze SG, Naji A, Grossman RA, Perloff LJ, Barker CF (1987) Percutaneous transluminal angioplasty. The procedure of choice in the hypertensive renal allograft recipeint with renal artery stenosis. Transplantation 43: 29–32.

Greminger P, Steiner A, Schneider E, Kuhlmann U, Steurer J, Siegenthaler W, Vetter W (1989) Cure and improvement of renovascular hypertension after percutaneous transluminal angioplasty of renal artery stenosis. Nephron 51: 362–366.

Grim CE (1981) Percutaneous transluminal dilatation: the treatment of choice for renal artery stenosis causing hypertension. Am J Kidney Dis 1: 186–187.

Grim CE, Luft FC, Yune HY, Klatte EC, Weinberger MH (1981) Percutaneous transluminal dilatation in the treatment of renal vascular hypertension. Ann Intern Med 95: 439–442.

Grim CE, Whitworth JA, Thomson KR, Hare WS, Kincaid-Smith PS (1985) Treatment of renal artery stenosis with percutaneous transluminal angioplasty. Australas Radiol 29: 42–49.

Grim CE, Yune HY, Donohue JP, Weinberger MH, Dilley R, Klatte EC (1986) Renal vascular hypertension. Surgery vs. dilation. Nephron 44 (Suppl 1): 96–100.

Grim CE, Yune HY, Donahue JP, Weinberger MH, Dilley R, Klatte EC (1982) Unilateral renal vascular hypertension: surgery vs. dilation. Vasa 11: 367–368.

Gross-Fengels W, Degenhardt S, Steinbrich W (1988) Early and late results of percutaneous transluminal angioplasty of renal artery stenoses. Radiologe 28: 387–394.

Grossman RA, Dafoe DC, Shoenfeld RB, Ring EJ, McLean GK, Oleaga JA, Freiman DB, Naji A, Perloff LJ, Barker CF (1982) Percutaneous transluminal angioplasty treatment of renal transplant artery stenosis. Transplantation 34: 339–343.

Gruenewald SM, Collins LT, Antico VF, Farlow DC, Fawdry RM (1989) Can quantitative renography predict the outcome of treatment of atherosclerotic renal artery stenosis? J Nucl Med 30: 1946–1954.

Gruenewald SM, Stewart JH, Crocker EF (1983) Advances in diagnosis and treatment of renovascular hypertension. Med J Aust 1: 572–574.

Gruentzig A, Kuhlmann U, Vetter W, Lutolf U, Meier B, Siegenthaler W (1978) Treatment of renovascular hypertension with percutaneous transluminal dilatation of a renal artery stenosis. Lancet 1: 801–802.

Grutzmacher P, Bussmann WD, Meyer TH, Starck E, Kollath J, Baum RP, Fassbinder W, Schoeppe W (1988) Non-operative revascularization of renal artery occlusion by transluminal angioplasty. Nephrol Dial Transplant 3: 130–137.

Gutierrez OH, Izzo JL Jr, Burgener FA (1981) Transluminal recanalization of an occluded renal artery: reversal of anuria in a patient with a solitary kidney. AJR 137: 1254–1256.

Guzzetta PC, Potter BM, Kapur S, Ruley EJ, Randolph J (1983) Reconstruction of the renal artery after unsuccessful percutaneous transluminal angioplasty in children. Am J Surg 145: 647–651.

Hagg A, Abers H, Eriksson I, Lorelius LE, Morlin C (1987) Fibromuscular dysplasia of the renal artery: management and outcome. Acta Chir Scand 153: 15–20.

Hagg A, Lorelius LE, Morlin C, Aberg H (1985) Percutaneous transluminal renal artery dilatation for fibromuscular dysplasia with special reference to the acute effects on the renin-angiotensin-aldosterone system and blood pressure. Scand J Urol Nephrol 19: 205–209.

Hagg A, Lorelius LE, Morlin C, Wide L (1988) Serial measurements of plasma renin activity, aldosterone and cortisol during percutaneous transluminal angioplasty of the renal artery in man. Acta Physiol Scand 134: 473–478.

Halley SE, White WB, Ramsby GR, Voytovich AE (1988) Renovascular hypertension in moyamoya syndrome. Therapeutic response to percutaneous transluminal angioplasty. REVIEW ARTICLE: 13 REFS. Am J Hypertens 1: 348–352.

Hariharan S, Pandey AP, Jacob CK, Shastry JC, Kirubakaran MG (1987) Nephrotic-range proteinuria with renal artery stenosis: its reversal after transluminal angioplasty (letter). Nephron 47: 77.

Hawkins IF Jr, Freeman JA, Pillsbury ND (1982) A new minicatheter and deflector technique for renal angioplasty. Radiology 145: 837–838.

Hayes JM, Risius B, Novick AC, Geisinger M, Zelch M, Gifford RW, Jr., Vidt DG, Olin JW (1988) Experience with percutaneous transluminal angioplasty for renal artery stenosis at the Cleveland Clinic. J Urol 139: 488–492.

Hayes PT, Siddle KJ, Harper J, Petrie JB (1982) Transluminal angioplasty of a transplant renal artery stenosis. Australas Radiol 26: 171–173.

Heeney DJ, Bookstein JJ, Carey PH, Rapoport S (1982) The role of para renal collaterals in assessing renal artery stenosis before and after percutaneous transluminal angioplasty. Cardiovasc Intervent Radiol 5: 71–78.

Heidler R, Zeitler E, Gessler U (1978) Percutaneous transluminal dilatation of stenosis behind AV-fistulas in hemodialysis patients. In: Zeitler E et al. (eds) Percutaneous Vascular Recanalization. Berlin Heidelberg New York, Springer, pp 142–144.

Hernandez Lezana A, Gallego Beuter J (1988) Percutaneous transluminal angioplasty in hypertensive patients with stenosis of the renal arteries. Rev Clin Esp 182: 347–349.

Heyborne KD, Schultz MF, Goodlin RC, Durham JD (1991) Renal artery stenosis during pregnancy: a review. Obstet Gynecol Surv 46: 509–514.

Hillman BJ, Ovitt TW, Capp MP, Prosnitz EH, Osborne RW Jr, Goldstone J, Zukoski CF, Malone JM (1982) The potential impact of digital video substraction angiography on screening for renovascular hypertension. Radiology 142: 577–579.

Hiramatsu K, Narimatsu Y (1988) The kidney and adrenal gland angiography: their therapeutic application in embolization and angioplasty. Rinsho Hoshasen 33: 1359–1375.

Hohnke C, Abendroth D, Schleibner S, Land W (1987) Vascular complications in 1,200 kidney transplantations. REVIEW ARTICLE: 3 REFS. Transplant Proc 19: 3691–3692.

Hollenberg NK (1987) The treatment of renovascular hypertension: surgery, angioplasty, and medical therapy with converting-enzyme inhibitors. Am J Kidney Dis 10 (1 Suppl 1): 52–60.

Holley KE, Hunt JC, Brown AL Jr, et al (1964) Renal artery stenosis: a clinical-pathologic study in normotensive and hypertensive patients. Am J Med 37: 14–22.

Hoorntje SJ, Donker AJ, Schuur KH, Boomsma JH (1982) Renal artery dilatation in a patient on captopril: changing a "two-kidney, two-clip hypertension" into a "two-kidney, one clip hypertension." Nephron 30: 56–59.

Houck WS (1979) Renovascular hypertension secondary to arterial fibrodysplasia: treatment by dilation using a Fogarty balloon. JAMA 242: 1396–1397.

Hovinga TK, De Jong PE, De Zeeuw D, Schuur KH, Van de Hem GK (1986) Short-term effects of percutaneous transluminal renal angioplasty on renal function in unilateral renal artery stenosis. Neth J Med 29: 347–351.

Hruby W (1989) Interventional uroradiology. Curr Opin Radiol 1: 290–292.

Hudgins LB, Gold RE, Gregory AW (1980) Percutaneous transluminal angioplasty - an alternative treatment for renovascular hypertension. South Med J 73: 810–812.

Hunter DW, So SK, Castaneda-Zuniga WR, Coleman CE, Sutherland DE, Amplatz K (1983) Failing or thrombosed Brescia-Cimino arteriovenous dialysis fistulas. Angiographic evaluation and percutaneous transluminal angioplasty. Radiology 149: 105–109.

Imanishi M, Ohta M, Akabane S, Kawamura M, Matsushima Y, Kojima S, Kuramochi M, Kimura K, Takamiya M, Ito K, et al (1991) Aspirin injection test to predict angioplasty outcome in unilateral renovascular hypertension: preliminary report. Clin Invest Med 14(6): 566–573.

Ingrisch H (1981) Diagnostik der nierenarterien-stenose durch angiotomographie. Fortschr Med 99: 774.

Ingrisch H, Hazlin M (1980) Perkutane transluminale angioplastik einer stenose in einem aortorenalen veneninterpositionstransplantat. ROEFO 133: 493–495.

Ingrisch H, Hegele T, Frey KW (1982) Angiographic control of renal artery stenoses 6 months following percutaneous transluminal angioplasty. Cardiovasc Intervent Radiol 5: 249–256.

Ingrisch H, Holzgrev H, Middleke M, Frey KW (1980) New developments in diagnosis and treatment of renovascular hypertension. Klin Wochenschr 58: 1105–1115.

Ishibashi M, Morita S, Umezaki N, Ohtake H (1988) Evaluation of renal first pass blood flow with a functional image technique in hypertensive patients. Eur J Nucl Med 14: 25–27.

Jeunemaitre X, Raynaud A, Pagny JY, Chatellier G, Julien J, Plouin PF,

Lagneau P, Corvol P (1988) Transluminal angioplasty in renovascular hypertension with renal insufficiency. Arch Mal Coeur 81 Spec No: 217–220.

Joffre F, Rousseau H, Bernadet P, Nomblot C, Montoy JC, Chemali R, Knight C (1992) Midterm results of renal artery stenting. Cardiovasc Intervent Radiol 15(5): 313–318.

Julien J, Jeunemaitre X, Raynaud A, Azizi M, Pagny JY, Plouin PF, Corvol P (1989) Influence of age on the outcome of percutaneous angioplasty in atheromatous renovascular disease. J Hypertens Suppl 7: S188–S189.

Kadir S, Russell RP, Kaufman SL, Williams GM, Burdick JF, White RI Jr, Soya-Grimm K (1984) Renal artery angioplasty. Technical considerations and results. ROFO 141: 378–383.

Kadir S, Watson A, Burrow C (1987) Percutaneous transcatheter recanalization in the management of acute renal failure due to sudden occlusion of the renal artery to a solitary kidney. Am J Nephrol 7: 445–449.

Kancharla SR, Kumar A, Curmally FM, Goyal BK (1991) Renal angioplasty in a case of renovascular hypertension presenting with stroke. J Assoc Physicians India 39(7): 580–581.

Kang HJ, Trethewey KL, Bauer J, Lee HT (1981) Percutaneous transluminal angioplasty in renal artery stenosis. Mo Med 78: 582–588.

Kaplan-Pavlobcic S, Koselj M, Obrez I, Luzar S, Licina A, Kolar B, Surlan M (1985) Percutaneous transluminal renal angioplasty: follow up studies on renovascular hypertension. Przegl Lek 42: 342–344.

Katafuchi T, Abe I, Kawasaki T, Muratani H, Omae T, Fukiyama K, Numaguchi Y (1981) A case of renovascular hypertension treated with percutaneous transluminal angioplasty. Jpn J Nephr 23: 789–797.

Katzen BT, Chang J, Lukowsky GH, Abramson EG (1970) Percutaneous transluminal angioplasty for treatment of renovascular hypertension. Radiology 131: 53–58.

Kazmers A, Moneta GL, Harley JD, Goldman ML, Clowes AW (1989) Treatment of acute renal artery occlusion after percutaneous transluminal angioplasty. J Vasc Surg 9: 487–492.

Khalilullah M, Tyagi S (1992) Percutaneous transluminal angioplasty in Takayasu arteritis. Heart Vessels 7(Suppl): 146–153.

Kim D, Porter DH, Siegel JB, Shapiro ME, Strom TB, Glotzer DJ (1991) Use of a reperfusion catheter after angioplasty dissection for salvage of ischemic renal allograft: case report. Cardiovasc Intervent Radiol 14: 179–182.

Kim PK, Spriggs DW, Rutecki GW, Reaven RE, Blend D, Whittier FC (1989) Transluminal angioplasty in patients with bilateral renal artery stenosis or renal artery stenosis in a solitary functioning kidney. AJR Am J Roentgenol 153: 1305–1308.

Kirste G, Wilms H, Matthias K (1990) Transluminal angioplasty as treatment for renal transplant artery stenosis [letter]. Transplantation 50: 357.

Klinge J, Mali WP, Puijlaert CB, Geyskes GG, Becking WB, Feldberg MA (1989) Percutaneous transluminal renal angioplasty: initial and long-term results. Radiology 171: 501–506.

Koga N, Sato T, Baba T, Ueda O, Okazaki H, Kohchi K, Norita H, Maw PR, Moriyama A (1989) Angioscopy in transluminal balloon and laser angioplasty in the management of chronic hemodialysis fistulae. ASAIO Trans 35: 193–196.

Koga T, Okuda S, Takishita S, Shigematsu A, Komota T, Fujishima M, Matsukuma A (1991) Renal failure due to cholesterol embolization following percutaneous transluminal renal angioplasty. Jpn J Med 30: 35–38.

Koga T, Ueno M, Tsuchihashi T, Tomita Y, Abe I, Muratani H, Takata Y, Takishita S, Kobayashi K, Fujishima M (1988) The effect of percutaneous transluminal angioplasty in renovascular hypertension and the renin-angiotensin system. Nippon Jinzo Gakkai Shi 30: 1265–1271.

Kopelman RI, McNutt RA, Pauker SG (1988) Use of decision analysis in a complicated case of renovascular hypertension [clinical conference]. Hypertension 12: 611–619.

Korogi Y, Takahashi M (1993) A double-guide-wire technique in renal angioplasty. A modified approach. Acta Radiol 34(2): 196–197.

Korogi Y, Takahashi M Bussaka H, Miyawaki M, Tokuda N (1985) Percutaneous transluminal angioplasty for renal branch stenosis: a report on a six-year-old boy. Br J Radiol 58: 77–78.

Kremer Hovinga TK, de Jong PE (1989) Results of percutaneous transluminal angioplasty in renal artery stenosis in 1978–1986 (letter). Ned Tijdschr Geneeskd 133: 998.

Kremer Hovinga TK, de Jong PE, de Zeeuw D, Donker AJ, Schuur KH, van der Hem GK (1986) Restenosis prevalence and long-term effects on renal function after percutaneous transluminal renal angioplasty. Nephron 44 (Suppl 1): 64–67.

Kudo K, Abe K, Yasujima M, Seino M, Sata M, Omata K, Hiwatari M, Kanazawa M, Yoshinaga K (1989) The clinical profiles of 78 patients with renovascular hypertension. Nippon Naika Gakkai Zasshi 78: 493–499.

Kuhlmann U, Greminger P, Gruentzig A, Schneider E, Pouliadis G, Luscher T, Steurer J, Siegenthaler W, Vetter W (1985) Long-term experience in percutaneous transluminal dilatation of renal artery stenosis. Am J Med 79: 692–698.

Kuhlmann U, Gruentzig A, Vetter W, Lutolf U, Meier B, Siegenthaler W (1978) Percutaneous transluminal dilatation: a new treatment of renovascular hypertension? Klin Wochenschr 56: 703–707.

Kuhlmann U, Gruentzig A, Vetter W, Siegenthaler W (1978) Renovaskular hypertonie: therapiedurch perkutane transluminale dilatation von nierenarterienstnosen. Schweiz Med Wochenschr 108: 1847–1850.

Kuhlmann U, Vetter W, Furrer J, Lutolf U, Siegenthaler W, Gruentzig A (1980) Renovascular hypertension: treatment by percutaneous transluminal dilatation. Ann Intern Med 92: 1–6.

Kuhlmann U, Vetter W, Gruentzig A, Schneider E, Pouliadis G, Steurer J, Siegenthaler W (1981) Percutaneous transluminal dilatation of renal artery stenosis: 2 years' experience. Clinic Sci 61: 481–483.

Kuhn FP, Kutkuhn B, Torsello G, Modder U (1991) Renal artery stenosis: preliminary results of treatment with the Strecker stent. Radiology 180: 367–372.

Kuiper KJ, de Jong PE, de Zeeuw D, Schuur KH, Van der Hem GK (1983) Restenosis of the renal artery after percutaneous transluminal renal angioplasty: an inevitable outcome? Proc Eur Dial Transplant Assoc 20: 538–545.

Kukharch VV, Arabidze GG, Matveeva LS, Shpilkin VM, Kungurts VV, Khalchev VM, Kutsenko AI, Saveliev VY, (1982) Transcutaneous intravascular balloon dilatation in patients with stenosis of the renal artery and arterial hypertension. Kardiologia 22: 38.

Kumagai H, Suzuki H, Matsukawa S, Ryuzaki M, Saruta T (1989) Captopril therapy following percutaneous transluminal angioplasty for bilateral renal artery stenosis. Arch Intern Med 149: 1973–1976.

Kupersmit MA (1981) Percutaneous transluminal angioplasty of the renal arteries. J Am Osteopath Assoc 81: 173–176.

Laasonen L, Edgren J, Forslund T, Eklund B (1985) Renal transplant artery stenosis and percutaneous transluminal angioplasty. Acta Radiol (Diagn) (Stockh) 26: 609–613.

Lacombe P, Mulot R, Labedan F, Jondeau G, Barre O, Chagnon S, Judet O, et al. (1992) Percutaneous recanalization of a renal artery in aortic dissection. Radiology 185(3): 829–831.

Lamki L, Spence JD, MacDonald AC, Roulston M (1986) Differential glomerular filtration rate in diagnosis of renovascular hypertension and follow-up of balloon angioplasty. Clin Nucl Med 11: 188–193.

Lang EV, Bookstein JJ (1989) Accelerated thrombolysis and angioplasty for hand ischemia in Buerger's disease. Cardiovasc Intervent Radiol 12: 95–97.

Lawrence PF, Miller FJ, Mineau DE (1981) Balloon catheter dilatation in patients with failing arteriovenous fistulas. Surgery 89: 439–442.

Lawson JD, Boerth R, Foster JH, Dean RH (1977) Diagnosis and management of renovascular hypertension in children. Arch Surg 112: 1307–1316.

Legge D (1984) Renal angioplasty. Ir Med J 77: 115–116.

Levin DC (1984) Percutaneous transluminal angioplasty of the renal arteries. JAMA 251: 759–763.

Levin DC, Murray P, Harrington DP (1982) New curved catheter for renal angioplasty. AJR 138: 359–360.

Levitt RG, Wholey M (1990) Renal arterial rupture complicating transluminal angioplasty [letter]. Radiology 176: 583–584.

Libertino JA (1991) Renovascular hypertension in elderly patients. Cardiol Clin 9: 543–545.

Logan AG, Steinhardt MI (1980) Restoration of renal function by unilateral percutaneous transluminal dilatation of stenosed renal artery. Can Med Assoc J 122: 910–912.

Lohr E, Bock KD, Eigler F, Verhagen V, Sievers K, Phillip T, Stuschke M (1991) Angioplasty of renal arteries: a report of ten year's experience. Angiology 42: 44–47.

Lohr E, Weichert HC, Funke-Volkers R, Strotges MW, Bildstein A (1982) Renal angioplasty: experiences with 94 patients. Urol Radiol 4: 211–214.

Lohr JW, MacDougall ML, Chonko AM, Diederich DA, Grantham JJ, Savin VJ, Wiesmann TB (1986) Percutaneous transluminal angioplasty in transplant renal artery stenosis: experience and review of the literature. Am J Kidney Dis 7: 363–367.

Lossef SV, Rackson ME, Sos TA (1990) Renal angioplasty using a TEGwire angioplasty balloon: technical note. Cardiovasc Intervent Radiol 13: 115–116.

Lucon AM, Sabbaga E, Borrelli M, deGoes GM (1984) Percutaneous transluminal dilatation of renal artery stenosis in transplanted kidney. Urology 24: 485–486.

Luft FC, Grim CE, Weinberger MH (1983) Intervention in patients with renovascular hypertension and renal insufficiency. J Urol 130: 654–656.

Lund G, Sinaiko A, Castaneda-Zuniga W, Cragg A, Salomonowitz E, Amplatz K (1984) Percutaneous transluminal angioplasty for treatment of renal artery stenosis in children. Eur J Radiol 4: 254–257.

Lundbom J, Ystgaard B, Myhre HO, Myhr G, Anda S, Wideroe T (1989) Surgical treatment of renal artery stenosis. Tidsskr Nor Laegeforen 109: 1971–1973.

Luscher TF, Greminger P, Kuhlmann, U, Siegenthaler W, Largiader F, Vetter W (1986) Renal venous renin determinations in renovascular hypertension. Diagnostic and prognostic value in unilateral renal artery stenosis treated by surgery or percutaneous transluminal angioplasty. Nephron 44 (Suppl 1): 17–24.

MacDonell RC Jr, Gerlock AJ Jr, Parris WC, Richie RE, Tallent MB, Johnson HK, Turner BI, Niblack GD (1980) Therapeutic angiography in renal transplant complications. Proc Clin Dial Transplant Forum 10: 145–149.

Madias NE (1982) Percutaneous transluminal renal angioplasty. Chest 81: 632–634.

Madias NE, Ball JT, Millan VG (1981) Percutaneous transluminal renal angioplasty in the treatment of unilateral atherosclerotic renovascular hypertension. Am J Med 70: 1078–1083.

Madias NE, Kwon OJ, Millan VG (1982) Percutaneous transluminal renal angioplasty. A potentially effective treatment for preservation of renal function. Arch Intern Med 142: 693–697.

Magalhaes AC, David E, Magalhaes A (1989) Percutaneous recanalization of a renal artery with restoration of renal function. J Radiol 70: 57–59.

Mahler F, Krneta A, Haertel M (1979) Treatment of renovascular hypertension by transluminal renal artery dilatation. Ann Intern Med 90: 56–57.

Mahler F, Probst P, Haertel M, Weidmann P, Krneta A (1982) Lasting improvement of renovascular hypertension by transluminal dilatation of atherosclerotic and nonatherosclerotic renal artery stenoses: a follow-up study. Circulation 65: 611–617.

Mahler F, Probst P, Weidmann P, Krneta A (1981) Transluminal dilatation of renal artery stenoses due to atherosclerosis and fibromuscular dysplasia: early results and follow-up of twelve consecutive cases. Ann Radiol (Paris) 24: 355–356.

Mahler F, Triller J, Weidmann P, Nachbur B (1986) Complications in percutaneous transluminal dilatation of renal arteries. Nephron 44 (Suppl 1): 60–63.

Main J, Loose H (1991) Angioplasty in atheromatous renovascular disease [letter]. Clin Radiol 44: 139–140.

Majeski JA, Munda R (1981) Hazard of percutaneous transluminal dilation in renal transplant arterial stenosis. Arch Surg 116: 1225–1226.

Mali WP, Puijlaert CB, Kouwenberg HJ, Klinge J, Donckerwolcke RA, Geijskes BG, Overbosch EH, Rosenbusch GJ, Ludwig WW, Feldberg MA (1987) Percutaneous transluminal renal angioplasty in children and adolescents. Radiology 165: 391–394.

Mallmann R, Roth FJ (1986) Treatment of neurofibromatosis associated renal artery stenosis with hypertension by percutaneous transluminal angioplasty. Clin Exp Hypertens (A) 8: 893–899.

Manly RJ, Belzer FO (1981) Spontaneous reversal of renal failure by renal artery recanalization. Arch Surg 116: 107–109.

Mann JF, Mehmel HC, Allenberg J, Ritz E, Kubler W (1985) Dilatation to avoid dialysis: angioplasty of an occluded renal artery with a coronary guiding catheter (letter). Lancet 1: 579.

Marshall FI, Hagen S, Mahaffy RG, Petrie JC, Roy-Chaudhury P, Russell

IT, Webster J (1990) Percutaneous transluminal angioplasty for atheromatous renal artery stenosis—blood pressure response and discriminant analysis of outcome predictors. Qu J Med 75: 483–489.

Martin EC, Mattern RF, Baer L, Fankuchen EI, Casarella WJ (1981) Renal angioplasty for hypertension: predictive factors for long term success. AJR 137: 921–924.

Martin LG, Casarella WJ, Alspaugh JP, Chuang VP (1986) Renal artery angioplasty: increased technical success and decreased complications in the second 100 patients. Radiology 159: 631–634.

Martin LG, Casarella WJ, Gaylord GM (1988) Azotemia caused by renal artery stenosis: treatment by percutaneous angioplasty. AJR 150: 839–844.

Martin LG, Cork RD, Kaufman SL (1992) Long-term results of angioplasty in 110 patients with renal artery stenosis. J Vasc Intervent Radiol 3(4): 619–626.

Martin LG, Price RB, Casarella WJ, Sones PJ, Wells JO Jr, Zellmer RA, Chuang VP, Silbiger ML Jr, Berkman WA (1985) Percutaneous angioplasty in clinical management of renovascular hypertension: initial and long-term results. Radiology 155: 629–633.

Martinez AG, Novick AC, Hayes JM (1990) Surgical treatment of renal artery stenosis after failed percutaneous transluminal angioplasty. J Urol 144: 1094–1096.

Martinez-Amenos A, Rama H, Sarrias X, Galceran J, Alsina J, Montanya X (1991) Percutaneous transluminal angioplasty in the treatment of renovascular hypertension. J Hum Hypertens 5: 97–100.

Masugi F, Ogihara T, Saeki S, Sakaguchi K, Kumahara Y (1988) Platelet-activating factor and anti-platelet-aggregating factor in acute reduction of blood pressure following percutaneous transluminal renal angioplasty in patients with renovascular hypertension. J Hum Hypertens 2: 111–116.

Masugi F, Ogihara T, Saeki S, Sakaguchi K, Kumahara Y, Satouchi K, Oda M, Saito K, Tokunaga K (1988) Endogenous platelet-activating factor and anti-platelet-activating factor in patients with renovascular hypertension. Life Sci 42: 455–460.

Matalon TA, Thompson MJ, Patel SK, Brunner MC, Merkel FK, Jensik SC (1992) Percutaneous transluminal angioplasty for transplant renal artery stenosis. J Vasc Intervent Radiol 3(1): 55–58.

Mathias K, Billmann P, Liebig R, Kropelin T, Thierfelder K (1980) Treatment of renovascular hypertension by catheter dilatation. Radiologe 20: 494–499.

Mathias K, Struck E, Schindera F, Urbanyi B (1981) Percutaneous treatment of renovascular hypertension. Pediatr Radiol 11: 154–156.

Matsumoto AH, Baum PA, Barth KH, Teitelbaum GP (1989) Triple catheter aortoiliac angioplasty in a patient with a horseshoe kidney: technical note. Cardiovasc Intervent Radiol 12: 334–336.

Maxwell DD, Mispireta LA (1982) Transfemoral renal artery embolectomy. Radiology 143: 653–654.

McAllister MD, Thompson WC 3d, Pabian CJ (1992) Percutaneous angioplasty for renovascular hypertension due to fibromuscular dysplasia. Am Fam Physician 46(4): 1225–1230.

McCann RL, Bollinger RR, Newman GE (1988) Surgical renal artery reconstruction after percutaneous transluminal angioplasty. J Vasc Surg 8: 389–394.

McCarron DA, Keller FS, Lundquist G, Kirk PE (1982) Transluminal angioplasty for renovascular hypertension complicated by pregnancy. Arch Intern Med 142: 1737–1739.

McCarthy S, Stein S (1980) Renovascular hypertension treated by percutaneous transluminal angioplasty. Conn Med 44: 788–799.

McCook TA, Mills SR, Kirks DR, Heaston DK, Seigler HF, Malone RB, Osofsky SG (1980) Percutaneous transluminal renal artery angioplasty in a 3 ½-year-old hypertensive girl. J Pediatr 97: 958–960.

McCormack LJ, Dustan HP, Meaney TF (1967) Selected pathology of the renal artery. Semin Roentgenol 2: 126–138.

McCormack LJ, Poutasse EF, Meaney TF, Noto TJ Jr, Dustan HP (1966) A pathologic-arteriographic correlation of renal arterial disease. Am Heart J 72: 188–198.

McDonald DN; Smith DC, Maloney MD (1988) Percutaneous transluminal renal angioplasty in the patient with a solitary functioning kidney. AJR 151: 1041–1043.

McDonald WJ (1981) Renal artery stenosis causing hypertension: the current status of classical surgical therapy versus percutaneous transluminal dilatation. Am J Kidney Dis 1: 185.

McKenzie WB, Palmer J, Wilcken DE (1982) Percutaneous angioplasty in the management of renovascular hypertension. Aust NZ J Med 12: 189–191.

McMullin ND, Reidy JF, Koffman CG, Rigden SP, Haycock G, Chantler C, Bewick M (1992) The management of renal transplant artery stenosis in children by percutaneous transluminal angioplasty. Transplantation 53(3): 559–563.

Meakins JL (1980) Percutaneous transluminal dilatation for post-transplantation renal artery stenosis. CMA 123: 711–712.

Meaney TF, Dustan HP, McCormack LJ (1968) Natural history of renal arterial disease. Radiology 91: 881–887.

Medina M, Butt KM, Gordon DH, Thanawala S, Solomon N (1981) A complication of percutaneous transluminal angioplasty in the transplanted kidney. Urol Radiol 3: 59–61.

Meholic AJ, Saddler MC, Hallin GW, Avasthi PS, Tzamaloukas AH (1992) The captopril renogram in percutaneous transluminal angioplasty of the renal arteries. Am J Physiol Imaging 7(1): 36–41.

Menges HW, Jaschke W, Henrich W, Haase H (1988) Significance of percutaneous transluminal angioplasty in the treatment of renovascular hypertension from the vascular surgery viewpoint. Vasa 23 (Suppl): 193–197.

Merkus JW, Huysmans FT, Hoitsma AJ, Buskens FG, Skotnicki SH, Koene RA (1993) Renal allograft artery stenosis: results of medical treatment and intervention. A retrospective analysis. Transplant Int 6(2): 111–115.

Michielsen PP, Verbist LM, Verpooten GA, Vereycken HA, De Schepper AM, De Broe ME (1987) Digital substraction angiography and percutaneous transluminal angioplasty in patients with renal transplant artery stenosis. Acta Clin Belg 42: 414–420.

Millan VG, Madias NE (1979) Percutaneous transluminal angioplasty for severe renovascular hypertension due to renal artery medial fibroplasia. Lancet I: 993–995.

Millan VG, Mast WE, Madias NE (1979) Nonsurgical treatment of severe hypertension due to renal artery intimal fibroplasia by percutaneous transluminal angioplasty. N Engl J Med 300: 1371–1373.

Miller GA, Ford KK, Braun SD, Newman GE, Moore AV Jr, Malone R, Dunnick NR (1985) Percutaneous transluminal angioplasty vs. surgery for renovascular hypertension. AJR 144: 447–450.

Mills SR, Wertman DE Jr, Grossman SH (1981) Renal cortical arteriovenous fistula complicating percutaneous renal angioplasty. AJR 137: 1251–1253.

Milutinovic J, Darcy M, Thompson KA (1990) Radiation-induced renovascular hypertension successfully treated with transluminal angioplasty: case report. Cardiovasc Intervent Radiol 13: 29–31.

Miner DG, Dunnick NR (1987) Percutaneous transluminal angioplasty of renal transplant artery stenosis. Invest Radiol 22: 524–526.

Minton MJ, McIvor J, Cappuccio FP, MacGregor GA, Newlands ES (1986) Renovascular hypertension following radiotherapy and chemotherapy treated by transluminal angioplasty. Clin Radiol 37: 399–401.

Miyajima E, Yamada Y, Yoshida Y, Matsukawa T, Shionoiri H, Tochikubo O, Ishii M (1991) Muscle sympathetic nerve activity in renovascular hypertension and primary aldosteronism. Hypertension 17: 1057–1062.

Modhe JM, Someshwar VR, Ramakantan R, Khanna UB, Punekar S (1988)

Post-transplant renal artery stenosis-percutaneous transluminal angioplasty (report of 3 cases). J Postgrad Med 34: 48–50B.

Morganti A (1989) Renal angioplasty: morphological and pathophysiological aspects. REVIEW ARTICLE: 16 REFS. Contrib Nephrol 69: 87–94.

Morganti A, Quorso P, Ferraris P, Lovaria A, Fruscio M, Saccheri S, Zanchetti A (1989) Time-course of the changes in blood pressure and in plasma renin activity during the first week after dilation of renal artery stenosis. J Hypertens 7(Suppl): S186–S187.

Morlin C, Fagius J, Hagg A, Lorelius LE, Niklasson F (1990) Continuous recording of muscle nerve sympathetic activity during percutaneous transluminal angioplasty in renovascular hypertension in man. J Hypertens 8: 239–244.

Mukai J, Sabel P (1986) Application of dynamic computed tomography to physiologic imaging of renal artery stenosis before and after angioplasty. Am J Physiol Imaging 1: 33–43.

Nakada T, Yanagi S, Katayama T (1982) Successful treatment of renovascular hypertension with percutaneous transluminal angioplasty. J Urol 127: 526–527.

Nardi L, Bosch J (1988) Recirculation: review, techniques for measurement and ability to predict hemoaccess stenosis before and after angioplasty. Blood Purif 6: 85–89.

Navarro-Lopez F, Urbano-Marquez A, Castaner A, Panes J, Botey A, Rozman YC (1981) Tratamiento de la hipertension vasculorrenal por dilatacion transluminal percutanea de la arteria renal estenotica. Med Clin (Barc) 77: 333–337.

Nguyen BD, Adatepe MH (1992) Renal artery stenosis in en-bloc pediatric renal transplant: demonstration by captopril-enhanced renal scintigraphy. J Nucl Med 33(2): 263–265.

Nicholas GG, DeMuth WE Jr (1984) Treatment of renal artery embolism. Arch Surg 119: 278–281.

Norling LL, Chevalier RL, Gomez RA, Tegtmeyer CJ (1992) Use of interventional radiology for hypertension due to renal artery stenosis in children. Child Nephrol Urol 12(2-3): 162–166.

Novick AC (1991) Management of renovascular disease. A surgical perspective. Circulation 83: I167–171.

Novick AC (1989) Current concepts in the management of renovascular hypertension and ischemic renal failure. Am J Kidney Dis 13: 33–37.

Novick AC (1988) Evaluation and preparation for surgical treatment of renal artery disease. REVIEW ARTICLE: 21 REFS. Ann Vasc Surg 2: 150–154.

O'Donovan RM, Gutierrez OH, Izzo JL Jr (1992) Preservation of renal function by percutaneous renal angioplasty in high-risk elderly patients: short-term outcome. Nephron 60(2): 187–192.

Ohta H, Takabatake T, Yamamoto Y, Ishida Y, Hara H, Ushiosi Y, Nakamura S, Kawabata M, Hashimoto N, Sasaki T, et al (1986) The long term effects of percutaneous transluminal angioplasty for treating patients with renovascular hypertension: case studies. Angiology 37: 535–542.

Oleaga JA, Grossman RA, McLean GK, Rosen RJ, Freiman DB, Ring EJ (1981) Arteriovenous fistula of a segmental renal artery branch as a complication of percutaneous angioplasty. AJR 136: 988–989.

Olin JW, Wholey M (1987) Rupture of the renal artery nine days after percutaneous transluminal angioplasty. JAMA 257: 518–520.

Olmer M, Noordally R, Berland Y, Casanova P, Coulange C, Rampal M (1988) Hypertension in renal transplantation. Kidney Int Suppl 25: 129–132.

Pak K, Konishi T, Wakabayashi Y, Tomoyoshi T (1987) Nephrectomy necessitated by percutaneous transluminal angioplasty for renovascular hypertension. Nippon Jinzo Gakkai Shi 29: 341–345.

Palmar AH, Defeyter IR, Vandenbogaerde JF (1989) Renal arterial stenosis as a cause of high output cardiac failure. Int J Cardiol 22: 404–406.

Paoline RM, Marcondes M, Widman A, Sabbaga E, Bernardes Silva H, Nissensweig I, De Almeida Magalhaes A (1981) Percutaneous transluminal angioplasty of renal artery stenosis. Acta Radiol (Diagn) (Stockh) 22: 571–575.

Pattison JM, Reidy JF, Rafferty MJ, Ogg CS, Cameron JS, Sacks SH, Williams DG (1992) Percutaneous transluminal renal angioplasty in patients with renal failure. Q J Med 85(307–308): 883–888.

Pauker SC, Kopelman RI (1989) Screening for renovascular hypertension. A which hunt. Hypertension 14: 258–260.

Pedersen EB, Jensen FT, Madsen B, Eiskjaer H, Nielsen JT, Rehling M (1992) Angiotensin-converting enzyme inhibitor renography in the diagnosis of renovascular hypertension. Studies before and after angioplasty. Nephrol Dial Transplant 7(12): 1178–1184.

Pedersen EB, Madsen B, Danielsen H, Jespersen B (1987) Experience with percutaneous transluminal renal angioplasty in renovascular hypertension. Acta Med Scand 714 (Suppl): 23–27.

Perry MO (1985) Intramural dissection of superior mesenteric artery. A complication of attempted renal artery balloon dilation. J Vasc Surg 2: 480–484.

Peters AM (1990) Renal artery stenosis, reno-vascular hypertension and predicting the blood pressure response to renal revascularization. REVIEW ARTICLE: 26 REFS. Nucl Med Commun 11: 1–5.

Pezzulli FA, Purnell FM, Dillon EH (1986) Acute posttraumatic hypertension in fibromuscular dysplasia of the renal artery. Subintimal hemorrhage treated by percutaneous transluminal angioplasty. NY State J Med 86: 100–102.

Pickering TG, Herman L, Devereux RB, Sotelo JE, James GD, Sos TA, Silane MF, Laragh JH (1988) Recurrent pulmonary edema in hypertension due to bilateral renal artery stenosis: treatment by angioplasty of surgical revascularization. Lancet 2: 551–552.

Pickering TG, Sos TA, Laragh JH (1984) Role of balloon dilatation in the treatment of renovascular hypertension. Am J Med 77: 61–66.

Pickering TG, Sos TA, Laragh JH, Bell GM (1988) Percutaneous angioplasty in renovascular hypertension (letter). Lancet 1: 234–235.

Pickering TG, Sos TA, Vaughan ED Jr, Case DB, Sealey JE, Harshfield GA, Laragh JH (1984) Predictive value and changes of renin secretion in hypertensive patients with unilateral renovascular disease undergoing successful renal angioplasty. Am J Med 76: 398–404.

Pickering TG, Sos TA, Vaughan ED, Jr., Laragh JH (1986) Differing patterns of renal vein renin secretion in patients with renovascular hypertension, and their role in predicting the response to angioplasty. Nephron 44 (Suppl 1): 8–11.

Plouin PF, Darne B, Chatellier G, Pannier I, Battaglia C, Raynaud A, Azizi M (1993) Restenosis after a first percutaneous transluminal renal angioplasty. Hypertension 21(1): 89–96.

Postma CT, van Oijen AH, Barentsz JO, de Boo T, Hoefnagels WH, Corstens FH, Thien T (1991) The value of tests predicting renovascular hypertension in patients with renal artery stenosis treated by angioplasty. Arch Int Med 151: 1531–1535.

Priest EM (1988) Treatment of shunt-produced edema [letter]. South Med J 81: 1204.

Priollet P, Blanchard B, Mourad JJ, Lazareth I, Melki JP, Laurian C, Cormier JM (1992) Treatment of radiation-induced renal artery stenosis: reconstructive surgery or angioplasty? [letter]. J Vasc Surg 16(3): 489–490.

Probst P, Mahler F, Krneta A, Descoeudres C (1982) Percutaneous transluminal dilatation for restoration of angioaccess in chronic hemodialysis patients. Cardiovasc Intervent Radiol 5: 257–259.

Probst P, Mahler F, Roesler H, Fuchs WA (1983) Renal artery stenosis and evaluation of the effect of endoluminal dilatation. Comparison of dynamic CT scanning and I-131-OIHA renogram. Invest Radiol 18: 264–271.

Puijlaert CB, Klinge J, Mali WP, Geyskes GG, Kouwenberg JJ (1989) Results of percutaneous transluminal angioplasty in renal artery stenosis during the period 1978–1986. Ned Tijdschr Geneeskd 133: 400–404.

Puijlaert CB, Mali WP, Rosenbusch G, van Straalen AM, Klinge J, Feldberg

MA (1986) Delayed rupture of renal artery after renal percutaneous transluminal angioplasty. Radiology 159: 635–637.

Puijlaert CBAJ, Boomsma JHB, Ruijs JHJ, Geyskes GG, Franken AH, Hoekstra A, Oei HY (1981) Transluminal renal artery dilatation in hypertension: technique, results, and complications in 60 cases. Urol Radiol 2: 201–210.

Puijlaert CBAJ, Boomsma JHBB, Ruijs JHI, Oei HY, Franken AH, Koekstra A, Geyskes GG (1981) Dilatation des stenoses arterielles renales a l'aide d'un catheter a ballonnet. Ann Radiol 24:

Puijlaert CBAJ, Geyskes GG, Oej HY, Ruijs JHJ, Boomsma JHB, Wustefeld PJ, Mali WPT (1982) Renal angioplasty in hypertension, technique, radiological and clinical results in 108 dilatations in 96 patients. In: Oliva L, Pires-Veiga JH (eds) Proceedings of the Second International Symposium on Interventional Radiology, Venice-Lido, 27 September 1981. Excerpta Medica, Amsterdam, pp 317–322 (International congress-series no 575).

Punekar S, Someshwar VR, Ramakantan R, Sobti MK, Gulanikar AG, Shah AM, Pardanani DS (1988) Surgery and balloon angioplasty in advanced renovascular hypertension (46 cases). J Postgrad Med 34: 61–66B.

Puylaert CB, Klinge J, Mali WP, Geyskes GG (1988) Results and complications of renal PTA. Ann Radiol (Paris) 31: 82–86.

Ramirez G, Bugni W, Farber SM, Curry AJ (1987) Incidence of renal artery stenosis in a population having cardiac catheterization. South Med J 80: 734–737.

Ramsay LE, Waller PC (1990) Blood pressure response to percutaneous transluminal angioplasty for renovascular hypertension: an overview of published series. BMJ 300: 569–572.

Rankin RN, Keown PA, Ulan RA, Stiller CR (1981) Percutaneous transluminal dilatation of transplant renal artery stenosis. Postgrad Med J 57: 300–303.

Raynaud A, Bedrossian J, Remy P, Brisset JM, Angel CY, Gaux JC (1986) Percutaneous transluminal angioplasty of renal transplant arterial stenoses. AJR 146: 853–857.

Reilly DT, Wood RF, Watkin EM (1981) Attempted balloon catheter dilation of transplant renal artery stenosis and subsequent operative correction. Transplantation 32: 444–445.

Reisfeld D, Matas AJ, Tellis VA, Sprayragen S, Bakal C, Soberman R, Glicklich D, Veith FJ (1989) Late follow-up of percutaneous transluminal angioplasty for treatment of transplant renal artery stenosis. Transplant Proc 21: 1955–1956.

Richter EI, Gruentzig A, Ingrisch H, Mahler F, Mathias K, Roth FJ, Sorensen A, Zeitler E (1979) Percutaneous dilatation of renal artery stenoses. Ann Radiol 23: 275–278.

Roberts JP, Ascher NL, Fryd DS, Hunter DW, Dunn DL, Payne WD, Sutherland DE, Castaneda-Zuniga W, Najarian JS (1989) Transplant renal artery stenosis. Transplantation 48: 580–583.

Robinson L, Gedroyc W, Reidy J, Saxton HM (1991) Renal artery stenosis in children. Clin Radiol 44(6): 376–382.

Rodkin RS, Bookstein JJ, Heeney DJ, Davis GB (1983) Streptokinase and transluminal angioplasty in the treatment of acutely thrombosed hemodialysis access fistulas. Radiology 149: 425–428.

Rodriguez-Perez JC, Maynar M, Rams A, Plaza C, Vega N, Alamo R, Reyes R, Fernandez A, Palop L (1989) Percutaneous transluminal angioplasty as best treatment in stenosis of vascular access for hemodialysis. Nephron 51: 192–196.

Rosler H, Thoni A, Mahler F (1985) Radionephrosraphic follow-up with hypertensive patients after angioplasty of renal artery stenosis. Cardiology (72 Suppl) 1: 13–21.

Rossi GP, Pessina AC, Semplicini A, Feltrin GP, Mozzata MG, Dissegna L, Dal Palu C (1986) Captopril-stimulated renin in the diagnosis of restenosis after percutaneous transluminal renal angioplasty. Jpn Heart J 27: 299–305.

Roubidoux MA, Dunnick NR, Knelson M, Debatin JF (1992) Renal revascularization: indications and results. Urol Radiol 14(1): 18–23.

Rudolphi DM (1990) Renovascular hypertension diagnosis to discharge: a case study. J Vasc Nurs 8: 6–10.

Russell RD (1982) Embolization and angioplasty to relieve malignant hypertension and azotemia in a renal transplant patient. Cardiovasc Intervent Radiol 5: 307–311.

Russo D, Iaccarino V, Conte G, Fuiano G, Niola R, Testa A, Mazzone P, Andreucci VE (1988) Treatment of severe renovascular hypertension by percutaneous transluminal renal angioplasty in patients with solitary functioning kidney. Effects on blood pressure and renal function. Nephron 50: 315–319.

Sanchez GR, Prebis JW, Gruskin AB, Black IF, Faerber EN, Mehta AV, Ring EJ, McLean GK (1983) Blood pressure response to dynamic exercise in adolescents before and after percutaneous transluminal renal artery angioplasty. Int J Pediatr Nephrol 4: 251–254.

Sandmann W (1992) How to choose the ideal therapy for renovascular hypertension. Ann Chir Gynaecol 81(2): 161–164.

Sasaki S, Imai Y, Abe K, Nihei M, Minami N, Munakata M, Sasaki H, Sekino H, Yoshinaga K (1988) The hypotensive mechanism of percutaneous transluminal dilatation (PID) in renovascular hypertension due to bilateral renal artery stenosis. Tohoku J Exp Med 154: 173–183.

Schwab SJ, Quarles LD, Middleton JP, Cohan RH, Saeed M, Dennis VW

(1988) Hemodialysis-associated subclavian vein stenosis. Kidney Int 33: 1156–1159.

Schwarten DE (1980) Percutaneous transluminal angioplasty of the renal artery. Cardiovasc Interven Radiol 3: 197–206.

Schwarten DE (1980) Transluminal angioplasty of renal artery stenosis: 70 experiences. AJR 135: 967–974.

Schwarten DE (1984) Percutaneous transluminal angioplasty of renal arteries: intravenous digital subtraction angiography for follow-up. Radiology 150: 369–373. Schwarten DE (1981) Percutaneous transluminal renal angioplasty. Urol Radiol 2: 193–200.

Schwarten DE, Yune Hym Klatte EC, Grim CE, Weinberger MH (1980) Clinical experience with percutaneous transluminal angioplasty (PTA) of stenotic renal arteries. Radiology 135: 601–604.

Scoble JE, Maher ER, Hamilton G, Dick R, Sweny P, Moorhead JF (1989) Atherosclerotic renovascular disease causing renal impairment: a case for treatment. Clin Nephrol 31: 119–122.

Serrallach N, Serrate R, Franco E, Munoz J, Aguilo F, Gutierrez R, Rius G, Montana X, Marco-Luque M, Cairols MA, et al (1985) Renal artery stenosis in transplanted kidney: management and results in six patients. Eur Urol 11: 31–35.

Setaro JF, Chen CC, Hoffer PB, Black HR (1991) Captopril renography in the diagnosis of renal artery stenosis and the prediction of improvement with revascularization. The Yale Vascular Center experience. Am J Hypertens 4(12 Pt 2): 698S–705S.

Sfakianakis GN, Bourgoignie JJ (1991) Renographic diagnosis of renovascular hypertension with angiotensin converting enzyme inhibition and furosemide. Am J Hypertens 4(12 Pt 2): 706S–710S.

Sharma S, Saxena A, Talwar KK, Kaul U, Mehta SN, Rajani M (1992) Renal artery stenosis caused by nonspecific arteritis (Takayasu's disease): results of treatment with percutaneous transluminal angioplasty. AJR 158(2): 417–422.

Sheehan JP (1983) Percutaneous transluminal renal artery angioplasty (PTRA) in hypertensive encephalopathy. Ir Med J 76: 187–188.

Sheikh KH, Davidson CJ, Newman GE, Kisslo KB, Schwab SJ (1991) Intravascular ultrasound assessment of the renal artery. Ann Int Med 115: 22–25.

Sherwood T (1988) Finding and dilating renal artery stenoses for hypertension. REVIEW ARTICLE: 6 REFS. Clin Radiol 39: 359–360.

Simonetti G, Rossi P, Passariello R, Caboni M, Castrucci M, Pesce B (1983) Percutaneous transluminal renal angioplasty in nephrovascular hypertension. Ann Radiol (Paris) 26: 483–491.

Simunic S, Winter-Fuduric I, Radanovic B, Bradic I, Marinovic B, Marinkovic M, Cavka K, Batinica S, Batinic D, Roglic M, Jr (1990) Percutaneous transluminal renal angioplasty (PTRA) as a method of therapy for renovascular hypertension in children. Eur J Radiol 10: 143–146.

Slater EE (1980) Renal artery angioplasty versus surgery: A hypertensionologist's dilemma. AJR 135: 961–962.

Slavis SA, Hodge EE, Novick AC, Maatman T (1990) Surgical treatment for isolated dissection of the renal artery. J Urol 144: 233–237.

Smith TP, Cragg AH, Castaneda F, Hunter DW (1989) Thrombosed polytetrafluoroethylene hemodialysis fistulas: salvage with combined thrombectomy and angioplasty. Radiology 171: 507–508.

Sniderman KW, Sos TA (1982) Percutaneous transluminal recanalization and dilation of totally occluded renal arteries. Radiology 124: 607–610.

Sniderman KW, Sos TA, Sprayregen S, Saddekni S, Cheigh JS, Tapia L, Tellis V, Veith FJ (1980) Percutaneous transluminal angioplasty in renal transplant arterial stenosis for relief of hypertension. Radiology 135: 23–26.

Sniderman KW, Sprayregen S, Sos TA, Saddekni S, Hilton S, Mollenkopf F, Soberman R, Cheigh JS, Tapia L, Stubenbord W, Tellis V, Veith FJ (1980) Percutaneous transluminal dilation in renal transplant arterial stenosis. Transplantation 30: 440–444.

Sos TA (1985) Percutaneous transluminal renal angioplasty for the treatment of renovascular hypertension. Am J Kidney Dis 5: A131–135.

Sos TA (1991) Angioplasty for the treatment of azotemia and renovascular hypertension in atherosclerotic renal artery disease. Circulation 83: I162–166.

Sos TA, Pickering TG, Saddekni S, Srur M, Case DB, Silane MF, Vaughan ED Jr, Laragh JH (1984) The current role of renal angioplasty in the treatment of renovascular hypertension. Urol Clin North Am 11: 503–513.

Sos TA, Pickering TG, Sniderman K, Saddekni S, Case DB, Silane MF, Vaughan Ed Jr, Laragh JH (1983) Percutaneous transluminal renal angioplasty in renovascular hypertension due to atheroma or fibromuscular dysplasia. N Engl J Med 309: 274–279.

Sos TA, Saddekni S, Pickering TG, Laragh JH (1986) Technical aspects of percutaneous transluminal angioplasty in renovascular disease. Nephron 44 (Suppl 1): 45–50.

Sos TA, Saddekni S, Sniderman KW, Weiner M, Beinart C, Pickering TG, Case DB, Vaughan ED Jr, Laragh JH (1982) Renal artery angioplasty: techniques and early results. Urol Radiol 3: 223–231.

Soulen MC, Benenati JF, Sheth S, Merton D, Rothgeb J (1991) Changes in renal artery Doppler indexes following renal angioplasty. J Vasc Intervent Radiol 2(4): 457–461; discussion 461–462.

Spijkerboer AM, Mali WP, Donckerwolcke RA (1992) Renal transplant artery stenosis in children: treatment with percutaneous transluminal angioplasty. Pediatr Radiol 22(7): 519–521.

Srur MF, Sos TA, Saddekni S, Cohn DJ, Rozenblit G, Wetter EB (1985) Intimal fibromuscular dysplasia and Takayasu's arteritis: delayed response to percutaneous transluminal renal angioplasty. Radiology 157: 657–660.

Staessen J, Wilms G, Baert A, Fagard R, Lijnen P, Suy R, Amery A (1988) Blood pressure during long-term converting-enzyme inhibition predicts the curability of renovascular hypertension by angioplasty. Am J Hypertens 1: 208–214.

Stanley P, Hieshima G, Mehringer M (1984) Percutaneous transluminal angioplasty for pediatric renovascular hypertension. Radiology 153: 101–104.

Stanley P, Senac MO, Bakody P, Malekzadeh MH (1983) Percutaneous transluminal dilatation for renal artery stenosis in a 22-month-old hypertensive girl. AJR 140: 983–984.

Strauss MH, Reeves RA, Marquez-Julio FH, Leenen FH (1984) Percutaneous transluminal renal angioplasty in renovascular hypertension (letter). N Engl J Med 310: 322–323.

Stribrna J, Zabka J, Belan A, Boruvka V, Kocandrle V, Kovac J, Zastava V, Karasova L, Janata V (1988) Percutaneous transluminal angioplasty of renal transplant artery stenosis in patients with rejection nephropathy. Nephrol Dial Transplant 3: 312–316.

Suzuki T, Saitoh F, Kawano Y, Abe H, Ashizawa A, Shimohara A, Kojima S, Kuramochi M, Itoh K, Omae T, et al (1989) Long-term results of percutaneous transluminal angioplasty in patients with renovascular hypertension: a follow-up study on renal function and renal size. Nippon Jinzo Gakkai Shi 31: 49–56.

Szostek M, Malek A, Kulesza A, Naumowski Z, Rowinski O (1987) Early results of percutaneous renal artery angioplasty in patients with renovascular hypertension. Cor Vasa 29: 217–221.

Tack C, Sos TA (1989) Radiologic diagnosis of renovascular hypertension and percutaneous transluminal renal angioplasty. REVIEW ARTICLE: 59 REFS. Semin Nucl Med 19: 89–100.

Takabatake T, Yamamoto Y, Takemori Y, Maekawa M, Ohta H, Arai S, Nomura G, Hattori N (1981) Treatment of renovascular hypertension with percutaneous transluminal angioplasty. Jpn J Nephr 23: 479–488.

Takahashi M, Miyawaki M, Bussaka H, Saito R (1985) Use of short-tapered catheters in combination with a balloon catheter for markedly stenotic renal and brachiocephalic arteries. Br J Radiol 58: 751–753.

Tan AT, Chia BL, Tan LK, Gwee HM (1983) Successful angioplasty of renal artery stenosis due to aorto-arteritis. Cardiology 70: 213–215.

Tani M, Mizuno K, Midorikawa H, Igari T, Egawa M, Niimura S, Fukuchi

S, et al. (1993) Thermal laser-assisted angioplasty of renal artery stenosis for renovascular hypertension. Cardiovasc Intervent Radiol 16(1): 52–54.

Taylor DC, Moneta GL, Strandness DE, Jr (1989) Follow-up of renal artery stenosis by duplex ultrasound. J Vasc Surg 9: 410–415.

Teates CD, Tegtmeyer CJ, Croft BY, Ayers CR (1983) Effects of percutaneous transluminal angioplasty on renal plasma flow. Semin Nucl Med 13: 245–257.

Tegtmeyer CJ (1982) Percutaneous transluminal renal angioplasty. The evolution of a procedure (editorial). Arch Intern Med 142: 1085–1086.

Tegtmeyer CJ (1984) Renal angioplasty. Proc Annu Meet Med Sect Am Counc Life Insur, pp 57–65.

Tegtmeyer CJ, Ayers CA, Wellons HA (1980) The axillary approach to percutaneous renal artery dilatation. Radiology 135: 775–776.

Tegtmeyer CJ, Brown J, Ayers CA, Wellons HA, Stanton LW (1981) Percutaneous transluminal angioplasty for the treatment of renovascular hypertension. JAMA 245: 2068–2070.

Tegtmeyer CJ, Elson J, Glass TA, Ayers CR, Chevalier RL, Wellons HA Jr, Studdard WE Jr (1982) Percutaneous transluminal angioplasty: the treatment of choice for renovascular hypertension due to fibromuscular dysplasia. Radiology 143: 631–637.

Tegtmeyer CJ, Kellum CD, Ayers C (1984) Percutaneous transluminal angioplasty of the renal artery. Results and long-term follow-up. Radiology 153: 77–84.

Tegtmeyer CJ, Kofler TJ, Ayers CA (1984) Renal angioplasty: current status. AJR 142: 17–21.

Tegtmeyer CJ, Myer R, Teates CD, Ayers CR, Carey RM, Wellons HA, Stanton LW (1980) Percutaneous transluminal dilatation of the renal arteries: the techniques and results. Radiology 135: 589–599.

Tegtmeyer CJ, Selby JB, Hartwell GD, Ayers C, Tegtmeyer V (1991) Results and complications of angioplasty in fibromuscular disease. Circulation 83: I155–161.

Tegtmeyer CJ, Sos TA (1986) Techniques of renal angioplasty. Radiology 161: 577–586.

Tegtmeyer CJ, Teates CD, Cringer N, Gandee RW, Ayers CR, Stoddard M, Wellons HA (1981) Percutaneous transluminal angioplasty in patients with renal artery stenosis. Radiology 140: 323–330.

Tenschert W, Langer K, Wiesmann W, Rolf N, Winterberg B, Paulus H, Zumkley H, Buchholz B, Lison AE (1988) Renovascular hypertension due to transplantation-induced stenosis of the iliac artery. Successful therapy with transluminal angioplasty. Schweiz Rundsch Med Prax 77: 274–276.

Thomas CP, Riad H, Johnson BF, Cumberland DC (1992) Percutaneous transluminal angioplasty in transplant renal arterial stenoses: a long-term follow-up. Transplant Int 5(3): 129–132.

Thomsen HS, Sos TA, Nielsen SL (1989) Renovascular hypertension. Diagnosis and intervention. REVIEW ARTICLE: 83 REFS. Acta Radiol 30: 113–120.

Tonkin IL, Stapleton FB, Roy S, 3d (1988) Digital subtraction angiography in the evaluation of renal vascular hypertension in children. Pediatrics 81: 150–158.

Tsukamoto Y, Komuro Y, Akutsu F, Fujii K, Marumo F, Kusano S, Kikawada R (1988) Orthostatic hypertension due to coexistence of renal fibromuscular dysplasia and nephroptosis. Jpn Circ J 52: 1408–1414.

Tubbs CB, Schreiner GC, Gumbiner C, Houser MT, Mardis HK, Smith JW (1985) Renovascular hypertension in a child: percutaneous transluminal renal artery angioplasty. Nebr Med J 70: 358–362.

Valvo E, Bedogna V, Gammaro L, Taddei G, Maso R, Cavaggioni M, Tonon M, Maschio G (1987) Systemic hemodynamics in renovascular hypertension: changes after revascularization with percutaneous transluminal angioplasty. J Hypertens 5: 629–632.

Vanmaele RG, D'Archambeau OC, Van Schil PE, Van Landuyt KA, De Schepper AM (1993) Ruptured balloon separation during percutaneous transluminal renal artery angioplasty. Eur J Vasc Surg 7(1): 104–106.

Van Olden RW, Weerdenburg JP, Gerlag PG (1989) Terminal kidney insufficiency caused by disseminated cholesterol emboli as a complication of intra-arterial manipulation. Ned Tijdschr Geneeskd 133: 835–838.

Verhelst JA, Daelemans RA, Vereycken HA, Lins RL (1989) Mesenteric infarction: a fatal complication of renal transluminal angioplasty. Acta Clin Belg 44: 336–338.

Vidt DG, Eisele G, Gephardt GN, Tubbs R, Novick AC (1989) Atheroembolic renal disease: association with renal arterial stenosis. Cleve Clin J Med 56: 407–413.

Viron B, Lacombe M, Raynaud A, Bindi P, Thibault P, Mignon F (1991) Delayed extensive arterial dissection after percutaneous transluminal angioplasty for transplant renal artery stenosis. Nephron 58: 351–353.

Von Eiff M, Baumgart P, Glaser J, Lison AE (1988) Renovascular hypertension. Med Klin 83: 381–384.

Von Polnitz A, Hofling B (1989) Percutaneous atherectomy of a recurrent renal transplant artery stenosis. Transplantation 48: 880–883.

Watson AR (1986) Renovascular hypertension: treatment choices. Clin Exp Hypertens 8: 879–885.

Weibull H, Bergqvist D, Jendteg S, Lindgren B, Persson U, Jonsson K, Bergentz SE (1991) Clinical outcome and health care costs in renal revascularization—percutaneous transluminal renal angioplasty versus reconstructive surgery. Br J Surg 78: 620–624.

Weibull H, Bergqvist D, Jonsson K, Hulthen L, Mannhem P, Bergentz SE (1991) Long-term results after percutaneous transluminal angioplasty of atherosclerotic renal artery stenosis—the importance of intensive follow-up. Eur J Vasc Surg 5: 291–301.

Weibull H, Bergqvist D, Jonsson K, Carlsson S, Takolander R (1987) Analysis of complications after percutaneous transluminal angioplasty of renal artery stenoses. Eur J Vasc Surg 1: 77–84.

Weibull H, Tornquist C, Bergqvist D, Nyman U, Takolander R, Karlsson S, Bergentz SE (1984) Reversible renal insufficiency after percutaneous transluminal angioplasty (PTA) of renal artery stenosis. Acta Chir Scand 150: 295–300.

Weigele JB (1991) Iliac artery stenosis causing renal allograft-mediated hypertension: angiographic diagnosis and treatment. AJR 157: 513–515.

Weinberger MH, Grim CE, Luft FC, Yune HY (1986) Percutaneous transluminal angioplasty in complicated renal vascular hypertension. Nephron 44 (Suppl 1): 51–53.

Weinberger MH, Yune HY, Grim CE, Luft FC, Klatte C, Donohue JP (1979) Percutaneous transluminal angioplasty for renal artery stenosis in a solitary functining kidney; an alternative to surgery in the high-risk patient. Ann Intern Med 91: 684–688.

Weisman ID, Ney AL, Andrisevic JH, Stanchfield W, Jr, Odland MD, Andersen RC (1988) Unusual transplant renal angioplasty complication: case report. Cardiovasc Intervent Radiol 11: 97–100.

White CJ, Ramee SR, Collins TJ, Dearing B, Rees AP, Granke K, Hollier LH (1991) Guiding catheter-assisted renal artery angioplasty. Cathet Cardiovasc Diagn 23: 10–13.

Whiteside CI, Cardella CJ, Yeung H, de Veber GA, Cook GT (1982) The role of percutaneous transluminal dilatation in the treatment of transplant renal artery stenosis. Clin Nephrol 17: 55–59.

Whiteside CI, Cardella CJ, Yeung H, Uldall PR, deVeber GA, Cook T (1981) Percutaneous transluminal dilatation for transplant renal artery stenosis. Kidney Int 19: 395.

Wikholm G (1983) Use of a modified lunderquist guide wire for percutaneous transluminal renal angioplasty. AJR 141: 605–606.

Wilms G, Baert AL, Amery AK, Staessen JA, Vermylen JG (1989) Short-term morphologic results of percutaneous transluminal renal angioplasty as determined with angiography. Radiology 170: 1019–1021.

Wilms G, Baert AL, Suy R, Nevelsteen A, Staessen J, Amery A (1989) Percutaneous transluminal renal angioplasty versus renovascular surgery: statistical, medical and economical considerations. J Belge Radiol 72: 173–179.

Wilms G, Staessen J, Baert AL, Michielsen P, Amery A (1989) Percutaneous transluminal renal angioplasty and renal function. Radiology 29: 195–200.

Wise KL, McCann RL, Dunnick NR, Paulson DF (1988) Renovascular hypertension. REVIEW ARTICLE: 91 REFS. J Urol 140: 911–924.

Yal:Cinkaya F, Tumer N, Ekim M, Sanlidilek U (1990) Fibromuscular dysplasia of the renal arteries treated with percutaneous transluminal renal angioplasty: a case report. Turk J Pediatr 32(4): 265–271.

Yune HY (1980) Percutaneous transluminal angioplasty of stenotic renal arteries. Diagn Radiol 135: 603–604.

Yune HY, Klatte EC, Grim CE, Weinberger MH (1980) Transluminal balloon dilatation of renal artery stenosis causing hypertension: 18 months experience. Clin Sci 59: 483s–485s.

Zaitoun R, Dorros G, Iyer SS, Lewin RF (1990) Percutaneous high-speed rotational atherectomy (Rotablator) of a restenosed ostial renal artery: a case report. Cathet Cardiovasc Diagn 20: 254–256.

Zajko AB, McLean GK, Grossman RA, Barker CF, Freiman DB, Ring EJ, Alavi A, Perloff LJ (1982) Percutaneous transluminal angioplasty and fibrinolytic therapy for renal allograft arterial stenosis and thrombosis. Transplantation 33: 447–450.

Zamboulis C, Karagiannis A, Douma S, Vogiatzis K, Doumas M, Byzantiades A, Metaxas P, Efremidis S (1989) Changes of plasma noradrenaline levels in the renal and systemic circulation after successful percutaneous transluminal angioplasty in renovascular hypertension. Clin Exp Hypertens 11: 449–458.

Zeitler E (1971) Angiographische probleme zur diagnostik und therapie der renovaskularen hypertonie. In: Denck H, Flora G, Hilbe G, Piza F (eds) Renovasculare Hypertonie. Vienna, Wiener Medizinische Akademie, pp 113–117.

Zheng DY, Liu LS, Dai RP (1988) Studies of hemodynamics with renal vein renin ratio before and after percutaneous transluminal renal angioplasty (PTRA). Chung Hua Nei Ko Tsa Chih 27: 554–556, 587–588.

Ziegelbaum M, Novick AC, Hayes J, Vidt DG, Risius B, Gifford RW, Jr. (1987) Management of renal arterial disease in the elderly patient. Surg Gynecol Obstet 165: 130–134.

Zimbler MS, Pickering TG, Sos TA, Laragh JH (1987) Proteinuria in renovascular hypertension and the effects of renal angioplasty. Am J Cardiol 59: 406–408.

VI. Tibioperoneal (Below Knee; Infrapopliteal)

Anonymous (1992) Second European Consensus Document on chronic critical leg ischemia. Eur J Vasc Surg 6(Suppl A): 1–32.

Bakal CW, Sprayregen S, Scheinbaum K, Cynamon J, Veith FJ (1990) Percutaneous transluminal angioplasty of the infrapopliteal arteries: results in 53 patients. AJR 154: 171–174.

Barton P, Karnel F, Schurawitzki H, Kretschmer G, Polterauer P (1990) Long-term results of interventional treatment of arteries below the knee [Ger]. Vasa 30: 181–185.

Bell PR, London NJ (1992) Aggressive arterial reconstruction for critical lower limb ischaemia (letter). Br J Surg 79(7): 718.

Bendick PJ, Price JL, Glover JL (1992) Limb perfusion. An objective measure of hemodynamic improvement after angioplasty. Arch Surg 127(7): 806–811.

Bergan JJ, Wilson SE, Wolf G, Deupree RH (1992) Unexpected, late cardiovascular effects of surgery for peripheral artery disease. Veterans Affairs Cooperative Study 199. Arch Surg 127(9): 1119–1123; discussion 1123–1124.

Brown KT, Moore ED, Getrajdman GI, Saddekni S (1993) Infrapopliteal angioplasty: long-term follow-up. J Vasc Intervent Radiol 4(1): 139–144.

Brown KT, Schoenberg NY, Moore ED, Saddekini S (1988) Percutaneous transluminal angioplasty of infrapopliteal vessels: Preliminary results and technical considerations. Radiology 169: 75–78.

Buckenham TM, Loh A, Dormandy JA, Taylor RS (1993) Infrapopliteal angioplasty for limb salvage. Eur J Vasc Surg 7(1): 21–25.

Bull PG, Mendel H, Hold M, Schlegl A, Denck H (1992) Distal popliteal and tibioperoneal transluminal angioplasty: long-term follow-up. J Vasc Intervent Radiol 3(1): 45–53.

Casarella WJ (1988) Percutaneous transluminal angioplasty below the knee: New techniques, excellent results. Radiology 169: 271–272.

Cheshire NJ, Wolfe JH (1992) ABC of vascular diseases. Critical leg ischaemia: amputation or reconstruction. BMJ 304(6822): 312–314.

Davies AH, Cole SE, Magee TR, Scott DJ, Baird RN, Horrocks M (1992) The effect of diabetes mellitus on the outcome of angioplasty for lower limb ischaemia. Diabetic Med 9(5): 480–481.

Dorros G, Hall P, Prince C (1993) Successful limb salvage after recanalization of an occluded infrapopliteal artery utilizing a balloon expandable (Palmaz-Schatz) stent. Cathet Cardiovasc Diagn 28(1): 83–88.

Dorros G, Lewin RF, Jamnadas P, Mathiak LM (1990) Below-the-knee angioplasty: tibioperoneal vessels, the acute outcome. Cathet Cardiovasc Diagn 19: 170–178.

Flueckiger F, Lammer J, Klein GE, Hausegger K, Pilger E, Waltner F, Aschauer M (1992) Percutaneous transluminal angioplasty of crural arteries. Acta Radiol 33(2): 152–155.

Goldman ML, Bertino RE, Nelson JA, Shaw DW, Intlekofer MJ, Clement TC, Sano A, Johansen KH (1988) Nonsurgical portacaval shunt by use of a radio-frequency hot tip guide wire. Radiology 169P(Suppl): 366.

Greenfield AJ (1980) Femoral, popliteal, and tibial arteries: Percutaneous transluminal angioplasty. AJR 135: 927–935.

Griffith CD, Harrison JD, Gregson RH, Makin GS, Hopkinson BR (1989) Transluminal iliac and angioplasty with distal bypass surgery in patients with critical limb ischaemia. J R Coll Surg Edinb 34: 253–255.

Hunink MG, Donaldson MC, Meyerovitz MF, Polak JF, Whittemore AD, Kandarpa K, Grassi CJ, et al. (1993) Risks and benefits of femoropopliteal percutaneous balloon angioplasty. J Vasc Surg 17(1): 183–192.

Kashdan BJ, Trost DW, Jagust MB, Rackson ME, Sos TA (1992) Retrograde approach for contralateral iliac and infrainguinal percutaneous transluminal angioplasty: experience in 100 patients. J Vasc Intervent Radiol 3(3): 515–521.

Kugel RD, Pereyra R (1989) Combined femorotibial bypass and distal intraoperative transluminal angioplasty. J Vasc Surg 4: 533–5.

Lipchik EO (1989) Arterial occlusive disease below the knee (letter). Radiology 171: 283.

London NJ, Sayers RD, Thompson MM, Naylor AR, Hrtshorne T, Ratliff DA, Bell PR, et al. (1993) Interventional radiology in the maintenance of infrainguinal vein graft patency. Br J Surg 80(2): 187–193.

Lu CT, Zarins CK, Yang CF, Turcotte JK (1982) Percutaneous transluminal angioplasty for limb salvage. Radiology 142: 337–431.

Mansell PI, Gregson R, Allison SP (1992) An audit of lower limb arteriography in diabetic patients. Diabet Med 9(1): 84–90.

Martorell F (1970) Arterial embolism of the popliteal artery and tibioperoneal trunk. Angiologia 22: 196–8.

Mosley JG, Gulati Sm, Raphael M, Marston A (1985) The role of percutaneous transluminal angioplasty for atherosclerotic disease of the lower extremities. Ann R Coll Surg Engl 67: 83–86.

Ratner SW, Reilly CH, Gudas CJ (1983) Percutaneous transluminal angioplasty in the treatment of ischemic disease of the lower extremity. J Foot Surg 22: 86–91.

Rollins NK, Sheffield EG, Andrews WS (1992) Portal vein stenosis complicating liver transplantation in children: percutaneous transhepatic angioplasty. Radiology 182(3): 731–734.

Saab MH, Smith DC, Aka PK, Brownlee RW, Killeen JD (1992) Percutaneous transluminal angioplasty of tibial arteries for limb salvage. Cardiovasc Intervent Radiol 15(4): 211–216.

Sanborn TA, Mitty HA, Train JS, Dan SJ (1989) Infrapopliteal and below-knee popliteal lesions: treatment with sole laser thermal angioplasty. Work in progress. Radiology 172: 89–93.

Schroeder J (1989) Catheter lysis and percutaneous transluminal angioplasty below the knee via the popliteal artery in a patient with femoral artery obstruction: technical note. Cardiovasc Intervent Radiol 12: 344–345.

Schwarten DE (1986) Extracardiac uses for the steerable coronary balloon systems. Ann Radiol 29: 120–126.

Schwarten DE (1991) Clinical and anatomical considerations for nonoperative therapy in tibial disease and the results of angioplasty. Circulation 83: I86–90.

Schwarten DE, Cutliff WB (1988) Arterial occlusive disease below the knee: Treatment with percutaneous transluminal angioplasty performed with low profile catheters and steerable guide wires. Radiology 169: 71–74.

Sharma S, Loya YS, Daxini BV (1992) Percutaneous balloon membranotomy combined with prolonged streptokinase infusion for management of inferior vena cava obstruction. Am Heart J 123(2): 515–518.

Sprayregen S, Sniderman KW, Sos TA, Vieux U, Singer A, Veith FJ (1980) Popliteal artery branches: percutaneous transluminal angioplasty. AJR 135: 945–950.

Tamura S, Sniderman KW, Beinart C, Sos TA (1982) Percutaneous transluminal angioplasty of the popliteal artery and its branches. Radiology 143: 645–648.

Veith FJ, Gupta SK, Wengerter KR, Goldsmith J, Rivers SP, Bakal CW, Dietzek AM, Cynamon J, Sprayregen S, Gliedman ML (1990) Changing arteriosclerotic disease pattterns and management strategies in lower-limb-threatening ischemia. Ann Surg 212: 402–412.

Wyffels PL, DeBord Jr (1990) Increased limb salvage. Distal tibial/peroneal artery thrombectomy/embolectomy in acute lower extremity ischemia. Am Surg 56: 468–475.

VII. Venous

Anderson PG, Bajaj RK, Baxley WA, Roubin GS (1992) Vascular pathology of balloon-expandable flexible coil stents in humans. J Am Coll Cardiol 19(2): 372–381.

Antonucci F, Salomonowitz E, Stuckman G, Stiefel M, et al (1992) Hemodialysis related venous stenoses: treatment with self-expanding endovascular prosthesis. Eur J Radiol 14(3): 195–200.

Antonucci F, Salomonowitz E, Stuckmann G, Stiefel M, Largiader J, Zollikofer CL (1992) Placement of venous stents: clinical experience with a self-expanding prosthesis. Radiology 183(2): 493–497.

Bar-Meir S, Rubinstein Z, Miller HI, Papo J, Morag B, et al (1984) Failure of balloon membranotomy of the inferior vena cava. Israel J Med Sci 20(7): 618–621.

Baron B, Kiproff PM, Khoury MB (1992) Local thrombolysis and percutaneous transluminal venoplasty for the venous complications of thoracic outlet syndrome: case report. Angiology 43(11): 957–960.

Becker GJ, Wenker JC, Rees CR, Reilly MK, Bendick PJ et al (1986) Percutaneous transluminal angioplasty and valvectomy in a failing in situ saphenous graft. 159(2): 431–433.

Benson LN, Yeatman L, Laks H (1985) Balloon dilatation for superior vena caval obstruction after the senning procedure. Cathet Cardiovasc Diagn 11(1): 63–68.

Bilodeau M, Rioux L, Willems B, Pomier-Layrargues G (1992) Transjugular intrahepatic portacaval stent shunt as a rescue treatment for life-threatening variceal bleeding in a cirrhotic patient with severe liver failure. Am J Gastroenterol 87(3): 369–371.

Brady HR, Fitzcharles B, Goldberg H, Huraib S, Richardson T, Simons M, Uldall PR (1989) Diagnosis and management of subclavian vein thrombosis occurring in association with subclavian cannulation for hemodialysis. Blood Purif 7: 210–217.

Cada E, Karnel F, Mayer G, Langle F, Schurawitzki H, Graf H (1989) Percutaneous transluminal angioplasty of failing arteriovenous dialysis fistulae. Nephrol Dial Transplant 4: 57–61.

Capek P, Cope C (1989) Percutaneous treatment of superior vena cava syndrome. AJR 152: 183–184.

Carrasco CH, Charnsangavej C, Wright KC, Wallace S, Gianturco C (1992) Use of the Gianturco self-expanding stent in stenoses of the superior and inferior venae cavae. J Vasc Intervent Radiol 3(2): 409–419.

Chatelain P, Meier B, Friedle B (1991) Stenting of superior vena cava and inferior vena cava for symptomatic narrowing after repeated atrial surgery for D-transposition of the great vessels. Br Heart J 66(6): 466–468.

Cope C (1986) Dilatation of mesocaval shunts. Annal Radiol 29(2): 178–180.

Dake MD, Zemel G, Dolmatch BL, Katzen BT (1990) The cause of superior vena cava syndrome: diagnosis with percutaneous atherectomy. Radiology 174: 957–959.

Daniell SJ, Dacie JE (1988) Percutaneous transluminal angioplasty of brachiocephalic vein stenoses in patients with dialysis shunts (letter). Radiology 169(1): 280–281.

Darcy MD, Vesely TM, Picus D, Middleton WD, Hicks ME (1992) Percutaneous revision of an acutely thrombosed transjugular intrahepatic portosystemic shunt. J Vasc Intervent Radiol 3(1): 77–80; discussion 81–82.

Davidson CJ, Newman GE, Sheikh KH, Kisslo K, Stack RS, Schwab SJ (1991) Mechanisms of angioplasty in hemodialysis fistula stenoses evaluated by intravascular ultrasound. Kidney Int 40: 91–95.

Deckelbaum LI (1989) Laser-assisted angioplasty of inferior vena caval obstructions: what's good for the artery is good for the vein. Hepatology 9(2): 338–339.

Dev V, Kaul U, Jain P, Reddy S, Sharma S, Pandey G, Rajani M (1989) Percutaneous transluminal balloon angioplasty for obstruction of the suprahepatic inferior vena cava and cavo-atrial graft stenosis. Am J Cardiol 64: 397–399.

Dev V, Kaul U, Sahni P, Sharma S (1992) Balloon angioplasty for complete obstruction of inferior vena cava: needle puncture followed by balloon dilatation. Cathet Cardiovasc Diagn 25(4): 320–322.

Driscoll DJ, Hesslein PS, Mullins CE (1982) Congenital stenosis of individual pulmonary veins: clinical spectrum and unsuccessful treatment by transvenous balloon dilation. Am J Cardiol 49(7): 1767–1772.

Elson JD, Becker GJ, Wholey MH, Ehrman KO (1991) Vena caval and central venous stenoses: management with Palmaz balloon-expandable intraluminal stents. J Vasc Intervent Radiol 2(2): 215–223.

Feifarek MJ, Appen RE, Strother CM (1982) Carotid-cavernous fistulae and their current therapy. Wisc Med J 81(6): 17–20.

Feigin RD, Glickson M, Varstending A, Lauria B, Gordon RL, Ring EJ, TurKaspa R (1990) Familial Budd-Chiari syndrome due to membranous obstruction of the right hepatic vein treated with transluminal angioplasty. Am J Gastroenterol 85: 94–97.

Fraschini G, Jadeja J, Lawson M, Holmes FA, Carrasco HC et al (1987) Local infusion of urokinase for the lysis of thrombosis associated with permanent central venous catheters in cancer patients. J Clin Oncol 5(4): 672–678.

Furui S, Sawada S, Irie T, Makita K, Yamauchi T, et al (1990) Hepatic inferior vena cava obstruction: treatment of two types with Gianturco expandable metallic stents (see comments). Radiology 176(3): 665–670.

Garfinkel HB, Rohr RE, Rottenberg RW (1984) Angioplasty of a stenotic aorto-renal artery saphenous vein bypass graft to a single kidney. Am J Kidney Dis 4(2): 171–174.

Gaux JC, Borquelot P, Raynaud A, Seurot M, Cattan S (1983) Percutaneous transluminal angioplasty of stenotic lesions in dialysis vascular accesses. Eur J Radiol 3: 189–193.

Gillams A, Dick R, Platts A, Irving D, Hobbs K (1991) Dilatation of the inferior vena cava using an expandable metal stent in Budd-Chiari syndrome. J Hepatol 13(2): 149–151.

Glanz S, Gordon D, Butt KM, Hong J, Adamson R, Sclafani SJ (1984) Dialysis access fistulas: treatment of stenoses by transluminal angioplasty. Radiology 152: 637–642.

Glanz S, Gordon DH, Lipkowitz GS, Butt KM, Hong J, Sclafani SJ (1988) Axillary and subclavian vein stenosis: percutaneous angioplasty. Radiology 168: 371–373.

Gmelin E, Winterhoff R, Rinast E (1989) Insufficient hemodialysis access fistulas: late results of treatment with percutaneous balloon angioplasty. Radiology 171: 657–660.

Gordon DH, Glanz S, Butt KM, Adamsons RJ, Koenig MA (1982) Treatment of stenotic lesions in dialysis access fistulas and shunts by transluminal angioplasty. Radiology 143: 53–58.

Gray RJ, Dolmatch BL, Buick MK (1992) Directional atherectomy treatment for hemodialysis access: early results. J Vasc Intervent Radiol 3(3): 497–503.

Gunther RW, Vorwerk D, Bohndorf K, Klose KC, Kistler D, Mann H, Sieberth HG, el-Din A (1989) Venous stenoses in dialysis shunts: treatment with self-expanding metallic stents. Radiology 170: 401–405.

Harville LE, Rivera FJ, Palmaz JC, Levine BA (1992) Variceal hemorrhage associated with portal vein thrombosis: treatment with a unique portal venous stent. Surgery 111(5): 585–590.

Hassell AB, Kelly AJ, Coward RA (1987) Balloon catheter angioplasty in subclavian-vein obstruction (letter). Nephrol Dialysis Transplant 2(4): 281–282.

Heidler R, Zeitler E, Gessler U (1978) Percutaneous transluminal dilatation of stenosis behind AV-fistulas in hemodialysis patients. In: Zeitler E et al. (eds) Percutaneous Vascular Recanalization. Berlin Heidelberg New York, Springer, pp 142–144.

Holemans JA, McIvor J, Brown EA (1992) Recurrent subclavian vein stenosis following successful angioplasty (letter). Nephrol Dialysis Transplant 7(3): 270–271.

Hosie KB, Bolia A, Watkin DF (1988) Treatment of Budd-Chiari syndrome by percutaneous transluminal angioplasty (letter). Lancet 2: 158–159.

Howd A, Loose H, Chamberlain J (1987) Transluminal angioplasty in the treatment of mesenteric vein graft stenosis. Cardiovasc Intervent Radiol 10(1): 43–45.

Hunter DW, So SK, Castaneda-Zuniga WR, Coleman CE, Sutherland DE, Amplatz K (1983) Failing or thrombosed Brescia-Cimino arteriovenous dialysis fistulas. Angiographic evaluation and percutaneous transluminal angioplasty. Radiology 149: 105–109.

Ida M, Arai K, Yoshikawa J, Takayama S, Miyamori H, et al (1986) Therapeutic hepatic vein angioplasty for Budd-Chiari syndrome. Cardiovasc Intervent Radiol 9(4): 187–190.

Ingram TL, Reid SH, Tisnado J, Cho SR, Posner MP (1988) Percutaneous transluminal angioplasty of brachiocephalic vein stenoses in patients with dialysis shunts. Radiology 166: 45–47.

Ishiguchi T, Fukatsu H, Itoh S, Shimamoto K, Sakuma S (1992) Budd-Chiari syndrome with long segmental inferior vena cava obstruction: treatment with thrombolysis, angioplasty, and intravascular stents. J Vasc Intervent Radiol 3(2): 421–425.

Jeans WD, Bourne JT, Read AE (1983) Treatment of hepatic vein and inferior vena caval obstruction by balloon dilatation. Br J Radiol 56(669): 687–689.

Kalman PG, Hobbs BB, Colapinto RF, Fenton SSA, Johnston KW (1980) Percutaneous transluminal dilatation of a stenotic arteriovenous bovine graft. Dial Transplant 9: 747, 778.

Koga N, Sato T, Baba T, Ueda O, Okazaki H, Kohchi K, Norita H, Maw PR, Moriyama A (1989) Angioscopy in transluminal balloon and laser angioplasty in the management of chronic hemodialysis fistulae ASAIO Trans 35: 193–196.

Kunkel JM, Machleder HI (1989) Spontaneous subclavian vein thrombosis: a successful combined approach of local thrombolytic therapy followed by first rib resection (letter). Surgery 106: 114.

LaBerge JM, Ferrell LD, Ring EJ, Gordon RL, Lake JR, Roberts JP, Ascher NL (1991) Histopathologic study of transjugular intrahepatic portosystemic shunts. J Vasc Intervent Radiol 2(4): 549–556.

Lamar R, Berg R, Rama K (1990) Femoral arteriovenous fistula as a complication of percutaneous transluminal coronary angioplasty. A report of five cases. Am Surg 56(11): 702–706.

Leipzig TJ, Mullan SF (1983) Deflation of metrizamide-filled balloon used to occlude a carotid-cavernous fistula: Case report. J Neurosurg 59(3): 524–528.

Lock JE, Bass JL, Castaneda-Zuniga W, Fuhrman BP, Rashkind WJ (1984)

Dilation angioplasty of congenital or operative narrowings of venous channels. Circulation 70(3): 457–464.

Lois JF, Hartzman S, McGlade CT, Gomes AS, Grant EC, Berquist W, Perrella RR, Busuttil RW (1989) Budd-Chiari syndrome: treatment with percutaneous transhepatic recanalization and dilation. Radiology 170: 791–793.

Loya YS, Sharma S, Amrapurka DN, Desai HG (1989) Complete membranous obstruction of inferior vena cava: case treated by balloon dilation. Cathet Cardiovasc Diagn 17: 164–167.

Machleder HI (1993) Evaluation of a new treatment strategy for Paget-Schroetter syndrome: spontaneous thrombosis of the axillary-subclavian vein. J Vasc Surg 17(2): 305–315; discussion 316–317.

Marache P, Asseman P, Jabinet JL, Prat A, Bauchart JJ, Aisenfarb JC, Lesenne M, et al. (1993) Percutaneous transluminal venous angioplasty in occlusive iliac vein thombosis resistant to thrombolysis. Am Heart J 125(2 Pt 1): 362–366.

Martin LG, Henderson JM, Millikan WJ Jr, Casarella WJ, Kaufman SL (1990) Angioplasty for long-term treatment of patients with Budd-Chiari syndrome. AJR 154: 1007–1010.

McCaughan JJ Jr, Walsh DB, Edgcomb LP, Garrett HE (1984) In vitro observations of greater saphenous vein valves during pulsatile and nonpulsatile flow and following lysis. J Vasc Surg 1(2): 356–361.

Mills SR, Wertman DE Jr, Grossman SH (1981) Renal cortical arteriovenous fistula complicating percutaneous renal angioplasty. Am J Roentgenol 137(6): 1251–1253.

Nagata Y, Kumada K, Yamada R, Abe W, Ozawa K (1989) Pulmonary thromboembolism following angioplasty for membranous occlusion of the vena cava: case report. Cardiovasc Intervent Radiol 12(6): 304–306.

Newman GE, Saeed M, Himmelstein S, Cohan RH, Schwab SJ (1991) Total central vein obstruction: resolution with angioplasty and fibrinolysis. Kidney Internat 39(4): 761–764.

Okrent D, Messersmith R, Buckman J (1991) Transcatheter fibrinolytic therapy and angioplasty for left iliofemoral venous thrombosis. J Vasc Intervent Radiol 2(2): 195–197.

Olcott EW, Ring EJ, Roberts JP, Ascher NL, Lake JR, et al (1990) Percutaneous transhepatic portal vein angioplasty and stent placement after liver transplantation: early experience. J Vasc Intervent Radiol 1(1): 17–22.

Parvin SD, Bolia AA (1989) Angioplasty for a failing vein graft. Eur J Vasc Surg 3: 283–284.

Perry SB, Rome J, Keane JF, Baim DS, Lock JE (1992) Transcatheter closure of coronary artery fistulas. J Am Coll Cardiol 20(1): 205–209.

Quinn SF, Schuman ES, Hall L, Gross GF, Uchida BT, Standage BA, Rosch

J, Ivancev K (1992) Venous stenoses in patients who undergo hemodialysis: treatment with self-expandable endovascular stents. Radiology 183(2): 499–504.

Ravikumar S, Stahl WM (1985) Intraluminal balloon catheter occlusion for major vena cava injuries. J Trauma 25(5): 458–460.

Reed JG, Goodman P, Nealon WH, Morettin LB (1992) Low-pressure balloon angioplasty of an occluded portacaval shunt. Hepatogastroenterology 39(2): 166–168.

Ricci E, Mortilla MG, Conigliaro R, Bertoni G, Bedogni G et al (1992) Portal vein filling: a rare complication associated with ERCP for endoscopic biliary stent placement (letter). Gastrointestinal Endosc 38(4): 524–525.

Ring EJ, Gordon RL, LaBerge JM, Shapiro HA (1991) Malignant biliary obstruction complicated by ascites: transjugular insertion of an expandable metallic endoprosthesis. Radiology 180(2): 579–581.

Rocchini AP, Cho KJ, Byrum C, Heidelberger K (1982) Transluminal angioplasty of superior vena cava obstruction in a 15-month-old child. Chest 82(4): 506–508.

Rodkin RS, Bookstein JJ, Heeney DJ, Davis GB (1983) Streptokinase and transluminal angioplasty in the treatment of acutely thrombosed hemodialysis access fistulas. Radiology 149: 425–428.

Rodriguez-Perez JC, Maynar M, Rams A, Plaza C, Vega N, Alamo R, Reyes R, Fernandez A, Palop L (1989) Percutaneous transluminal angioplasty as best treatment in stenosis of vascular access for hemodialysis. Nephron 51: 192–196.

Rollins NK, Sheffield EG, Andrews WS (1992) Portal vein stenosis complicating liver transplantation in children: percutaneous transhepatic angioplasty. Radiology 182(3): 731–734.

Rosch J, Petersen BD, Hall LD, Ivancev K (1990) Interventional treatment of hepatic arterial and venous pathology: a commentary. Cardiovasc Intervent Radiol 13(3): 183–188.

Rose BS, Van Aman ME, Simon DC, Sommer BG, Ferguson RM, Henry ML (1988) Transluminal balloon angioplasty of infrahepatic caval anastomotic stenosis following liver transplantation: case report. Cardiovasc Intervent Radiol 11: 79–81.

San Nicolo M, Achammer T, Flora G (1990) Duodenal fistula after reconstruction of the inferior vena cava with an externally stented PTFE graft. J Cardiovasc Surg 31(3): 382–384.

Sanders RJ, Haug C (1990) Subclavian vein obstruction and thoracic outlet syndrome: a review of etiology and management. Ann Vasc Surg 4: 397–410.

Sato M, Yamada R, Tsuji K, Kishi K, Terada M, et al (1990) Percutaneous transluminal angioplasty in segmental obstruction of the hepatic inferior vena cava: long-term results. Cardiovasc Intervent Radiol 13(3): 189–192.

Sawada S, Fujiwara Y, Koyama T, Kobayashi M, Tanigawa N, et al (1992) Application of expandable metallic stents to the venous system. Acta Radiologica 33(2): 156–159.

Schwab SJ, Quarles LD, Middleton JP, Cohan RH, Saeed M, Dennis VW (1988) Hemodialysis-associated subclavian vein stenosis. Kidney Int 33: 1156–1159.

Sharma S, Loya YS, Daxini BV (1992) Percutaneous balloon membranotomy combined with prolonged streptokinase infusion for management of inferior vena cava obstruction. Am Heart J 123(2): 515–518.

Sherry CS, Diamond NG, Meyers TP, Martin RL (1986) Successful treatment of superior vena cava syndrome by venous angioplasty. AJR 147: 834–835.

Shetty PC, Bok LR, Burke MW, Sharma RP (1986) Balloon dilation of the femoral vein expediting percutaneous Greenfield vena caval filter placement. Radiology 161: 275.

Shiomi S, Kuroki T, Takashima Y, Masaki K, Jomura L, Ueda T, Ikeoka N, Kobayashi K, Ochi H (1992) Course before and after treatment of a patient with Budd-Chiari syndrome monitored by iodine-123-iodoamphetamine scintigraphy per os and per rectum. J Nucl Med 33(5): 744–747.

Smith TP, Cragg AH, Castaneda F, Hunter DW (1989) Thrombosed polytetrafluoroethylene hemodialysis fistulas: salvage with combined thrombectomy and angioplasty. Radiology 171: 507–508.

Sniderman KW, Morse SS, Rapoport S, Ross GR (1985) Hemobilia following transhepatic biliary drainage: occlusion of an hepatoportal fistula by balloon tamponade. Radiology 154(3): 827.

Sparano J, Chang J, Trasi S, Bonanno C (1987) Treatment of the Budd-Chiari syndrome with percutaneous transluminal angioplasty. Case report and review of the literature. Am J Med 82: 821–828.

Spinowitz BS, Carsen G, Meisell R, Charytan C (1983) Percutaneous transluminal dilatation of vascular access. Nephron 35: 201–204.

Sprayregen S, Veith FJ (1983) Vein graft angioplasty with nonballoon catheters. Radiology 146(1): 224–225.

Sprayregen S, Veith FJ, Bakal CW (1988) Catheterization and angioplasty of the nonopacified peripheral autogenous vein bypass graft. Arch Surg 123(8): 1009–1012.

Stack RS, Stack RK, Morris KG, Bauman RP, Shadoff N, et al (1986) Temporary balloon occlusion of the inferior vena cava for immediate reversal of acute pulmonary edema. Am J Cardiol 57(10): 886–887.

Strumpf RK, Mehta SS, Ponder R, Heuser RR (1992) Palmaz-Schatz stent implantation in stenosed saphenous vein grafts: clinical and angiographic follow-up. Am Heart J 123(5): 1329–1336.

Teng GJ, He SC, Cai XL (1993) Percutaneous transluminal angioplasty of inferior vena cava and hepatic veins for Budd-Chiari syndrome [letter]. AJR 160(2): 423-424.

Uflacker R, Alves MA, Cantisani GG, Souza HP, Wagner J, et al (1985) Treatment of portal vein obstruction by percutaneous transhepatic angioplasty. Gastroenterology 88(1 Pt 1): 176–180.

Wakao F, Takayasu K, Muramatsu Y, Nawano S, Moriyama N (1990) MR evaluation of Budd-Chiari syndrome treated by percutaneous transluminal angioplasty (letter). AJR 154: 1350–1351.

Walker HS, Rholl KS, Register TE, van Breda A (1990) Percutaneous placement of a hepatic vein stent in the treatment of Budd-Chiari syndrome. J Vasc Intervent Radiol 1(1): 23–27.

Walpole HT Jr, Lovett KE, Chuang VP, West R, Clements SD Jr (1988) Superior vena cava syndrome treated by percutaneous transluminal balloon angioplasty. Am Heart J 115: 1303–1304.

Whittemore AD, Donaldson MC, Polak JF, Mannick JA (1991) Limitations of balloon angioplasty for vein graft stenosis. J Vasc Surg 14(3): 340–345.

Wright KC (1990) Percutaneous transcatheter stent placement (editorial; comment). Radiology 176(3): 620–621.

Yamada R, Sato M, Kawabata M, Nakatsuka H, Nakamura K, et al (1983) Segmental obstruction of the hepatic inferior vena cava treated by transluminal angioplasty. Radiology 149(1): 91–96.

Yang XL, Chen CR, Cheng TO (1992) Nonoperative treatment of membranous obstruction of the inferior vena cava by percutaneous balloon transluminal angioplasty. Am Heart J 124(2): 405–412.

Yankes JR, Uglietta JP, Grant J, Braun SD (1988) Percutaneous transhepatic recanalization and thrombolysis of the superior mesenteric vein. AJR 151: 289–290.

Zajko AB, Claus D, Clapuyt P, Esquivel CO, Moulin D, Starzl TE, De Ville De Goyet J, Otte JB (1989) Obstruction to hepatic venous drainage after liver transplantation: treatment with balloon angioplasty. Radiology 170: 763–765.

Zajko AB, McLean GK, Freiman DB, Oleaga JA, Ring EJ (1981) Percutaneous puncture of venous bypass grafts for transluminal angioplasty. AJR 137(4): 799–802.

Zemel G, Becker GJ, Bancroft JW, Benenati JF, Katzen BT (1992) Technical advances in transjugular intrahepatic portosystemic shunts. Radiographics 12(4): 615–622; discussion 623–624.

Zemel G, Katzen BT, Becker GJ, Benenati JF, Sallee DS (1991) Percutaneous transjugular portosystemic shunt. JAMA 266: 390–393.

Zemel G, Katzen BT, Dake MD, Benenati JF, Lempert TE, Moskowitz L (1990) Directional atherectomy in the treatment of stenotic dialysis access fistulas. J Vasc Intervent Radiol 1(1): 35–38.

Zollikofer CL, Largiader I, Bruhlmann WF, Uhlschmid GK, Marty AH (1988) Endovascular stenting of veins and grafts: preliminary clinical experience. Radiology 167(3): 707–712.

Section 2

Commentary (PTA)

I. Complications

Anonymous (1991) Balloon dilatation of native aortic coarctation [letter]. Int J Cardiol 31: 363–369.

Adams PS Jr (1984) Iliac artery-ureteral fistula developing after dilatation and stent placement. Radiology 153: 647–648.

Agrawal SK, Pinheiro L, Roubin GS, Hearn JA, Cannon AD, Macander PJ, Barnes JL, et al. (1992) Nonsurgical closure of femoral pseudoaneurysms complicating cardiac catheterization and percutaneous transluminal coronary angioplasty. J Am Coll Cardiol 20(3): 610–615.

Alcaraz A, Talbot-Wright R, Alvarez-Vijande R, Cugat E, Bielsa O, Carretero P (1989) Prolonged anuria after failed percutaneous transluminal angioplasty in a kidney transplant patient solved by surgery. Eur Urol 16: 317–319.

Armstrong MW, Torrie EP, Galland RB (1992) Consequences of immediate failure of percutaneous transluminal angioplasty. Ann R Coll Surg Engl 74(4): 265–268.

Ashenburg RJ, Blair RJ, Rivera FJ, Weigele JB (1990) Renal arterial rupture complicating transluminal angioplasty: successful conservative management. Radiology 174: 983–985.

Avery JK (1986) Sharing responsibilities. J Tenn Med Assoc 79: 298.

Bachenheimer LC, Green CE, Rosing DR, Wallace RB (1988) Surgical removal of the intracoronary portion of a fractured angioplasty guidewire. Am J Cardiol 61: 946–947.

Bakal CW, Sprayregen S, Scheinbaum K, Cynamon J, Veith FJ (1990) Percutaneous transluminal angioplasty of the infrapopliteal arteries: results in 53 patients. AJR Am J Roentgenol 154: 171–174.

Balaji S, Oommen R, Rees PG (1991) Fatal aortic rupture during balloon dilatation of recoarctation. Br Heart J 65: 100–101.

Becker GJ, Palmaz JC, Rees CR, Ehrman KO, Lalka SG, Dalsing MC, Cikrit DF, McLean GK, Burke DR, Richter GM, et al (1990) Angioplasty-induced dissections in human iliac arteries: management with Palmaz balloon-expandable intraluminal stents. Radiology 176: 31–38.

Belli AM (1991) Complications of peripheral PTA [editorial]. Br J Hosp Med 45: 67.

Belli AM, Cumberland DC, Knox AM, Procter AE, Welsh CL (1990) The complication rate of percutaneous peripheral balloon angioplasty. Clin Radiol 41: 380–383.

Bennett IC, Downes MO, Collins RE (1989) Distal bowel infarction following angioplasty of the internal iliac artery. Br J Radiol 62: 489–490.

Benson LN, Freedom RM, Wilson GJ, Halliday WC (1986) Cerebral complications following balloon angioplasty of coarctation of the aorta. Cardiovasc Intervent Radiol 9: 184–186.

Berger T, Sorensen R, Konrad J (1986) Aortic rupture: a complication of transluminal angioplasty. AJR 146: 373–374.

Bergqvist D, Jonsson K, Weibull H (1987) Complications after percutaneous transluminal angioplasty of peripheral and renal arteries. REVIEW ARTICLE: 75 REFS. Acta Radiol 28: 3–12.

Beyer-Enke SA, Zeitler E (1989) Angioplasty and angioscopy. Curr Opin Radiol 1: 183–185.

Block PC, Elmer D, Fallon JT (1982) Release of atherosclerotic debris after transluminal angioplasty. Circulation 65: 950–952.

Borrero E (1989) "Mechanical" obstruction of the superficial femoral artery with the coronary angioplasty introducer sheath. South Med J 82: 753–755.

Brandt B 3rd, Marvin WJ Jr, Rose EF, Mahoney LT (1987) Surgical treatment of coarctation of the aorta after balloon angioplasty. J Thorac Cardiovasc Surg 94: 715–719.

Brewer ML, Kinnison ML, Perler BA, White RI, Jr (1988) Blue toe syndrome: treatment with anticoagulants and delayed percutaneous transluminal angioplasty. Radiology 166: 31–36.

Brummitt CF, Kravitz GR, Granrud GA, Herzog CA (1989) Femoral endarteritis due to Staphylococcus aureus complicating percutaneous transluminal coronary angioplasty. Am J Med 86: 822–824.

Casarella WJ, Martin LG (1988) Failed percutaneous transluminal renal angioplasty: experience with lesions requiring operative intervention [letter]. J Vasc Surg 7: 821–822.

Castaneda-Zuniga WR, Tadavarthy SM, Laerum F, Amplatz K (1984) "Pseudo" intramural injection following percutaneous transluminal angioplasty. Cardiovasc Intervent Radiol 7: 104–108.

Chong WK, Cross FW, Raphael MJ (1990) Iliac artery rupture during percutaneous angioplasty. REVIEW ARTICLE: 10 REFS. Clin Radiol 41: 358–359.

Cikrit DF, Helikson MA, Nichols WK, Silver D (1991) Complete external iliac artery disruption after percutaneous aortic valvuloplasty in two young children: successful repair with hypogastric artery transposition. Surgery 109: 623–626.

Connolly JE, Kwaan JHM, McCart PM (1981) Complications after percutaneous transluminal angioplasty. Am J Surg 142: 60–66.

Cooper JC, Woods DA, Spencer P, Procter AE (1991) The development of an infected false aneurysm following iliac angioplasty. Br J Radiol 64: 759–760.

Coy KM, Park JC, Fishbein MC, Laas T, Diamond GA, Adler L, Maurer G, et al. (1992) In vitro validation of three-dimensional intravascular ultrasound for the evaluation of arterial injury after balloon angioplasty [see comments]. J Am Coll Cardiol 20(3): 692–700.

Creasy TS, McMilan PM (1987) False aneurysm after percutaneous transluminal angioplasty (letter). Br J Surg 74: 1069.

Davies RP, Voyvodic F (1992) Percutaneous retrieval of a partially expanded iliac artery stent: case report. Cardiovasc Intervent Radiol 15(2): 120–122.

Deligonul U, Gabliani G, Kern MJ, Vandormael M (1988) Percutaneous brachial catheterization: the hidden hazard of high brachial artery bifurcation. Cathet Cardiovasc Diagn 14: 44–45.

Dell'Aria JC, Petrilli R, Schwartz E (1988) Acute occlusion of the left renal artery manifested by hypertensive crisis. J Emerg Med 6: 23–27.

DeMonte F, Peerless SJ, Rankin RN (1989) Carotid transluminal angioplasty with evidence of distal embolization. Case report [see comments]. Comment in: J Neurosurg 71: 301. J Neurosurg 70: 138–141.

Dixon GD, Anderson S, Crouch TT (1986) Renal arterial rupture secondary to percutaneous transluminal angioplasty treated without surgical intervention. Cardiovasc Intervent Radiol 9: 83–85.

Dolmatch BL, Rholl KS, Moskowitz LB, Dake MD, van Breda A, Kaplan JO, Katzen BT (1989) Blue toe syndrome: treatment with percutaneous atherectomy. Radiology 173: 799–804.

Dorros G, Hall P, Prince C (1993) Successful limb salvage after recanalization of an occluded infrapopliteal artery utilizing a balloon expandable (Palmaz-Schatz) stent. Cathet Cardiovasc Diagn 28(1): 83–88.

Dorros G, Jamnadas P, Lewin RF, Sachdev N (1989) Percutaneous aspiration of a thromboembolus. Cathet Cardiovasc Diagn 17: 202–206.

Drummer E, Furey K, Hollman J (1987) Rupture of a saphenous vein bypass graft during coronary angioplasty. Br Heart J 58: 78–81.

Dwyer ML, Colombo A, Bozzi G (1989) Retrieval technique of a PTCA guidewire. G Ital Cardiol 19: 170–172.

Erbel R, Bednarczyk I, Pop T, Todt M, Henrichs KJ, Brunier A, Thelen M, Meyer J (1990) Detection of dissection of the aortic intima and media after angioplasty of coarctation of the aorta. An angiographic, computer tomographic, and echocardiographic comparative study. Circulation 81: 805–814.

Esente P, Giambartolomei A (1989) On percutaneous aspiration of a coronary thrombus [letter; comment]. Cathet Cardiovasc Diagn 18: 199.

Fellmeth BD, Bookstein JJ, Lurie AL, Dillard JP (1990) Rapid progression of peripheral vascular disease after diagnostic angiography [see comments]. Comment in Radiology 175: 33. Radiology 175: 71–74.

Ferns GA, Stewart-Lee AL, Anggard EE (1992) Arterial response to mechanical injury: balloon catheter de-endothelialization. Atherosclerosis 92(2-3): 89–104.

Fitzgerald PJ, Ports TA, Yock PG (1992) Contribution of localized calcium deposits to dissection after angioplasty. An observational study using intravascular ultrasound (see comments). Circulation 86(1): 64–70.

Flandroy P, Lenelle J, Collignon J, Stevenaert A (1988) Carotid cavernous fistula associated with Fogarty catheter angioplasty. AJNR 9: 1242.

Fletcher JP, Kershaw LZ (1988) Outcome in patients with failed percutaneous transluminal angioplasty for peripheral vascular disease. J Cardiovasc Surg (Torino) 29: 733–735.

Fontes VF, Esteves CA, Braga SL, da Silva MV, E Silva MA, Sousa JE, de Souza JA (1990) It is valid to dilate native aortic coarctation with a balloon catheter. Int J Cardiol 27: 311–316.

Fraedrich G, Beck A, Bonzel T, Schlosser V (1987) Acute surgical intervention for complications of percutaneous transluminal angioplasty. Eur J Vasc Surg 1: 197–203.

Franco CD, Goldsmith J, Veith FJ, Calligaro KD, Gupta SK, Wengerter KR (1993) Management of arterial injuries produced by percutaneous femoral procedures. Surgery 113(4): 419–425.

Frazee BW, Flaherty JP (1991) Septic endarteritis of the femoral artery following angioplasty. Rev Infect Dis 13: 620–623.

Gardiner GA Jr, Meyerovitz MF, Stokes KR, Clouse ME, Harrington DP, Bettmann MA (1986) Complications of transluminal angioplasty. Radiology 159: 201–208.

Ghosh PK, Alber G, Schistek R, Unger F (1989) Rupture of guide wire during percutaneous transluminal coronary angioplasty. Mechanics and management. J Thorac Cardiovasc Surg 97: 467–469.

Ginsburg R, Thorpe P, Bowles CR, Wright AM, Wexler L (1989) Pull-through approach to percutaneous angioplasty of totally occluded common iliac arteries. Radiology 172: 111–113.

Grabenwoger F, Dock W, Pinterits F (1987) Olbert dilatation catheter system: complication due to inexpert handling. Cardiovasc Intervent Radiol 10:168–170.

Greenfield AJ (1991) Hot-tip laser. Results and complications. Circulation 83: I94–96.

Grosse-Vorholt R, Groos G (1981) Komplizierter Verlauf einer perkutanen GefaBrekanalisation. Radiologe 21: 84–86.

Guzzetta PC, Potter BM, Kapur S, Ruley EJ, Randolph J (1983) Reconstruction of the renal artery after unsuccessful percutaneous transluminal angioplasty in children. Am J Surg 145: 647–651.

Hamada Y, Matsuda Y, Takashiba K, Ohno H, Fujii B, Ebihara H, Hyakuna

E (1989) Difficult deflation of Probe balloon due to twisting the system. Cathet Cardiovasc Diagn 18: 12–14.

Haraphongse M, Rossall RE (1989) Large air embolus complicating coronary angioplasty. Cathet Cardiovasc Diagn 17: 168–171.

Hillis LD (1990) Efficacy and safety of coronary balloon angioplasty and directional atherectomy [editorial; comment]. Circulation 82: 305–307.

Ho SY, Somerville J, Yip WC, Anderson RH (1988) Transluminal balloon dilation of resected coarcted segments of thoracic aorta: histological study and clinical implications. Int J Cardiol 19: 99–105.

Hollenberg NK (1991) Implications of thrombosis and vasospasm in peripheral vascular disease. J Cardiovasc Pharm 17 (Suppl 5): S21–28.

Hontz RA, Tripp MD, Kline LP (1991) Stents keep occluded vessels open. Rn 54: 50–4.

Horvath L, Illes I, Varro J (1978) Complications of the transluminal angioplasty excluding the puncture site complications. In: Zeitler E, et al (eds) Percutaneous Vascular Recanalization. Berlin, Heidelberg, New York, Springer, chap 19, pp 126–139.

Ino T, Benson LN, Freedom RM, Barker GA, Aipursky A, Rowe RD (1988) Thrombolytic therapy for femoral artery thrombosis after pediatric cardiac catheterization. Am Heart J 115: 633–639.

Isner JM (1988) Excimer laser angioplasty: pygmalion makes it to the ball. Lasers Surg Med 8: 447–449.

Jackson S (1987) Femoral neuropathy secondary to heparin induced intrapelvic hematoma. A case report and review of the literature. Orthopedics 10: 1049–1052.

Jacobs MJ, Gregoric ID, Reul GJ (1992) Profunda femoral artery pseudoaneurysm after percutaneous transluminal procedures manifested by neuropathy. J Cardiovasc Surg 33(6): 729–731.

Jenkins DM, Newton WD (1991) Atheroembolism. Am Surg 57: 588–590.

Jensen SR, Voegeli DR, Crummy AB, Turnipseed WD, Acher CW, Goodson S (1985) Iliac artery rupture during transluminal angioplasty: treatment by embolization and surgical bypass. AJR 145: 381–382.

Jorgensen B, Meisner S, Holstein P, Tonnesen KH (1990) Early rethrombosis in femoropopliteal occlusions treated with percutaneous transluminal angioplasty. Eur J Vasc Surg 4: 149–152.

Joseph N, Levy E, Lipman S (1987) Angioplasty-related iliac artery rupture: treatment by temporary balloon occlusion. Cardiovasc Intervent Radiol 10: 276–279.

Joshi SV, Desai R, Agarwal N, Thakker J, Parikh S, Someshwar V, Magotra R (1988) Successful management of ruptured suprarenal aortic aneurysm with left artery stenosis (a case report). J Postgrad Med 34: 105–107.

Joyce DH, McGrath LB (1990) Pseudo-aneurysm formation following balloon angioplasty for recurrent coarctation of the aorta. Cathet Cardiovasc Diagn 20: 133–135.

Juilli'ere Y, Danchin N, Amrein D, Suty-Selton C, Cherrier F (1991) Proximal rupture and intracoronary entrapment of a rotating device during low-speed rotational coronary angioplasty. Cathet Cardiovasc Diagn 23: 34–36.

Kadir S, White RI Jr, Kaufman SL, et al: (1982) Prevention of thromboembolic complications of angioplasty of critical patient selection. 82nd Annual Meeting, Am Roentgen Ray Soc, New Orleans.

Kahn JK, Hartzler GO (1990) The spectrum of symptomatic coronary air embolism during balloon angioplasty: causes, consequences, and management. Am Heart J 119: 1374–1377.

Katzen BT, Chang J (1979) Percutaneous transluminal angioplasty (PTA) with the Gruentzig balloon catheter: technical problems encountered in the first forty patients. Cardiovasc Intervent Radiol 2: 3–7.

Kaufman J, Moglia R, Lacy C, Dinerstein C, Moreyra A (1989) Peripheral vascular complications from percutaneous transluminal coronary angioplasty: a comparison with transfemoral cardiac catheterization. Am J Med Sci 297: 22–25.

Kazmers A, Moneta GL, Harley JD, Goldman ML, Clowes AW (1989) Treatment of acute renal artery occlusion after percutaneous transluminal angioplasty. J Vasc Surg 9: 487–492.

Kempczinski RF (1979) Lower extremity arterial emboli from ulcerating atherosclerotic plaques. JAMA 241: 807–810.

Khoury M, Batra S, Berg R, Rama K, Kozul V (1992) Influence of arterial access sites and interventional procedures on vascular complications after cardiac catheterizations. Am J Surg 164(3): 205–209.

Kim D, Porter DH, Siegel JB, Shapiro ME, Strom TB, Glotzer DJ (1991) Use of a reperfusion catheter after angioplasty dissection for salvage of ischemic renal allograft: case report. Cardiovasc Intervent Radiol 14: 179–182.

Koga T, Okuda S, Takishita S, Shigematsu A, Komota T, Fujishima M, Matsukuma A (1991) Renal failure due to cholesterol embolization following percutaneous transluminal renal angioplasty. Jpn J Med 30: 35–38.

Korogi Y, Takahashi M, Bussaka H, Hatanaka Y (1992) Percutaneous transluminal angioplasty: pain during balloon inflation. Br J Radiol 65(770): 140–142.

Krabill KA, Bass JL, Lucas RV Jr, Edwards JE (1987) Dissecting transverse aortic arch aneurysm after percutaneous transluminal balloon dilation angioplasty of an aortic coarctation. Pediatr Cardiol 8: 39–42.

Kresowik TF, Khoury MD, Miller BV, Winniford MD, Shamma AR, Sharp

WJ, Blecha MB, Corson JD (1991) A prospective study of the incidence and natural history of femoral vascular complications after percutaneous transluminal coronary angioplasty. J Vasc Surg 13: 328–333.

Kumar S, Mandalam KR, Rao VR, Subramanyan R, Gupta AK, Joseph S, Unni M, Rao AS (1989) Percutaneous transluminal angioplasty in nonspecific aortoarteritis (Takayasu's disease): experience of 16 cases. Cardiovasc Intervent Radiol 12: 321–325.

Kumpe DA, Zwerdlinger S, Griffin DJ (1988) Blue digit syndrome: treatment with percutaneous transluminal angioplasty. Radiology 166: 37–44.

Lablanche JM, Fourrier JL, Gommeaux A, Becquart J, Bertrand ME (1989) Percutaneous aspiration of a coronary thrombus [see comments]. Comment in: Cathet Cardiovasc Diagn 18: 199. Cathet Cardiovasc Diagn 17: 97–98.

Lachance DH, Daube JR (1991) Acute peripheral arterial occlusion: electrophysiologic study of 32 cases. Muscle Nerve 14: 633–9.

Laerum F, Castaneda WR, Amplatz KA (1983) Complications of transluminal angioplasty. In: Castaneda WR (ed) Transluminal Angioplasty. New York, Thieme-Stratton, pp 41–44.

Laerum F, Castaneda-Zuniga WR, Rysavy J, Moore R, Amplatz K (1982) The site of wall rupture in transluminal angioplasty: an experimental study. Radiology 144: 760–770.

Lassar TA (1991) Avoidance of vascular complications during transfemoral catheterization [letter; comment]. Cathet Cardiovasc Diagn 22: 156.

Law P, Dacie JE (1989) Avulsed Olbert balloon: an avoidable complication of percutaneous transluminal angioplasty. Clin Radiol 40: 88–90.

Lee TC, Hartzler GO, Rutherford BD, McConahay DR (1990) Removal of an occlusive coronary dissection flap by using an atherectomy catheter. Cathet Cardiovasc Diagn 20: 185–188.

Lemarbre L, Hudon G, Coche G, Bourassa MG (1987) Outpatient peripheral angioplasty: survey of complications and patients' perceptions. AJR 148: 1239–1242.

Lembo NK, King SB 3d, Roubin GS, Black AJ, Douglas JS Jr (1991) Effects of nonionic versus ionic contrast media on complications of percutaneous transluminal coronary angioplasty. Am J Cardiol 67: 1046–1050.

Levitt RG, Wholey MH (1990) Renal arterial rupture complicating transluminal angioplasty [letter]. Radiology 176: 583–584.

Linskey ME, Horton JA, Rao GR, Yonas H (1991) Fatal rupture of the intracranial carotid artery during transluminal angioplasty for vasospasm induced by subarachnoid hemorrhage. Case report. J Neurosurg 74: 985–990.

Little T (1992) Prolonged coronary splinting in the management of acute coronary closure. Cathet Cardiovasc Diagn 25(3): 213–217.

Lois JF, Takiff H, Schechter MS, Gomes AS, Machleder HI (1985) Vessel rupture by balloon catheters complicating chronic steroid therapy. AJR 144: 1073–1074.

Lord RS, Graham AR, Benn IV (1986) Radiologic control of operative carotid dilatation. Aneurysm formation following balloon dilatation. J Cardiovasc Surg (Torino) 27: 158–162.

Maat L, van Herwerden LA, van den Brand M, Bos E (1991) An unusual problem during surgical removal of a broken guidewire. Ann Thorac Surg 51; 829–830.

Mahler F, Triller J, Weidmann P, Nachbur B (1986) Complications in percutaneous transluminal dilatation of renal arteries. Nephron 44 (Suppl) 1: 60–63.

Mandalam KR, Rao VR, Neelakandhan KS, Kumar S, Unnikrishnan M, Mukhopadhyay S (1992) Hyperperfusion syndrome following balloon angioplasty and bypass surgery or aortic arch vessels: a report of 3 cases. Cardiovasc Intervent Radiol 15(2): 108–112.

Maouad J, Guermonprez JL (1988) Percutaneous femoral transluminal angioplasty of a right brachial artery occluded after Sones coronary angiography. Cathet Cardiovasc Diagn 14: 165–168.

Margolis JR, Mogensen L, Mehta S, Chen CY, Krauthamer D (1991) Diffuse embolization following percutaneous transluminal coronary angioplasty of occluded vein grafts: the blush phenomenon. Clin Cardiol 14(6): 489–493.

Mark DB, Hlatky MA, O'Connor CM, Pryor DB, Wall TC, Honan MB, Phillips HR, 3d, Califf RM (1988) Administration of thrombolytic therapy in the community hospital: established principles and unresolved issues. J Am Coll Cardiol 12(6 Suppl A): 32A–43A.

Marsa RJ, Jang GD (1991) Avoidance of vascular complications during transfemoral catheterization [letter]. Cathet Cardiovasc Diagn 22: 77.

Martinez AG, Novick AC, Hayes JM (1990) Surgical treatment of renal artery stenosis after failed percutaneous transluminal angioplasty. J Urol 144: 1094–1096.

Marx GR, Allen HD, Ovitt TW, Hanson W (1988) Balloon dilation angioplasty of Blalock-Taussig shunts. Am J Cardiol 62: 824–827.

Marx J (1990) Holding the line against heart disease [news]. Science 248: 1491–1493.

Matsumoto AH, Barth KH, Teitelbaum GP (1990) Percutaneous management of emboli associated with hot tip laser-assisted angioplasty. Cardiovasc Intervent Radiol 13: 71–74.

McCann RL, Bollinger RR, Newman GE (1988) Surgical renal artery reconstruction after percutaneous transluminal angioplasty. J Vasc Surg 8: 389–394.

McCann RL, Schwartz LB, Pieper KS (1991) Vascular complications of cardiac catheterization. J Vasc Surg 14: 375–381.

McDermott JC, Crummy AB, Voegeli DR, Starck EE (1987) Complications of transluminal angioplasty (letter). Radiology 162: 286–288.

McEniery PT, Grigera F, Chambers J, Franco I, Hollman J (1988) Balloon inflation following injection of contrast material through the distal lumen of the USCI balloon catheter. Cathet Cardiovasc Diagn 14: 59–62.

Medina M, Butt KM, Gordon DH, Thanawala S, Solomon N (1981) A complication of percutaneous transluminal angioplasty in the transplanted kidney. Urol Radiol 3: 59–61.

Messina LM, Brothers TE, Wakefield TW, Zelenock GB, Lindenauer SM, Greenfield LJ, Jacobs LA, Fellows EP, Grube SV, Stanley JC (1991) Clinical characteristics and surgical management of vascular complications in patients undergoing cardiac catheterization: interventional versus diagnostic procedures. J Vasc Surg 13: 593–600.

Mikolich JR, Hanson MW (1988) Transcatheter retrieval of intracoronary detached angioplasty guidewire segment. Cathet Cardiovasc Diagn 15: 44–46.

Mills SR, Wertman DE Jr, Grossman SH (1981) Renal cortical arteriovenous fistula complicating percutaneous renal angioplasty. AJR 137: 1251–1253.

Molpus WM, McCowan TC, Eidt JF (1991) External iliac artery rupture during angioplasty: control by balloon tamponade. South Med J 84: 1138–1139.

Moran CG, Ruttley MS (1987) Development of a false aneurysm following percutaneous transluminal angioplasty. Br J Surg 74: 652.

Morse MH, Jeans WD, Cole SE, Grier D, Ndlovu D (1991) Complications in percutaneous transluminal angioplasty: relationships with patient age. Br J Radiol 64: 5–9.

Muller DW, Shamir KJ, Ellis SG, Topol EJ (1992) Peripheral vascular complications after conventional and complex percutaneous coronary interventional procedures. Am J Cardiol 69(1): 63–68.

Murphy TP, Cronan JJ, Paolella LP, Dorfman GS, Francis WW (1987) Arterial rupture without balloon rupture during percutaneous transluminal angioplasty. J Vasc Surg 6: 528–530.

Nukta E, Meier B, Urban P, Muller T (1990) Circumferential rupture and entrapment of a balloon-on-a-wire device during coronary angioplasty. Cathet Cardiovasc Diagn 20: 123–125.

Oleaga JA, Grossman RA, McLean GK, Rosen RJ, Freiman DB, Ring EJ (1981) Arteriovenous fistula of a segmental renal artery branch as a complication of percutaneous angioplasty. AJR 136: 988–989.

Olin JW, Wholey M (1987) Rupture of the renal artery nine days after percutaneous transluminal angioplasty. JAMA 257: 518–520.

Oweida SW, Roubin GS, Smith RB 3d, Salam AA (1990) Postcatheterization vascular complications associated with percutaneous transluminal coronary angioplasty. J Vasc Surg 12: 310–315.

Owen ER, Moussa SA, Lewis JD, Wilkins RA (1990) Peripheral laser assisted angioplasty: results, complications and follow-up. J R Coll Surg Edinb 35: 75–79.

Pak K, Konishi T, Wakabayashi Y, Tomoyoshi T (1987) Nephrectomy necessitated by percutaneous transluminal angioplasty for renovascular hypertension. Nippon Jinzo Gakkai Shi 29: 341–345.

Palmar AH, Defeyter IR, Vandenbogaerde JF (1989) Renal arterial stenosis as a cause of high output cardiac failure. Int J Cardiol 22: 404–406.

Parker DJ (1990) Does angioplasty need on-site surgical cover? A surgeon's view. Br Heart J 64: 1–2.

Perkins SB, Kennally KM (1989) The hidden danger of internal hemorrhage (continuing education credit). Nursing 19: 34–42.

Perry MO (1985) Intramural dissection of superior mesenteric artery. A complication of attempted renal artery balloon dilation. J Vasc Surg 2: 480–484.

Pezzulli FA, Purnell FM, Dillon EH (1986) Acute posttraumatic hypertension in fibromuscular dysplasia of the renal artery. Subintimal hemorrhage treated by percutaneous transluminal angioplasty. NY State J Med 86: 100–102.

Piessens JH, Stammen F, Vrolix MC, Glazier JJ, Benit E, De Geest H, Willems JL (1993) Effects of an ionic versus a nonionic low osmolar contrast agent on the thrombotic complications of coronary angioplasty. Cathet Cardiovasc Diagn 28(2): 99–105.

Pitney MR, Cumpston N (1991) A solution to the problem of an unexpanded Palmaz-Schatz stent following balloon rupture. Cathet Cardiovasc Diagn 24(4): 246–247.

Price BA (1990) Management of critical ischaemia by transluminal iliac angioplasty with distal bypass surgery [letter]. J R Coll Surg Edinb 35: 132.

Price J, Hands LJ, Fletcher EW (1989) Removal of a nondeflating balloon angioplasty catheter after percutaneous aspiration (letter). AJR Am J Roentgenol 152: 1347.

Priest EM (1988) Treatment of shunt-produced edema (letter). South Med J 81: 1204.

Puijlaert CB, Mali WP, Rosenbusch G, van Straalen AM, Klinge J, Feldberg MA (1986) Delayed rupture of renal artery after renal percutaneous transluminal angioplasty. Radiology 159: 635–637.

Puylaert CB, Klinge J, Mali WP, Geyskes GG (1988) Results and complications of renal PTA. Ann Radiol (Paris) 31: 82–86.

Rao PS (1991) Fatal aortic rupture during balloon dilatation of recoarctation [letter]. Br Heart J 66: 406–407.

Rao PS (1991) Pseudoaneurysm following balloon angioplasty? [letter]. Cathet Cardiovasc Diagn 23: 150–152.

Rao PS, Chopra PS (1991) Role of balloon angioplasty in the treatment of aortic coarctation. Ann Thorac Surg 52: 621–631.

Rao PS, Thapar MK, Galal O, Wilson AD (1990) Follow-up results of balloon angioplasty of native coarctation in neonates and infants. Am Heart J 120 (6 Pt 1): 1310–1314.

Ravimandalam K, Rao VR, Kumar S, Gupta AK, Joseph S, Unni M, Rao AS (1991) Obstruction of the infrarenal portion of the abdominal aorta: results of treatment with balloon angioplasty. AJR 156: 1257–1260.

Reed H, Shandall A, Ruttley M (1991) Iliac artery rupture during percutaneous angioplasty [letter; comment]. Clin Radiol 43: 142–143.

Ritter SB (1989) Coarctation and balloons: inflated or realistic? J Am Coll Cardiol 13: 696–699.

Rizzo TF, Werres R, Ciccone J, Karanam R, Shah S (1988) Entrapment of an angioplasty balloon catheter: a case report. Cathet Cardiovasc Diagn 14: 255–257.

Rosenthal D, Pesa FA, Gottsegen WL, Crew JR, Moss CA, Walsky R, Pallos LL (1991) Thermal laser-assisted balloon angioplasty of the superficial femoral artery: a multicenter review of 602 cases. J Vasc Surg 14: 152–159.

Rosenthal D, Wheeler WG 3d, Seagraves A, Erdoes L, Lamis PA, Jones M, Clark MD, Pallos LL (1991) Nd:YAG iliac and femoropopliteal laser angioplasty: results with large probes as "sole therapy." J Cardiovasc Surg 32: 186–191.

Rosenthal E, Montarello JK, Palmer T, Curry PV (1989) Coronary artery thermal damage during percutaneous "hot tip" laser-assisted angioplasty. Am J Cardiol 64: 116–120.

Roth FJ, Rieser R, Scheffler A, Krings W (1991) Intra-arterial fibrinolytic therapy of chronic arterial occlusions. Semin Thromb Hemost 17: 39–47.

Samson RH, Sprayregen S, Veith FJ, Scher LA, Gupta SK, Ascer E (1984) Management of angioplasty complications, unsuccessful procedures and early and late failures. Ann Surg 199: 234–240.

Sanborn TA, Cumberland DC, Greenfield AJ, Motarjeme A, Schwarten DE, Leachman DR, Ferris EJ, Myler RK, McCowan TC, Tatpati D, et al (1989) Peripheral laser-assisted balloon angioplasty. Initial multicenter experience in 219 peripheral arteries. Arch Surg 124: 1099–1103.

Sanyal SK, Wilson N, Twum-Danso K, Abomelha A, Sohel S (1990) Moraxella endocarditis following balloon angioplasty of aortic coarctation. Am Heart J 119: 1421–1423.

Schlosser V, Spillner G, Mathias K (1979) Komplikationen nach perkutaner transluminaler GefaBrekanalisation (PTR) und ihre chirurgische Behandlung. Vasa 8: 324–328.

Schroder TM, Puolakkainen PA, Hahl J, Ramo OJ (1989) Fatal air embolism as a complication of laser-induced hyperthermia. Lasers Surg Med 9: 183–185.

Schroeder J, Papachrysanthou C, Huhmann W (1991) Embolization of a rubber disc from a hemostasis valve: technical note. Cardiovasc Intervent Radiol 14: 132–133.

Schuur KH, Vencken LM (1981) Arterial hypertension treated by angioplasty (Dotter), a serious complication. Diagn Imaging 50: 47–51.

Schwab SJ, Raymond JR, Saeed M, Newman GE, Dennis PA, Bollinger RR (1989) Prevention of hemodialysis fistula thrombosis. Early detection of venous stenoses. Kidney Int 36: 707–711.

Schwartz RA, Kerns DB, Mitchell DG (1991) Color Doppler ultrasound imaging in iatrogenic arterial injuries. Am J Surg 162: 4–8.

Selby JB Jr, Oliva VL, Tegtmeyer CJ (1992) Circumferential rupture of an angioplasty balloon with detachment from the shaft: case report. Cardiovasc Intervent Radiol 15(2): 113–116.

Sethi GK, Ferguson TB, Jr, Miller G, Scott SM (1989) Entrapment of broken guidewire in the left main coronary artery during percutaneous transluminal coronary angioplasty. Ann Thorac Surg 47: 455–457.

Sharma S, Gupta AK, Dev V (1992) Aortic dissection following transluminal angioplasty of the thoracic aorta in nonspecific aortoarteritis. Int J Cardiol 35(2): 264–267.

Shaw TR (1990) Does angioplasty need on-site surgical cover? A physician's view. Br Heart J 64: 3–4.

Sheikh KH, Adams DB, McCann R, Lyerly HK, Sabiston DC, Kisslo J (1989) Utility of Doppler color flow imaging for identification of femoral arterial complications of cardiac catheterization. Am Heart J 117: 623–628.

Shim WH, Jang YS, Lee JT, Lee KS (1988) A case of occult splenic abscess following percutaneous transluminal coronary angioplasty (PTCA): an unrecognized complication of PTCA. Yonsei Med J 29: 89–93.

Simonetti G (1984) Iliac artery rupture during transluminal angioplasty (letter). AJR 142: 1295.

Simonetti G, Rossi P, Passariello R, Faraglia V, Spartera C, Pistolese R, Fiorani P (1983) Iliac artery rupture: a complication of transluminal angioplasty. AJR 140: 989–990.

Sise MJ, Shackford SR, Rowley WR, Pistone FJ (1989) Claudication in young adults: a frequently delayed diagnosis. J Vasc Surg 10: 68–74.

Skillman JJ, Kim D, Baim DS (1988) Vascular complications of percutaneous femoral cardiac interventions. Incidence and operative repair. Arch Surg 123: 1207–1212.

Slavis SA, Hodge EE, Novick AC, Maatman T (1990) Surgical treatment for isolated dissection of the renal artery. J Urol 144: 233–237.

Smith DC, Durkos JL (1982) An improved ruptured-balloon retrieval set. Radiology 144: 430–431.

Sniderman KW, Bodner L, Saddekni S, Srur M, Sos TA (1984) Percutaneous embolectomy by transcatheter aspiration. Work in progress. Radiology 150: 357–361.

Staller BJ, Maleki M (1989) Percutaneous transluminal angioplasty for innominate artery stenosis and total occlusion of subclavian artery in Takayasu's-type arteritis. Cathet Cardiovasc Diagn 16: 91–94.

Starck EE, McDermott JC, Crummy AB, Turnipseed WD, Acher CW, Burgess JH (1985) Percutaneous aspiration thromboembolectomy. Radiology 156: 61–66.

Sutters M, Al-Kotoubi MA, Mathias CJ, Peart S (1987) Diuresis and syncope after renal angioplasty in a patient with one functioning kidney. Br Med J (Clin Res) 295: 527–528.

Svigals PJ, McLean GK, Davis JE, Meranze SG, Burke DR (1986) Transient hypertension after percutaneous transluminal renal artery angioplasty. Radiology 161: 293–294.

Talasz H, Genser N, Mair J, Dworzak EA, Friedrich G, Moes N, Muhlberger V, Puschendorf B (1992) Side-branch occlusion during percutaneous transluminal coronary angioplasty. Lancet 339(8806): 1380–1382.

Tani LY, Orsmond GS, Boucek MM, Shaddy RE (1993) Acute life-threatening hypertension following balloon angioplasty of native coarctation of the aorta. Am Heart J 125(3): 907–908.

Tegtmeyer CJ, Bezirdjian DR (1981) Removing the stuck, ruptured angioplasty balloon catheter. Radiology 139: 231–232.

Tegtmeyer CJ, Hartwell GD, Selby JB, Robertson R Jr, Kron IL, Tribble CG (1991) Results and complications of angioplasty in aortoiliac disease [comments]. Circulation 83: I53–60.

Tegtmeyer CJ, Selby JB, Hartwell GD, Ayers C, Tegtmeyer V (1991) Results and complications of angioplasty in fibromuscular disease. Circulation 83: I155–161.

Teirstein PS, Hartzler GO (1987) Nonoperative management of aortocoronary saphenous vein graft rupture during percutaneous transluminal coronary angioplasty. Am J Cardiol 60: 377–388.

The SH, Wilson RA, Gussenhoven EJ, Pieterman H, Bom K, Roelandt JR, van Urk H (1992) Extrinsic compression of the superficial femoral artery at the adductor canal: evaluation with intravascular sonography. AJR 159(1): 117–120.

Tonnesen KH, Sager P, Karle A, Henriksen L, Jorgensen B (1988) Percutaneous transluminal angioplasty of the superficial femoral artery by retrograde catheterization via the popliteal artery. Cardiovasc Intervent Radiol 11: 127–131.

Train JS, Dan SJ, Mitty HA, Dikman SH, Harrington EB, Miller CM, Jacobson JH 2nd (1988) Occlusion during iliac angioplasty: a salvageable complication. Radiology 168: 131–135.

Trerotola SO, Kuhlman JE, Fishman EK (1990) Bleeding complications of femoral catheterization: CT evaluation. Radiology 174: 37–40.

Ueda M, Fujimoto T, Ogawa N, Shoji S (1989) An autopsy case of cholesterol embolism following percutaneous transluminal coronary angioplasty and aortography. Acta Pathol 39: 203–206.

Vallance P (1989) EDRF and microvascular constriction after angioplasty (letter). Lancet 1: 1139.

Van Andel GJ (1980) Arterial occlusion following angiography. Br J Radiol 53: 747–753.

Van Beers B, Roche A, Cauquil P (1988) Transluminal angioplasty of a stenotic surgical splenorenal shunt. Acta Radiol 29: 327–329.

Verhelst JA, Daelemans RA, Vereycken HA, Lins RL (1989) Mesenteric infarction: a fatal complication of renal transluminal angioplasty. Acta Clin Belg 44: 336–338.

Verstraete M, Hess H, Mahler F, Mietaschk A, Roth FJ, Schneider E, Baert AL, Verhaeghe R (1988) Femoro-popliteal artery thrombolysis with intra-arterial infusion of recombinant tissue-type plasminogen activator: report of a pilot trial. Eur J Vasc Surg 2: 155–159.

Vidt DG, Eisele G, Gephardt GN, Tubbs R, Novick AC (1989) Atheroembolic renal disease: association with renal arterial stenosis. Cleve Clin J Med 56: 407–413.

Villarica J, Gross RC (1986) Treatment of angioplasty-related iliac-artery rupture without bypass surgery (case report). AJR 147: 389–390.

Viron B, Lacombe M, Raynaud A, Bindi P, Thibault P, Mignon F (1991) Delayed extensive arterial dissection after percutaneous transluminal angioplasty for transplant renal artery stenosis. Nephron 58: 351–353.

Vive J, Bolia A (1992) Aneurysm formation at the site of percutaneous transluminal angioplasty: a report of two cases and a review of the literature. Clin Radiol 45(2): 125–127.

Vorwerk D, Guenther RW (1990) Mechanical revascularization of occluded iliac arteries with use of self-expandable endoprostheses. Radiology 175: 411–415.

Vrolix M, Vanhaecke J, Piessens J, De Geest H (1988) An unusual case of guide wire fracture during percutaneous transluminal coronary angioplasty. Cathet Cardiovasc Diagn 15: 99–102.

Wang SP, Chiang BN (1987) Thrombus formation in the ascending aorta: a complication of angioplasty. Cathet Cardiovasc Diagn 13: 50–53.

Watson LE (1987) Snare loop technique for removal of broken steerable PTCA wire. Cathet Cardiovasc Diagn 13: 44–49.

Waugh JR, Sacharias N (1992) Arteriographic complications in the DSA era. Radiology 182: 243–246.

Wayne DA, Muizelaar PJ (1989) Acute lumbosacral epidural abscess after percutaneous transluminal angioplasty. Am J Med 87: 478.

Webb JG, Dodek AA, Allard M, Carere R, Marsh I (1992) 'Salvage atherectomy' for discrete arterial dissections resulting from balloon angioplasty. Can J Cardiol 8(5): 481–486.

Weber H, Enders S, Hessel S (1991) Thermal effects and histologic changes from Nd:YAG laser irradiation on normal and diseased aortic tissue using a novel angioplasty catheter with a mobile optical fiber: an in vitro assessment. Angiology 42: 597–606.

Weibull H, Bergqvist D, Jonsson K, Karlsson S, Takolander R (1987) Analysis of complications after percutaneous transluminal angioplasty of renal artery stenoses. Eur J Vasc Surg 1: 77–84.

Weibull H, Bergqvist D, Jonsson K, Karlsson S, Takolander R (1987) Complications after percutaneous transluminal angioplasty in the iliac, femoral, and popliteal arteries. J Vasc Surg 5: 681–686.

Weisman ID, Ney AL, Andrisevic JH, Stanchfield W Jr, Odland MD, Andersen RC (1988) Unusual transplant renal angioplasty complications: case report. Cardiovasc Intervent Radiol 11: 97–100.

Weitz Z, Gafter U, Chagnac A, Levi J (1987) Cholesterol emboli in atherosclerotic patients: reports of four cases occurring spontaneously or complicating angioplasty and aortorenal bypass. J Am Geriatr Soc 35: 357–359.

White RI, Jr, Rizer DM, Shuman KR, White EJ, Adams PE, Kinnison ML, Mitchell SE, Osterman FA, Jr (1988) Streamlining operation of an admitting service for interventional radiology. Radiology 168: 127–130.

Wiener RS, Ong LS (1989) Local infection after percutaneous transluminal coronary angioplasty: relation to early repuncture of ipsilateral femoral artery. Cathet Cardiovasc Diagn 16: 180–181.

Williams DM, Simon HJ, Marx MV, Starkey TD (1992) Acute traumatic aortic rupture: intravascular US findings. Radiology 182: 247–249.

Wyman RM, Safian RD, Portway V, Skillman JJ, McKay RG, Baim DS (1988) Current complications of diagnostic and therapeutic cardiac catheterization. J Am Coll Cardiol 12: 1400–1406.

Yeon EB, Cemaletin NS, Moses JW, McCrossan J (1990) Successful percutaneous removal of retained probe balloon wire during coronary angioplasty. Am Heart J 119: 1201–1205.

Yune HY, Klatte EC (1980) Circumferential tear of percutaneous transluminal angioplasty catheter balloon. AJR 135: 395–396.

Yune HY, Klatte EC, Grim CE, Weinberger MH (1980) Transluminal balloon dilatation of renal artery stenosis causing hypertension: 18 months experience. Clin Sci 59: 483s–485s.

Zarins CK, Lu CT, Gewertz BL, Lyon RT, Rush DS, Glagov S (1982) Arterial disruption and remodeling following balloon dilatation. Surgery 92: 1086–1095.

Zeitler E (1978) Complications in and after PTR. In: Zeitler E, et al (eds) Percutaneous Vascular Recanalization. Berlin, Heidelberg, New York, Springer, pp 120–125.

II. Pathology and Physiology

Anderson PG, Bajaj RK, Baxley WA, Roubin GS (1992) Vascular pathology of balloon-expandable flexible coil stents in humans. J Am Coll Cardiol 19(2): 372–381.

Annexton M (1978) Burrowing through blocked arteries with a balloon 'relocates' plaques. JAMA 240: 1117–1119.

Ashley S, Brooks SG, Gehani AA, Thorley P, Parkin A, Kester RC, Rees MR (1991) Isotope limb blood flow measurement in patients undergoing peripheral laser angioplasty. J Biomed Eng 13: 221–224.

Blinder RA, Randall PA (1982) The Bell-Thompson rule as an aid for peripheral percutaneous transluminal angioplasty. Radiology 145: 845.

Block PC (1984) Mechanism of transluminal angioplasty. Am J Cardiol 53: 69C-71C.

Block PC, Baughman KL, Pasternak RC, Fallon JT (1980) Transluminal angioplasty: correlation of morphologic and angiographic findings in an experimental model. Circulation 61: 778–785.

Block PC, Fallon JT, Elmer D (1980) Experimental angioplasty: lessons from the laboratory. AJR 135: 907–912.

Block PC, Myler RK, Stertzer S, Fallon JT (1981) Morphology after transluminal angioplasty in human beings. N Engl J Med 305: 382–385.

Bodrog I, Mohacsy J, Urai L (1986) Light and electron microscopic study of pathomorphological changes on the arterial wall after transluminal angioplasty. Int Angiol 5: 13–19.

Bollinger A, Gruentzig A, Schlumpf M, Casty M (1978) Ultrasound techniques for followup of hemodynamic changes after transluminal dilatation or recanalization. In: Zeitler E, et al (eds) Percutaneous Vascular Recanalization. Springer, Berlin Heidelberg New York, chap. 12, pp 78–85.

Brady AJ, Warren JB (1991) Angioplasty and restenosis [editorial]. Br Med J 303: 729–730.

Brevetti G, Angelini C, Rosa M, Carrozzo R, Perna S, Corsi M, Matarazzo A, Marcialis A (1991) Muscle carnitine deficiency in patients with severe peripheral vascular disease. Circulation 84: 1490–1495.

Brewster DC (1991) Acute peripheral arterial occlusion. Cardiol Clin 9: 497–513.

Bulkley BH, Hutchins GM (1977) Accelerated "atherosclerosis." A morphologic study of 97 saphenous vein coronary artery bypass grafts. Circulation 55: 163–169.

Castaneda-Zuniga WR, Amplatz K, Laerum F, Formanek A, Sibley R, Edwards J, Vlodaver A (1981) Mechanics of angioplasty: an experimental approach. Radiographics 1: 1–14.

Castaneda-Zuniga WR, Formanek A, Tadavarthy M, Vlodaver Z, Edwards JE, Zollikofer C, Amplatz K (1980) The mechanism of balloon angioplasty. Radiology 135: 565–571.

Castaneda-Zuniga WR, Sibley R, Amplatz K (1984) The pathologic basis of angioplasty. Angiology 35: 195–205.

Charoenkul V, Tey PH, Ahmed A, Peirce EC 2d, McElhinney AL (1982) Hemodynamic improvement after percutaneous transluminal angioplasty. Mt Sinai J Med (NY) 49: 468–471.

Chin AK, Kinney TB, Rurik GW, Shoor PM, Fogarty TJ (1984) A physical measurement of the mechanisms of transluminal angioplasty. Surgery 95: 196–201.

Clouse ME, Tomashefski JF, Reinhold RE, Gostello P (1981) Mechanical effect of balloon angioplasty: case report with histology. AJR 137: 869–871.

Cragg A, Einzig S, Rysavy J, Castaneda-Zuniga W, Borgwardt B, Amplatz K (1983) Effect of aspirin on angioplasty-induced vessel wall hyperemia. AJR 140: 1233–1238.

Cragg AH, Einzig S, Rysavy A, Castaneda-Zuniga WR, Borgwardt B, Amplatz K (1983) The vasa vasorum and angioplasty. Radiology 148: 75–80.

Cunningham DA, Kumar B, Siegel BA, Gilula LA, Totty WG, Welch MJ (1984) Aspirin inhibition of platelet deposition at angioplasty sites: demonstration by platelet scintigraphy. Radiology 151: 487–490.

Demer LL, Ariani M, Siegel RJ (1991) High intensity ultrasound increases distensibility of calcific atherosclerotic arteries. JACC 18: 1259–1262.

Dotter CT (1978) Transluminal angioplasty—pathologic basis. In: Zeitler E, et al (eds) Percutaneous Vascular Recanalization. Springer, Berlin Heidelberg New York, chap. 2, pp 3–12.

Ebner H, Wex P, Dragojevic D (1989) The mechanism of angioplasty—endoscopic and morphometric investigations in an experimental model. Eur J Vasc Surg 3: 543–547.

Erbel R, Bednarczyk I, Pop T, Todt M, Henrichs KJ, Brunier A, Thelen M, Meyer J (1990) Detection of dissection of the aortic intima and media after angioplasty of coarctation of the aorta. An angiographic, computer tomographic, and echocardiographic comparative study. Circulation 81: 805–814.

Fallon JT (1980) Pathology of arterial lesions amenable to percutaneous transluminal angioplasty. AJR 135: 913–916.

Faxon DP, Sanborn TA, Haudenschild CC (1987) Mechanism of angioplasty and its relation to restenosis. Am J Cardiol 60: 5B–9B.

Faxon DP, Weber VJ, Haudenschild C, Gottsman SB, McGovern WA, Ryan TJ (1982) Acute effects of transluminal angioplasty in three experimental models of atherosclerosis. Arteriosclerosis 2: 125–133.

Fellmeth BD, Bookstein JJ, Lurie AL, Dillard JP (1990) Rapid progression of peripheral vascular disease after diagnostic angiography [see comments]. Comment in: Radiology 175: 33. Radiology 175: 71–74.

Ferns GA, Raines EW, Sprugel KH, Motani AS, Reidy MA, Ross R (1991) Inhibition of neointimal smooth muscle accumulation after angioplasty by an antibody to PDGF. Science 253: 1129–1132.

Ferns GA, Stewart-Lee AL, Anggard EE (1992) Arterial response to mechanical injury: balloon catheter de-endothelialization. Atherosclerosis 92(2–3): 89–104.

Flanigan DP, Schuler JJ, Spigos DG, Lim LT (1982) Anatomic and hemodynamic evaluation of percutaneous transluminal angioplasty. Surg Gynecol Obstet 154: 181–185.

Fletcher JP, Kershaw LZ (1988) Outcome in patients with failed percutaneous transluminal angioplasty for peripheral vascular disease. J Cardiovasc Surg (Torino) 29: 733–735.

Gardner AW, Skinner JS, Cantwell BW, Smith LK (1991) Progressive vs single-stage treadmill tests for evaluation of claudication. Med Sci Sports Exerc 23: 402–408.

Gruentzig A, Schlumpf M, Wellauer J, Bollinger A (1974) Results of transluminal vascular canalization after Dotter surveillance using Doppler ultrasonic pressure measurement (Abstract). ASCA 249–251.

Harker LA (1987) Role of platelets and thrombosis in mechanisms of acute occlusion and restenosis after angioplasty. REVIEW ARTICLE: 118 REFS. Am J Cardiol 60: 20B-28B.

Haudenschild CC (1989) Pathogenesis of restenosis. REVIEW ARTICLE: 28 REFS. Z Kardiol 78(Suppl3): 28–34.

Haudenschild CC (1990) Pathogenesis of restenosis. A correlation of clinical observations with cellular responses. Z Kardiol 79 (Suppl 3): 17–22.

Hieshima GB, Higashida RT, Halbach VV (1990) Intravascular treatment of aneurysms. Clin Neurosurg 36: 338–343.

Hollman J (1991) What does pathology teach us about recurrent stenosis after coronary angioplasty? [editorial; comment]. J Am Coll Cardiol 17: 440–441.

Hornstra G (1989) Influence of dietary fish oil on arterial thrombosis and atherosclerosis in animal models and in man. REVIEW ARTICLE: 59 REFS. J Intern Med 225(Suppl): 53–59.

Imai Y, Abe K, Sasaki S, Munakata M, Minami N, Sakuma H, Hashimoto J, et al. (1992) Circadian blood pressure variation in patients with renovascular hypertension or primary aldosteronism. Clin Exp Hypertension 14(6)(Part A): 1141–1167.

Isner JM, Pickering JG, Mosseri M (1992) Laser-induced dissections: pathogenesis and implications for therapy (editorial; comment). J Am Coll Cardiol 19(7): 1619–1621.

Janevski BK, Breslau PJ, Jorning PJ (1986) More accurate assessment of stenotic lesions in percutaneous transluminal angioplasty. Int Angiol 5: 97–103.

Johnson DE, Braden L, Simpson JB (1990) Mechanism of directed transluminal atherectomy. Am J Cardiol 65: 389–391.

Kadir S, Hill-Zobel RL, Tsan ME (1983) Evaluation of arterial injury due to balloon angioplasty by In-labelled platelets. Nuklearmedizin 22: 324–328.

Karsch KR, Haase KK, Wehrmann M, Hassenstein S, Hanke H (1991) Smooth muscle cell proliferation and restenosis after stand alone coronary excimer laser angioplasty [comments]. J Am Coll Cardiol 17: 991–994.

Kinney TB, Chin AK, Rurik GW, Finn JC, Shoor PM, Hayden WG, Fogarty TJ (1984) The physical mechanisms of transluminal angioplasty: a mechanical pathophysiological correlation. Radiology 153: 85–89.

Kremer Hovinga TK, de Jong PE, de Zeeuw D, Donker AJ, Schuur KH, van der Hem GK (1986) Restenosis prevalence and long-term effects on renal function after percutaneous transluminal renal angioplasty. Nephron 44 (Suppl 1): 64–67.

Krone R (1981) Morphology after transluminal angioplasty (letter). N Engl J Med 305: 1652.

Laerum F, Vlodaver Z, Castaneda-Zuniga WR, Edwards JE, Amplatz K (1982) The mechanism of angioplasty: dilatation of iliac cadaver arteries with intravascular pressure control. ROFO 136: 573–576.

Laifer LI, O'Brien KM, Stetz ML, Gindi GR, Garrand TJ, Deckelbaum LI (1989) Biochemical basis for the difference between normal and atherosclerotic arterial fluorescence. Circulation 80: 1893–1901.

Lau CS, Scott N, Shaw JW, Belch JJ (1991) Increased activity of oxygen free radicals during reperfusion in patients with peripheral arterial disease undergoing percutaneous peripheral artery balloon angioplasty. Int Angiol 10(4): 244–246.

Laufer G, Wollenek G, Hohla K, Horvat R, Henke KH, Buchelt M, Wutzl G, Wolner E (1988) Excimer laser-induced simultaneous ablation and spectral identification of normal and atherosclerotic arterial tissue layers. Circulation 78: 1031–1039.

Leaf A (1988) Effects of n-3 fatty acids on reocclusion after angioplasty. REVIEW ARTICLE: 23 REFS. Semin Thromb Hemost 14: 290–292.

Lee BI, Becker GJ, Waller BF, Barry KJ, Connolly RJ, Kaplan J, Shapiro AR, Nardella PC (1989) Thermal compression and molding of atherosclerotic vascular tissue with use of radiofrequency energy: implications for radiofrequency balloon angioplasty. JACC 13: 1167–1175.

Lee G, Ikeda RM, Joye JA, Bogren HG, DeMaria AN, Mason DT (1980) Evaluation of transluminal angioplasty of chronic coronary artery stenosis. Value and limitations assessed in fresh human cadaver hearts. Circulation 61: 77–83.

Lee WM, Lee RT (1975) Advanced coronary atherosclerosis in swine produced by combination of balloon catheter injury and cholesterol feeding. Exp Mol Pathol 23: 491.

Leiboff R, Bren G, Katz R, Korkegi R, Ross A (1983) Determinants of transstenotic gradients observed during angioplasty: an experimental model. Am J Cardiol 52: 1311–1317.

Leu HJ, Gruentzig A (1978) Histopathologic aspects of transluminal recanalization. In: Zeitler E, et al (eds) Percutaneous Vascular Recanalization. Springer, Berlin Heidelberg New York, chap. 7, pp 39–50.

Lewis VD, 3d, Meranze SG, McLean GK, O'Neill JA, Jr, Berkowitz HD, Burke DR (1988) The midaortic syndrome: diagnosis and treatment [see comments]. Comment in: Radiology 1989 Feb;170(2): 571–572. Radiology 167: 111–113.

Lie JT, Lawrie GM, Morris GC Jr (1977) Aortocoronary bypass saphenous vein graft atherosclerosis. Anatomic study of 99 vein grafts from normal and hyperlipoproteinemic patients up to 75 months postoperatively. Am J Cardiol 40: 906–913.

Link DP, Foerster JM, Lantz Bo MT, Holcroft JW (1981) Assessment of peripheral blood flow in man by video dilution technique: a preliminary report. Invest Radiol 16: 298–304.

Linskey ME, Horton JA, Rao GR, Yonas H (1991) Fatal rupture of the intracranial artery during transluminal angioplasty for vasospasm induced by subarachnoid hemorrhage. Case report. J Neurosurg 74: 985–990.

Liu MW, Roubin GS, King SB, 3d (1989) Restenosis after coronary angioplasty. Potential biologic determinants and role of intimal hyperplasia. REVIEW ARTICLE: 100 REFS. Circulation 79: 1374–1387.

Lyon RT, Zarins CK, Lu CT, Yang CF, Glagov S (1987) Vessel, plaque, and lumen morphology after transluminal balloon angioplasty. Quantitative study in distended human arteries. Arteriosclerosis 7: 306–314.

Marshall M, Hess H (1978) New findings concerning pathogenesis and non-surgical treatment of peripheral arterial diseases. Vasa 7: 49–53.

McKean SC (1991) Preoperative evaluation of patients with peripheral vascular disease. Cardiol Clin 9: 475–481.

Minar E. Ehringer H, Ahmadi R, Dudczak R, Porenta G (1987) Platelet deposition at angioplasty sites and platelet survival time after PTA in iliac and femoral arteries: investigations with indium-111-oxine labelled platelets in patients with ASA (1.0 g/day)-therapy. Thromb Haemost 58: 718–723.

Mohacsy J, Bodrog I, Urai L (1984) Pathomorphology of the arterial wall following tansluminal recanalization. Light and electron microscopic study. Ann Radiol (Paris) 27: 357–360.

Moneta GL, Schneider E, Jager K, Brulisauer M, Thuring-Vollenweider U, Bollinger A (1988) Laser Doppler flux and vasomotion in patients before and after transluminal angioplasty for limb salvage. Vasa 17: 26–31.

Morin JF, Johnston KW, Wasserman L, Andrews D (1986) Factors that determine the long-term results of percutaneous transluminal dilatation for peripheral arterial occlusive disease. J Vasc Surg 4: 68–72.

Myles JL, Ratliff NB, Hollman J, Zaidi A, Tan TB (1988) Mechanisms of vessel injury during percutaneous transluminal angioplasty of saphenous vein bypass grafts and coronary arteries. Am J Cardiovasc Pathol 2: 133–136.

Neiman HL, Bergan JJ, Yao JST, Brandt TD, Greenberg M, O'Mara CS (1982) Hemodynamic assessment of transluminal angioplasty for lower extremity ischemia. Radiology 143: 639–643.

Ohta M, Kusaba A, Shrestha DR, Koja K, Kina M, Shiroma H, Ohmine Y (1991) Popliteal artery entrapment syndrome. Report of two cases. J Cardiovasc Surg 32: 697–701.

O'Mara CS, Neiman HL, Flinn WR, Herman RJ, Yao JST, Bergan JJ (1981) Hemodynamic assessment of transluminal angioplasty for lower extremity ischemia. Surgery 89: 106–117.

Pierangeli LF (1981) La desobstruction endoluminale par voie percutanee des stenoses arterielles. Ann Radiol (Paris) 24: 170–177.

Potkin BN, Roberts WC (1988) Effects of percutaneous transluminal coronary angioplasty on atherosclerotic plaques and relation of plaque composition and arterial size to outcome. Am J Cardiol 62: 41–50.

Probst R, Pachinger O, Sinzinger H, Kaliman J (1983) Release of prostaglandins after percutaneous transluminal coronary angioplasty. Circulation 68 (Suppl III): 144.

Rosner NH, Doris PE (1986) Persistent plaque following successful angioplasty: demonstration by Doppler duplex. J Ultrasound Med 5: 107–109.

Rousseau H, Joffre J, Puel J, Imbert C, Puech JL, Duboucher C, Wallstent H (1987) Percutaneous vascular stent: experimental studies and preliminary clinical results in peripheral arterial diseases. Int Angiol 6: 153–161.

Saffitz JE, Totty WG, McClennan BL, Gilula LA (1981) Percutaneous transluminal angioplasty. Radiological-pathological correlation. Radiology 141: 651–654.

Salles-Cunha SX, Andros G, Dulawa LB, Harris RW, Oblath RW (1989) Changes in peripheral hemodynamics after percutaneous transluminal angioplasty. J Vasc Surg 10: 338–342.

Samson RH, Sprayregen S, Veith FJ, Gupta SK, Ascer E, Scher LA (1984)

Inadequacy of the noninvasive hemodynamic evaluation of percutaneous transluminal angioplasty. Am J Surg 147: 212–215.

Sanborn TA (1989) Recanalization of arterial occlusions: pathologic basis and contributing factors. J Am Coll Cardiol 13: 1558–1560.

Sanborn TA, Faxon DP, Waugh D, Small DM, Haudenschild C, Gottsman SB, Ryan TJ (1982) Transluminal angioplasty in experimental atherosclerosis. Analysis for embolization using an in vivo perfusion system. Circulation 66: 917–922.

Saner HE, Gobel FL, Salomonowitz E, Erlien DA, Edwards JE (1985) The disease-free wall in coronary atherosclerosis: Its relation to degree of obstruction. JACC 6: 1096.

Schlegl A, Muzika N, Olbert F (1986) Non-invasive tests in ischemic disease of the lower limb before and after percutaneous transluminal angioplasty. Ann Radiol (Paris) 29: 130–132.

Scott RF, Imai H, Makita T, Thomas WA, Reiner JM (1980) Lining cell and intimal smooth muscle cell response and Evans blue staining in abdominal aorta of young swine after denudation by balloon catheter. Exp Mol Pathol 33: 185–202.

Sise MJ, Shackford SR, Rowley WR, Pistone FJ (1989) Claudication in young adults: a frequently delayed diagnosis. J Vasc Surg 10: 68–74.

Smith G, Train J, Mitty H, Jacobson J (1992) Hip pain caused by buttock claudication. Relief of symptoms by transluminal angioplasty. Clin Orthop (284): 176–180.

Smyth D (1991) Cardiology update. Restenosis after coronary angioplasty. Nurs Standard 5: 53–54.

Sprecher DL, Mikat EM, Stack R, Sutherland K, Schneider J, Bashore T, Hackel DB (1989) Histopathologic examination of material from angioplasty balloon catheters used in vivo in human coronary arteries. Atherosclerosis 75: 237–244.

Staiger J, Mathias K, Friederick H, Heiss HW, Konrad S, Spillner G (1980) Peripheral occlusive disease: influence of platelets aggregation inhibitor on the one year patency rate after catheter dilatation therapy (Dotter). Herz/Kreislaufforsch 12: 383–386.

Strauss AL, Roth FJ, Rieger H (1993) Noninvasive assessment of pressure gradients across iliac artery stenoses: duplex and catheter correlative study. J Ultrasound Med 12(1): 17–22.

Tennant M, McGeachie JK (1992) A biological basis for re-stenosis after percutaneous transluminal angioplasty: possible underlying mechanisms. Aust N Z J Surg 62(2): 135–141.

Valentine RJ, MacGillivray DC, DeNobile JW, Snyder DA, Rich NM (1990) Intermittent claudication caused by atherosclerosis in patients aged forty years and younger. Surgery 107: 560–565.

Vallance P (1989) EDRF and microvascular constriction after angioplasty [letter]. Lancet 1: 1139.

Vorwerk D, Zolotas G, Hessel S, Adam G, Wondrazek F, Gunther RW (1991) In vitro ablation of normal and diseased vascular tissue by a fiber-transmitted holmium laser. Invest Radiol 26: 660–664.

Waller BF (1985) Coronary luminal shape and the arc of disease-free wall: morphologic observations and clinical relevance (editorial comment). JACC 6: 1100.

Waller BF (1985) Morphologic observations in coronary arteries, aortocoronary saphenous vein bypass grafts and infant aortae following balloon angioplasty procedures. Herz 10: 255–268.

Waller BF (1986) Pathology of new interventions used in the treatment of coronary heart disease. Curr Probl Cardiol 11: 666–760.

Waller BF (1987) The pathology of transluminal balloon angioplasty used in the treatment of coronary heart disease. Hum Pathol 18: 476.

Waller BF (1988) Pathology of new interventional procedures in coronary disease. REVIEW ARTICLE: 110 REFS. Cardiovasc Clin 18: 63–122.

Waller BF (1989) "Crackers, breakers, stretchers, drillers, scrapers, shavers, burners, welders and melters"—the future treatment of atherosclerotic coronary artery disease? A clinical-morphologic assessment. REVIEW ARTICLE: 109 REFS. J Am Coll Cardiol 13: 969–987.

Waller BF, Dillon JC, Cowley MH (1983) Plaque hematoma and coronary dissection with percutaneous transluminal angioplasty (PTCA) of severely stenotic lesions: morphologic coronary observations in 5 men within 30 days of PTCA (Abstract). Circulation (Suppl III) 68: III-144.

Waller BF, Roberts WC (1981) Amount of luminal narrowing in bypassed and nonbypassed native coronary arteries in necropsy patients dying early or late after aortocoronary bypass operations. In: Mason DT, Collins JT Jr, (eds) Myocardial Revascularizaitons. Medical and Surgical Advances in Coronary Disease. New York, Yorke Medical, pp 503–513.

Waller BF, Rothbaum DA, Gorfinkel HJ, Ulbright TM, Linnemeier TJ, Berger SM (1984) Morphologic observations after percutaneous transluminal balloon angioplasty of early and late aortocoronary saphenous vein bypass grafts. JACC 4: 784–792.

Wholey MH (1988) Advances in balloon technology and reperfusion devices for peripheral circulation. REVIEW ARTICLE: 25 REFS. Am J Cardiol 61: 87G–95G.

Wilson SE, White GH, Wolf G, Cross AP (1990) Proximal percutaneous balloon angioplasty and distal bypass for multilevel arterial occlusion. Veterans Administration Cooperative Study No. 199. Ann Vasc Surg 4: 351–355.

Wolf GL, LeVeen RF, Ring EJ (1984) Potential mechanisms of angioplasty. Cardiovasc Interventional Radiol 7: 11–17.

Wolinsky H, Lin CS (1991) Use of the perforated balloon catheter to infuse marker substances into diseased coronary artery walls after experimental postmortem angioplasty. J Am Coll Cardiol 17: 174B–178B.

Woods BO (1991) Clinical evaluation of the peripheral vasculature. Cardiol Clin 9: 413–427.

Yamanashi WS, Patil AA, Hill DL, Lepage JR, Yassa NA, Valentine JL, Lester PD (1988) Precision surgery with an electromagnetically induced current convergence probe application in aneurysm treatment, angioplasty, and brain tumor resection in in vivo and in vitro models. Med Instrum 22: 205–216.

Yao JS, Flinn WR (1982) Initial hemodynamic changes after balloon dilatation in peripheral arterial occlusive disease. Vasa 11: 305–308.

Yoshida S, Yabe Y, Nakano H, Muramatsu T, Noike H (1991) Multivessel PTCA using the hugging balloon technique based on single guide catheter and dual balloon-on-a-wire systems. Cathet Cardiovasc Diagn 23: 37–41.

Zocholl G, Jungbluth A, Dux M, Shild H, Thelen M (1988) Does velocity of dilatation influence the result of dilatation? A postmortem study. Invest Radiol 23: 905–909.

Zollikofer CL, Cragg AH, Einzig S, et al (1983) Prostaglandins and angioplasty: an experimental study in canine arteries. Radiology 149: 681–685.

III. Reviews

A symposium: Interventional cardiology at a crossroad: diagnostics and therapeutics. (1988) March 26, 1988, Atlanta, Georgia. Am J Cardiol 62: 1K-29K.

A symposium: Interventional Cardiology: 1987. (1988) June 8–9, 1987, Sonoma, California. Proceedings. Am J Cardiol 61: 1G-117G.

Al-Kutoubi MA (1992) ABC of vascular diseases. Percutaneous transluminal angioplasty. BMJ 304(6818): 45–47.

Aaberg RA, Flaherty R, Smith RB (1991) Renal artery occlusive disease. Crit Care Nurs Clin North Am 3: 507–514.

Abbott WM (1980) Percutaneous transluminal angioplasty: surgeon's view. AJR 135: 917–920.

Ahn SS, Moore WS (1992) Endovascular surgery. Surg Annu 24: 107–142.

Ameli FM, Stein M, Provan JL, St. Louis EL, Legrand L (1989) Percutaneous transluminal angioplasty without anticoagulation. Ann Vasc Surg 3: 244–247.

Anderson JB, Wolinski AP, Wells IP, Wilkins DC, Bliss BP (1986) The impact of percutaneous transluminal angioplasty on the management of peripheral vascular disease. Br J Surg 73: 17–19.

Anonymous (1991) Cardiology and the quality of medical practice. The Cardiology Working Group [comments]. JAMA 265: 482–485.

Anonymous (1991) Second European Consensus Document on chronic critical leg ischemia. Circulation 84 (4 Suppl): IV1–26.

Anonymous (1992) Second European Consensus Document on chronic critical leg ischemia. Eur J Vasc Surg 6(Suppl A): 1–32.

Appenzeller T (1989) Balloon trial. Sci Am 260: 32, 35.

Athanasoulis CA (1980) Medical progress; therapeutic applications of angiography (second of two parts). N Engl J Med 302: 1174–1179.

Athanasoulis CA (1980) Percutaneous transluminal angioplasty: general principles. AJR 135: 893–900.

Athanasoulis CA (1980) Therapeutic applications of angiography. N Engl J Med 302:(Part 1) 1117–1125.

Banerjee A (1992) Boring arteries: television and tubes, a new peripheral vascular surgery? Br J Hosp Med 48(5): 242–244.

Barnathan ES, Hirshfeld JW Jr (1988) Adjunctive pharmacologic treatment. Cardiovasc Clin 19: 41–78.

Barnes RW (1989) Who took the "p" out of statistics? (editorial). J Vasc Surg 10: 100–102.

Barnes RW (1982) Indications for percutaneous transluminal angioplasty from the viewpoint of the surgeon. Vasa 11: 261–264.

Bartlett JE, Pfieffer RP (1981) Percutaneous transluminal angioplasty. Mo Med 78: 123–125.

Bass JL (1986) Percutaneous balloon dilation angioplasty of pulmonary artery branch stenosis. Cardiovasc Intervent Radiol 9: 299–302.

Becker GJ, Katzen BT (1988) Peripheral angioplasty and the newer circulatory interventions: whose responsibility? AJR 150: 1235–1239.

Becker GJ, Katzen BT, Dake MD (1989) Noncoronary angioplasty. Radiology 170: 921–940.

Becker GJ, Rowe DM, Holden RW, Dalsing MC, Bendick PJ (1986) Percutaneous transluminal angioplasty for vasculogenic impotence. Indiana Med 79: 256–262.

Becker RC (1991) Seminars in thrombosis, thrombolysis and vascular biology. 1. The vascular endothelium. Cardiology 78: 13–22.

Belli AM (1992) Arterial and venous stents: current developments (editorial). Br J Hosp Med 47(6): 407, 409.

Bergan JJ (1981) Introduction to the symposium on transluminal angioplasty. Arch Surg 116: 804–805.

Bergentz SE, Jonsson K (1983) Percutaneous transluminal angioplasty. A review. Acta Chir Scand 149: 641–649.

Bergentz SE, Jonsson K (1987) The role of percutaneous transluminal angioplasty in infrarenal redo surgery. REVIEW ARTICLE: 24 REFS. Acta Chir Scand 538: 144–147.

Black TJ (1979) Percutaneous transluminal angioplasty, a nonoperative treatment of occlusive vascular disease. J Maine Med Assoc 70: 318–332.

Block PC (1986) Transluminal angioplasty and atherosclerosis: does angioplasty accelerate or decelerate atherosclerosis? Prog Clin Biol Res 219: 51–58.

Bollinger A (1978) Appraisal of the therapy. In: Zeitler E et al. (eds) Percutaneous vascular recanalization. Berlin Heidelberg New York, Springer, chap 32, pp 194–195.

Bollinger A, Schneider E, Kuhlmann U, Pouliadis G, Brunner U (1982) Percutaneous transluminal angioplasty (PTA): state of the art and future perspectives. Vasa 11: 369–372.

Borio R, Chiocchini S, Lupattelli L, Barzi FM (1988) Personnel and patient doses during percutaneous transluminal angioplasty (PTA). Rays 13: 59–64.

Brewster DC (1991) Acute peripheral arterial occlusion. Cardiol Clin 9: 497–513.

Brown MM (1992) Balloon angioplasty for cerebrovascular disease. Neurol Res 14(2 Suppl): 159–163.

Burnett JR, Walsh JA, Howard PR, Phillips PJ, Fon GT, Dupont PA, Foreman RK, James MJ, Kneller PN (1987) Transluminal balloon angioplasty in diabetic peripheral vascular disease. Aust NZ J Surg 57: 307–309.

Butt KMH, Freidman EI, Kuntz SL (1976) Angioaccess. Curr Probl Surg 13: 1–67.

Cambria RP, Faust G, Gusberg R, Tilson MD, Zucker KA, Modlin IM (1987) Percutaneous angioplasty for peripheral arterial occlusive disease. Correlates of clinical success. Arch Surg 122: 283–287.

Campbell WB (1986) Angioplasty for intermittent claudication (editorial). Br Med J (Clin Res) 293: 1047–1048.

Campbell WB, Higgins JR, Barker CS, Von Eichstorff P, Fletcher EW (1988) Grading for angioplasty. Clin Radiol 39: 516–518.

Campbell WB, Jeans WD, Cole SE, Baird RN (1983) Percutaneous transluminal angioplasty for lower limb ischaemia. Br J Surg 70: 736–739.

Cantelmo NL, LoGerfo FW (1982) A technique of angioplasty of the profunda and superficial femoral arteries. Surg Gynecol Obstet 154: 564–565.

Casarella WJ (1986) Noncoronary angioplasty. Curr Probl Cardiol 11: 141–174.

Casarella WJ (1988) Percutaneous transluminal angioplasty below the knee: new techniques, excellent results (editorial). Radiology 169: 271–272.

Castaneda-Zuniga WR, Amplatz K, Laerum F, Formanek A, Sibley R, Edwards J, Vlodaver A (1981) Mechanics of angioplasty: an experimental approach. Radiographics 1: 1–14.

Castaneda-Zuniga WR, Formanek A, Lillehei RC, Tadavarthy M, Amplatz K (1981) Nonsurgical treatment of Takayasu's disease. Cardiovasc Intervent Radiol 4: 245–248.

Castaneda-Zuniga WR, Formanek A, Tadavarthy M, Vlodaver Z, Edwards JE, Zollikofer C, Amplatz K (1980) The mechanism of balloon angioplasty. Radiology 135: 565–571.

Castellanos A, Pereiras R (1980) Counter-current aortography. Rev Cubana Cardiol 2: 187.

Cheshire NJ, Wolfe JH (1992) ABC of vascular diseases. Critical leg ischaemia: amputation or reconstruction. BMJ 304(6822): 312–314.

Consigny PM (1986) Prevention of restenosis after transluminal angioplasty. Prog Clin Biol Res 219: 59–73.

Cooke RH, Kent KM (1989) Angioplasty, restenosis, and antiplatelet therapy. Transplant Proc 21: 3685.

Cope C (1986) Dilatation of mesocaval shunts. Ann Radiol (Paris) 29: 178–180.

Corsaro MC (1983) Balloon catheters: rising to the occasion. J Oper Room Res Inst 3: 42–45.

Couch NP (1980) Percutaneous transluminal angioplasty: Cardiovasc Intervent Radiol 3: 219–221.

Cox JL, Gotlieb AI (1986) Restenosis following percutaneous transluminal angioplasty: clinical, physiologic and pathological features. REVIEW ARTICLE: 39 REFS. Can Med Assoc J 134: 1129–1132.

Cox JL, Jacobs CP (1987) Laser-assisted angioplasty. Treating peripheral vascular disease. AORN J 46: 835–846.

Cragg AH, Einzig S, Rysavy A, Castaneda-Zuniga WR, Borgwardt B, Amplatz K (1983) The vasa vasorum and angioplasty. Radiology 148: 75–80.

Creasy TS, McMillan PJ, Fletcher EW, Collin J, Morris PJ (1990) Is percutaneous transluminal angioplasty better than exercise for claudication? Preliminary results from a prospective randomised trial. Eur J Vasc Surg 4: 135–140.

Crowley RJ, von Behren PL, Couvillon LA, Jr, Mai DE, Abele JE (1989) Optimized ultrasound imaging catheters for use in the vascular system. Int J Card Imaging 4: 145–151.

Cumberland DC (1982) Percutaneous transluminal angioplasty (letter). Br J Hosp Med 27: 94.

Cumberland DC (1983) Percutaneous transluminal angioplasty: a review. Clin Radiol 34: 25–38.

Cumberland DC (1988) Peripheral angioplasty: 10 years on (editorial). Clin Radiol 39: 573–574.

Curry R, Johnston L (1982) Percutaneous transluminal angioplasty. Ulster Med J 51: 59–66.

Dacie JE (1981) Percutaneous transluminal angioplasty. Br J Hosp Med 26: 314, 320–324, 326.

Dake MD (1990) Peripheral angiography, angioplasty, atherectomy, laser techniques, thrombolysis, and stents, Curr Opin Radiol 2: 239–249.

Dalman RL, Taylor LM Jr, Porter JM (1990) Will interventional angiology replace vascular surgery? Acta Chir Scand 555: 25–35.

Dash H (1987) Have balloon, will travel: expanded indications for nonoperative intravascular balloon dilation? (editorial). J Am Coll Cardiol 9: 387–388.

Denck H, Hold M, Russe O, Kobinia G (1978) Indications for PTR from the surgical point of view. In: Zeitler E et al. (eds) Percutaneous Vascular Recanalization. Berlin Heidelberg New York, Springer, chap 30, pp 183–188.

Dorne HL, Satin R, Palayew MJ (1986) Method for determining arterial entry site for catheter (letter). AJR 146: 175.

Dorros G (1984) The brachial artery method to peripheral transluminal angioplasty. Cathet Cardiovasc Diagn 10: 115–127.

Dorros G, Lewin RF, Jamnadas P, Mathiak LM (1990) Peripheral transluminal angioplasty of the subclavian and innominate arteries utilizing the brachial approach: acute outcome and follow-up. REVIEW ARTICLE: 17 REFS. Cathet Cardiovasc Diagn 19: 71–76.

Dotter CT (1980) Transluminal angioplasty: a long view. Radiology 135: 561–564.

Dotter CT (1982) Two decades of transluminal angioplasty. An overview. J Mal Vasc 7 (Suppl 4): 357–361.

Dotter CT (1983) Transluminal angioplasty. In: Abrams HL (ed) Angiography, 3rd ed. Boston, Little Brown.

Dotter CT (1983) Transluminal angioplasty, method, indications and role in therapy. Proceedings of vascular surgery course, June 1982, Minneapolis. In: Delaney JP (ed) Advances in vascular surgery. Chicago, Yearbook Med Publishers, pp 143–149.

Dotter CT, Judkins MP (1989) Transluminal treatment of arteriosclerotic obstruction. Description of a new technic and a preliminary report of its application. Radiology 172: 904–920.

Dotter CT, Judkins MP, Frische LH, Rosch J (1967) Nonoperative treatment of arterial occlusive disease: a radiologically facilitated technique. Radiol Clin North Am 5: 531–542.

Dotter CT, Judkins MP, Rosch J (1969) Transluminal angioplasty in arteriosclerotic obstruction of the lower extremities. Med Times 97: 95–108.

Dotter CT, Rosch J (1971) Transluminal angioplasty: the catheter treatment of peripheral arterial obstruction. In: Dale WA (ed) Management of Arterial Occlusive Disease. Chicago, Yearbook Publishing Company, Chicago, pp 257–267.

Dotter CT, Rosch J, Judkins MP (1968) Transluminal dilatation of atherosclerotic stenosis. Surg Gynecol Obstet 127: 794–804.

Doubilet P, Abrams HL (1984) The cost of underutilization. Percutaneous transluminal angioplasty for peripheral vascular disease. N Engl J Med 310: 95–102.

Doyle DL (1990) Update on laser angioplasty. Can Med Assoc J 142: 1391.

Dunnick NR, Sfakianakis GN (1991) Screening for renovascular hypertension. Radiol Clin North Am 29: 497–510.

Ebner H, Wex P, Dragojevic D (1989) The mechanism of angioplasty—endoscopic and morphometric investigations in an experimental model. Eur J Vasc Surg 3: 543–547.

Erbel R, Bednarczyk I, Pop T, Todt M, Henrichs KJ, Brunier A, Thelen M, Meyer J (1990) Detection of dissection of the aortic intima and media after angioplasty of coarctation of the aorta. An angiographic, computer tomographic, and echocardiographic comparative study. Circulation 81: 805–814.

Faulkner K, Love HG, Sweeney JK, Bardsley RA (1986) Radiation doses and somatic risk to patients during cardiac radiological procedures. Br J Radiol 59: 359–363.

Faxon DP (1989) Probing the frontiers of angioplasty (editorial). Mayo Clin Proc 64: 360–362.

Faxon DP, Sanborn TA, Haudenschild CC (1987) Mechanism of angioplasty and its relations to restenosis. REVIEW ARTICLE: 26 REFS. Am J Cardiol 60: 5B-9B.

Fellmeth BD, Bookstein JJ, Lurie AL, Dillard JP (1990) Rapid progression of peripheral vascular disease after diagnostic angiography [see comments]. Comment in: Radiology 175: 33. Radiology 175: 71–74.

Ferns GA, Stewart-Lee AL, Anggard EE (1992) Arterial response to mechanical injury: balloon catheter de-endothelialization. Atherosclerosis 92(2–3): 89–104.

Fischell TA, Stadius ML (1991) New technologies for the treatment of obstructive arterial disease. Cathet Cardiovasc Diagn 22: 205–233.

Fletcher JP, Kershaw LZ (1988) Outcome in patients with failed percutaneous transluminal angioplasty for peripheral vascular disease. J Cardiovasc Surg (Torino) 29: 733–735.

Fletcher JP, Little JM, Fermanis GG, Simmons K (1986) Percutaneous transluminal angioplasty for severe lower extremity ischaemia. Aust NZ J Surg 56: 121–125.

Fletcher JP, Little JM, Kershaw LZ (1987) The changing pattern of vascular surgery: the effect of percutaneous transluminal angioplasty. Aust NZ J Surg 57: 221–224.

Forrester JS, Fishbein M, Helfant R, Fagin J (1991) A paradigm for restenosis based on cell biology: clues for the development of new preventive therapies. J Am Coll Cardiol 17: 758–769.

Fowkes FG, Housley E, Cawood EH, Macintyre CC, Ruckley CV, Prescott RJ (1991) Edinburgh Artery Study: prevalence of asymptomatic and symptomatic peripheral arterial disease in the general population. Int J Epidemiol 20: 384–392.

Freeney P (1971) Transluminal angioplasty. Bull Mason Clin 31: 9–15.

Freiman DB, McLean GK, Oleaga JA, Ring EJ (1981) Percutaneous transluminal angioplasty. In: Ring EJ, McLean GK (eds) Interventional Radiology: Principles and Techniques, 2. Boston, Little Brown, pp 117–243.

Friedman SG (1989) Charles Dotter: interventional radiologist. Radiology 172: 921–924.

Gallino A, Mahler F, Probst P (1983) Progression to total occlusion of lower limb artery stenoses selected for percutaneous transluminal angioplasty (letter). Lancet 1: 59–60.

Gallino A, Mahler F, Probst P, Nachbur B (1984) Percutaneous transluminal angioplasty of the arteries of the lower limbs: a 5 year follow-up. Circulation 70: 619–623.

Gaskin TA; Isobe JH, Ballard JW (1983) Transluminal angioplasty in a community hospital: a surgeon's viewpoint. South Med J 76: 1116–1117.

Gaylord GM, Pritchard WF, Chuang VP, Casarella WJ, Sprawls P (1988) The geometry of triple-balloon dilation. Radiology 166: 541–545.

Goldberg S, Savage M, Zalewski A (1988) Developmental background, technique, and future challenges. Cardiovasc Clin 19: 3–40.

Goldsmith MF (1992) Cerebral percutaneous transluminal angioplasty in second year of trials [news]. J Am Med Assoc 268(21): 3039–3040.

Goldsmith MF (1991) Antistenosis approaches revisited, or rating the artery openers anew [news]. JAMA 266: 3397–3398.

Goodkind J, Coombs V, Golobic RA (1993) Excimer laser angioplasty. Heart Lung 22(1): 26–35.

Gordon RL, Horev G, Shifrin EG, Beer G, Katz S (1980) Early experience with balloon catheter angioplasty. Isr J Med S 16: 686–691.

Graor RA, Gray BH (1992) Nonsurgical restoration of pulsatile arterial flow. Cardiovasc Clin 22(3): 217–229.

Greenfield AJ (1988) Angioplasty for peripheral vascular disease. Hosp Pract 23: 13, 16, 18.

Gruentzig A (1981) Percutaneous transluminal angioplasty (Editorial). AJR 136: 216–217.

Gruentzig A, Zeitler E (1978) Cooperative study of results of PTR in twelve different clinics. In: Zeitler E et al. (eds) Percutaneous vascular recanalization. Springer, Berlin Heidelberg New York, chapt 17, pp 118–119.

Guidoin R, Couture J, Assayed F, Gosselin C (1988) New frontiers of vascular grafting. REVIEW ARTICLE: 117 REFS. Int Surg 73: 241–249.

Hagen P, Wang Z, Mikat EM, Hacket DB (1981) Antiplatelet therapy reduces aortic intimal hyperplasia distal to small diameter vascular prostheses (PTFE) in non-human primates. Ann Surg 195: 328–339.

Halfman Francy M, Coburn C (1990) Techniques in cardiac care: lasers, stents, and atherectomy devices. REVIEW ARTICLE: 128 REFS. AACN Clin Issues Crit Care Nurs 1: 87–109.

Hall LT (1990) Endovascular surgery: an overview. REVIEW ARTICLE: 25 REFS. Prog Cardiovasc Nurs 5: 43–49.

Hare WS, Thomson KR, Field PL, Robertson DB (1981) Balloon dilatation in the treatment of early intermittent claudication. Med J Aust 2: 331–333.

Harker LA (1987) Role of platelets and thrombosis in mechanisms of acute occlusion and restenosis after angioplasty. REVIEW ARTICLE: 118 REFS. Am J Cardiol 60: 20B-28B.

Harries J (1982) Interventional radiology—a new subspecialty. S Afr Med J 61: 585–586.

Harrison JK, Sheikh KH, Davidson CJ, Kisslo KB, Leithe ME, Himmelstein SI, Kanter RJ, Bashore TM (1990) Balloon angioplasty of coarctation of the aorta evaluated with intravascular ultrasound imaging. J Am Coll Cardiol 15: 906–909.

Hartnell GG (1991) Conventional angioplasty versus percutaneous transluminal laser angioplasty (letter). Circulation 84: 2204–2205.

Haudenschild CC (1989) Pathogenesis of restenosis. REVIEW ARTICLE: 28 REFS. Z Kardiol 78(Suppl3): 28–34.

Hertzer NR (1991) The natural history of peripheral vascular disease. Implications for its management. Circulation 83: I12–19.

Hibberd AD (1983) Percutaneous transluminal angioplasty: a vascular surgeon's viewpoint. Australas Radiol 27: 303–304.

Hirschl M, Urbanek A, Tischler R (1991) Outpatient percutaneous transluminal angioplasty: preconditions and results. Wien Klin Wochenschr 103(22): 673–677.

Holmes DR Jr, Bresnahan JF (1991) Interventional cardiology. Cardiol Clin 9: 115–134.

Holmes DR Jr, Vlietstra RE, Reiter SJ, Bresnahan DR (1990) Advances in interventional cardiology. REVIEW ARTICLE: 79 REFS. Mayo Clin Proc 65: 565–583.

Hornstra G (1989) Influence of dietary fish oil on arterial thrombosis and atherosclerosis in animal models and in man. REVIEW ARTICLE: 59 REFS. J Intern Med 225(Suppl): 53–59.

Hruby W (1989) Interventional uroradiology. Curr Opin Radiol 1: 290–292.

Hudon G, Goulet C (1981) Angioplastie transluminale percutanee: Principles et revue de la Litterature. Union Med Can 111: 3–10.

Ida M, Arai K, Yoshikawa J, Takayama S, Miyamori H, Toya T, Yanagi S, Miura S, Fujisawa M, Matsui O (1986) Therapeutic hepatic vein angioplasty for Budd-Chiari syndrome. Cardiovasc Intervent Radiol 9: 187–190.

Ike BW (1983) Intervention radiology in a small center hospital. Diagn Imaging 52: 104–112.

Isner JM, Salem DN (1984) The persistent enigma of percutaneous angioplasty. Int J Cardiol 6: 391–400.

Jacobson HG (1981) Diagnostic radiology; Interventional radiology. JAMA 245: 2220.

Jacobson HG (1982) Radiology: Interventional radiology. JAMA 247: 2220–2221.

Jamieson C (1988) The management of intermittent claudication. Practitioner 232: 613–616.

Jeans WD, Danton RM, Baird RN, Horrocks M (1986) A comparison of the costs of vascular surgery and balloon dilatation in lower limb ischaemic disease. Br J Radiol 59: 453–456.

Jeans WD, Danton RM, Baird RN, Horrocks M (1986) The effects of introducing balloon dilatation into vascular surgical practice. Br J Radiol 59: 457–459.

Johnson DE, Braden L, Simpson JB (1990) Mechanism of directed transluminal atherectomy. Am J Cardiol 65: 389–391.

Johnston KW, Colapinto RF; Baird RJ (1982) Transluminal dilation. An alternative? Arch Surg 117: 1604–1610.

Jones BA, Maggisano R, Robb C, Saibil EA, Witchell SJ, Harrison AW (1985) Transluminal angioplasty: results in high-risk patients with advanced peripheral vascular disease. Can J Surg 28: 150–152.

Joyce E (1981) Transluminal angioplasty: pro/con. Miami Med 51: 9–11.

Kadir S, Smith GW, White RI Jr, Kaufman SL, Barth KH, Williams GM, O'Mara CS; Burdick JF (1982) Percutaneous transluminal angioplasty as an adjunct to the surgical management of peripheral vascular disease. Ann Surg 195: 786–795.

Kantoch M, Ruzyo W, Dabrowski M (1988) Transluminal dilation techniques in the management of congenital obstructive cardiovascular disease. Mater Med Pol 20: 103–113.

Katzen BT (1980) Intervention diagnostic and therapeutic procedures. Berlin Heidelberg New York, Springer.

Kaufman SL (1987) Intrathoracic interventional vascular techniques in congenital cardiovascular disease. REVIEW ARTICLE: 52 REFS. J Thorac Imaging 2: 1–10.

Khayata M, Aymard A, Guichard JP, Merland JJ (1992) Interventional neuroradiology. Curr Opin Radiol 4(1): 71–78.

King SB 3d (1991) Role of new technology in balloon angioplasty. Circulation 84: 2574–2579.

Kinney TB, Chin AK, Rurik GW, Finn JC, Shoor PM, Hayden WG, Fogarty

TJ (1984) The physical mechanisms of transluminal angioplasty: a mechanical pathophysiological correlation. Radiology 153: 85–89.

Kinnison ML, Steinberg EP, Powe NR, Anderson GF (1988) Reducing the cost of using contrast media: a look at discarded volumes. Radiology 166: 367–370.

Kinnison ML, White RI Jr, Bowers WP, Dunlap ED (1985) Cost incentives for peripheral angioplasty. AJR 145: 1241–1244.

Korogi Y, Takahashi M, Bussaka H, Hatanaka Y (1992) Percutaneous transluminal angioplasty: pain during balloon inflation. Br J Radiol 65(770): 140–142.

Kramer PH, Vacek JL (1990) Peripheral vascular disease. Treatment with balloon angioplasty. Postgrad Med 87: 77–80, 83–86, 89–90.

Krone R (1981) Morphology after transluminal angioplasty (letter). N Engl J Med 305: 1652.

Kumpe DA, Jones DN (1982) Percutaneous transluminal angioplasty: radiologic viewpoint. Appl Radiol 11: 29–40.

Kumpe DA, Zwerdlinger S, Griffin DJ (1988) Blue digit syndrome: treatment with percutaneous transluminal angioplasty. Radiology 166: 37–44.

Laifer LI, O'Brien KM, Stetz ML, Gindi GR, Garrand TJ, Deckelbaum LI (1989) Biochemical basis for the difference between normal and atherosclerotic arterial fluorescence. Circulation 80: 1893–1901.

Lally ME, Johnston KW, Andrews D (1984) Percutaneous transluminal dilatation of peripheral arteries: an analysis of factors predicting early success. J Vasc Surg 1: 704–709.

Lamerton A (1986) Percutaneous transluminal angioplasty. Br J Surg 73: 91–97.

Lau CS, Scott N, Shaw JW, Belch JJ (1991) Increased activity of oxygen free radicals during reperfusion in patients with peripheral arterial disease undergoing percutaneous peripheral artery balloon angioplasty. Int Angiol 10(4): 244–246.

Lavanier GL, Sacks D, Robinson ML (1992) Acute limb ischemia. Emerg Med Clin North Am 10(1): 103–119.

Leaf A (1988) Effects of n-3 fatty acids on reocclusion after angioplasty. REVIEW ARTICLE: 23 REFS. Semin Thromb Hemost 14: 290–292.

Lee C, Stein S (1980) Percutaneous transluminal angioplasty: interventional radiology. Conn Med 44: 214–215.

Lee WM, Lee RT (1975) Advanced coronary atherosclerosis in swine produced by combination of balloon catheter injury and cholesterol feeding. Exp Mol Pathol 23: 491.

Legge D (1984) Percutaneous transluminal angioplasty in peripheral vascular disease. Ir Med J 77: 85–87.

Lemarbre L, Hudon G, Coche G, Bourassa MG (1987) Outpatient peripheral angioplasty: survey of complications and patients' perceptions. AJR 148: 1239–1242.

LePage JR, Lewis JE, Ruiz OF, Yamanashi WS, Padron GM Hood CH (1987) Angiopyroplasty using electromagnetically induced focused heat. Angiology 38: 520–523.

Levin DC, Harrington DP, Bettmann MA, Garnic JD, Torman H, Murray P, Boxt LM, Geller SC (1984) Equipment choices, technical aspects and pitfalls of percutaneous transluminal angioplasty. Cardiovasc Intervent Radiol 7: 1–10.

Levin DC, Matteucci T (1990) "Turf battles" over imaging and interventional procedures in community hospitals: survey results (comments). Radiology 176: 321–324.

Lewis JE (1989) Percutaneous transluminal angioplasty. Adjunctive treatment of ischemic ulcers. Int J Dermatol 28: 134–135.

Lewis VD, 3d, Meranze SG, McLean GK, O'Neill JA, Jr, Berkowitz IID, Burke DR (1988) The midaortic syndrome: diagnosis and treatment [see comments]. Comment in: Radiology 1989 Feb;170(2): 571–572. Radiology 167: 111–113.

Liang GC, Nemickas R, Madayag M (1989) Multiple percutaneous transluminal angioplasties and low dose pulse methotrexate for Takayasu's arteritis. J Rheumatol 16: 1370–1373.

Lipchik EO (1989) Arterial occlusive disease below the knee (letter). Radiology 171: 283.

Lu C, Zarins CK, Yang C, Sottiurai V (1982) Approach to transluminal angioplasty in patients with groin scarring or vascular grafts. Radiology 143: 395–398.

Mansell PI, Gregson R, Allison SP (1992) An audit of lower limb arteriography in diabetic patients. Diabetic Med 9(1): 84–90.

Martin EC, Diamond NG, Casarella WJ (1980) Percutaneous transluminal angioplasty in non-atherosclerotic disease. Radiology 135: 27–33.

Martin LG, Cork RD, Kaufman SL (1992) Long-term results of angioplasty in 110 patients with renal artery stenosis. J Vasc Intervent Radiol 3(4): 619–626.

Martin LG, Henderson JM, Millikan WJ, Jr, Casarella WJ, Kaufman SL (1990) Angioplasty for long-term treatment of patients with Budd-Chiari syndrome. AJR Am J Roentgenol 154: 1007–1010.

McAllister MD, Thompson WC 3d, Pabian CJ (1992) Percutaneous angioplasty for renovascular hypertension due to fibromuscular dysplasia. Am Fam Physician 46(4): 1225–1230.

McLean L, Jeans WD, Horrocks M, Baird RN (1987) The place of percutaneous transluminal angioplasty in the treatment of patients having angiography for ischaemic disease of the lower limb. Clin Radiol 38: 157–160.

McMillan PJ, Collin J, Fletcher EW (1988) Intraoperative transluminal balloon dilatation permits simpler safer reconstructive surgery. Clin Radiol 39: 91–93.

Menges HW, Jaschke W, Trede M (1988) Percutaneous transluminal angioplasty: the surgeon's role. World J Surg 12: 788–797.

Messmer BJ (1987) Personal view: balloon, where do you fly? Eur Heart J 8: 1170–1171.

Millward S. Jaward A, Gooding J, Wyant D (1987) Outpatient peripheral angioplasty (letter). AJR 149: 1292–1293.

Mitchell SE, Kan JS, White RI Jr (1985) Interventional techniques in congenital heart disease. Semin Roentgenol 20: 290–311.

Morettin LB, Schreiber MH (1980) Interventional radiology: an alternative to surgery. Tex Med 76: 4344.

Motarjeme A, Keifer JW, Zuska AJ (1980) Percutaneous transluminal angioplasty and case selection. Radiology 135: 573–581.

Mortarjeme A, Keifer JW, Zuska AJ (1981) Percutaneous transluminal angioplasty as a complement to surgery. Radiology 141: 341–346.

Murie JA (1988) Percutaneous transluminal angioplasty and vascular surgery for lower limb ischaemia (editorial). Br J Surg 75: 1051–1052.

Neiman HL, Brandt TD, Greenberg M (1981) Percutaneous transluminal angioplasty: an angiographer's viewpoint. Arch Surg 116: 821–828.

Novelline RA (1980) Percutaneous transluminal angioplasty: newer applications. AJR 135: 983–988.

O'Byrne P, Blakeney C, Ham R, Murfitt J (1988) Transluminal balloon dilatation (letter). Clin Radiol 39: 464–465.

O'Keeffe ST, Persson AV (1991) Use of noninvasive vascular laboratory in diagnosis of venous and arterial disease. Cardiol 9: 429–442.

O'Keeffe ST, Woods BO, Beckmann CD (1991) Percutaneous transluminal angioplasty of the peripheral arteries. Cardiol Clin 9: 515–522.

O'Neill DM (1984) Percutaneous transluminal angioplasty: development, technique, and application. Radiol Technol 55: 10–17.

O'Neill WW (1992) Mechanical rotational atherectomy. Am J Cardiol 69(15): 12F–18F.

Paskin LS (1982) Percutaneous transluminal angioplasty in peripheral vascular disease. Radiography 48: 129–133.

Peeters FLM (1979) A non-surgical method for the treatment of intermittent claudication: so-called catheter angioplasty. Radiol Clin 41: 350–359.

Perry SB, Keane JF, Lock JE (1988) Interventional catheterization in pediatric congenital and acquired heart disease. REVIEW ARTICLE: 81 REFS. Am J Cardiol 61: 109G-117G.

Peterkin GA, Belkin M, Cantelmo NK, Guben J, Greenfield AJ, Johnson WC, Menzoian JO (1990) Combined transluminal angioplasty and infra-inguinal reconstruction in multilevel atherosclerotic disease. Am J Surg 160: 277–279.

Pfeiffer RB, String ST (1986) Adjunctive use of the balloon dilatation catheter during vascular reconstructive procedures. J Vasc Surg 3: 841–845.

Plouin PF, Darne B, Chatellier G, Pannier I, Battaglia C, Raynaud A, Azizi M (1993) Restenosis after a first percutaneous transluminal renal angioplasty. Hypertension 21(1): 89–96.

Priest EM (1988) Nonsurgical management of peripheral vascular disease: state of the art. J Tenn Med Assoc 81: 731–735.

Puijlaert CBAJ (1980) Historical introduction. In: Veiga-Pires JA, da Silva H, Oliva L (eds) Intervention Radiology. Proceedings of 1st International Symposium on Interventional Radiology. Algarve, Portugal, May 29-June 2, 1979. Excerpta Medica, Amsterdam, pp 25–28.

Rao PS (1989) Balloon angioplasty and valvuloplasty in infants, children, and adolescents. REVIEW ARTICLE: 225 REFS. Curr Probl Cardiol 14: 417–497.

Rees M, Gehani AA, Richens D (1988) Percutaneous dynamic removal of atheroma (letter). Lancet 1: 174.

Reidy JF (1987) Angioplasty in peripheral vascular disease. REVIEW ARTICLE: 14 REFS. Postgrad Med J 63: 435–438.

Reilly DT, Packer SG, Morrison N, Van Rij AM (1988) Percutaneous transluminal angioplasty for the ischaemic lower limb: the early Dunedin experience. N Z Med J 101: 129–132.

Rich S (1980) Percutaneous transluminal angioplasty nonsurgical therapy of occlusive arterial disease. Postgrad Med 68: 217–224.

Ring EJ, Ehrenfeld WK (1988) Percutaneous transluminal angioplasty (letter). J Vasc Surg 8: 92.

Ring EJ, McLean GK (1980) Interventional Radiology: Principles and Techniques. Boston, Little Brown.

Ring EJ, McLean GK, Freiman DB (1982) Selected techniques in percutaneous transluminal angioplasty. AJR 139: 767–773.

Roberts B (1982) Balloon angioplasty in the treatment of peripheral vascular disease. J Cardiovasc Surg (Torino) 23: 225–228.

Roberts B, McLean GK (1986) Role of percutaneous angioplasty in the treatment of peripheral arterial disease. Adv Surg 19: 329–354.

Roberts B, Ring EJ (1982) Current status of percutaneous transluminal angioplasty. Surg Clin North Am 62: 357–372.

Rocchini AP, Kveselis D (1984) The use of balloon angioplasty in the pediatric patient. Pediatr Clin North Am 31: 1293–1305.

Rogers PN, Vallance R (1983) Marathon run after Gruntzig dilatation (letter). Lancet 1: 417.

Rooke TW, Stanson AW, Johnson CM, Sheedy PF 2nd, Miller WE, Hollier LH, Osmundson PJ (1987) Percutaneous transluminal angioplasty in the lower extremities: a 5-year experience. Mayo Clin Proc 62: 85–91.

Rothman A, Perry SB, Keane JF, Lock JE (1990) Early results and follow-up of balloon angioplasty for branch pulmonary artery stenoses. J Am Coll Cardiol 15: 1109–1117.

Rubinstein ZJ, Morag B, Itzchak A (1980) Interventional therapeutic procedures in radiology. Isr J Med Sci 16: 831–842.

Rush DS, Gewertz BL, Lu CT, Ball DG, Zarins CK (1983) Limb salvage in poor-risk patients using transluminal angioplasty. Arch Surg 118: 1209–1212.

Saddekni S, Sniderman KW, Hilton S, Sos TA (1980) Percutaneous transluminal angioplasty of nonatherosclerotic lesions. AJR 135: 975–982.

Saffitz JE, Totty WG, McClennan BL, Gilula LA (1981) Percutaneous transluminal angioplasty. Radiological-pathological correlation. Radiology 141: 651–654.

Salles-Cunha SX, Andros G, Dulawa LB, Harris RW, Oblath RW (1989) Changes in peripheral hemodynamics after percutaneous transluminal angioplasty. J Vasc Surg 10: 338–342.

Sanborn TA (1989) Recanalization of arterial occlusions: pathologic basis and contributing factors. J Am Coll Cardiol 13: 1558–1560.

Schlegl A, Muzika N, Olbert F (1986) Non-invasive tests in ischemic disease of the lower limb before and after percutaneous transluminal angioplasty. Ann Radiol (Paris) 29: 130–132.

Schoop W (1978) Indications for PTR from the angiologic point of view. In: Zeitler E et al. (eds) Percutaneous Vascular Recanalization. Berlin Heidelberg New York, Springer, chap 29, pp 175–182.

Schwarten DE (1986) Extracardiac uses for the "steerable" coronary balloon angioplasty systems. Ann Radiol (Paris) 29: 120–126

Scobie TK (1986) Transluminal angioplasty: indications and overview. Can J Surg 29: 90–92.

Scobie TK (1987) Current status of transluminal angioplasty. Can J Surg 30: 175–178.

Seeger JM, Abela GS, Silverman SH, Jablonski SK (1989) Initial results of laser recanalization in lower extremity arterial reconstruction. J Vasc Surg 9: 10–17.

Sigwart U (1989) Transluminal angioplasty in arterial disease: new developments. Helv Chir Acta 55: 783–790.

Simmons K (1984) Investigators widen inquiry into percutaneous angioplasty application (news). JAMA 251: 301–302.

Sise MJ, Shackford SR, Rowley WR, Pistone FJ (1989) Claudication in young adults: a frequently delayed diagnosis. J Vasc Surg 10: 68–74.

Smith SM, Galland RB (1992) Late presentation of femoral artery complications following percutaneous cannulation for cardiac angiography or angioplasty. J Cardiovasc Surg 33(4): 437–439.

Society of Cardiovascular and Interventional Radiology: credentials criteria for peripheral, renal, and visceral percutaneous transluminal angioplasty. (1988) Radiology 167: 452.

Sos TA, Sniderman KW (1981) Percutaneous transluminal angioplasty. Semin Roentgenol 16: 26–41.

Spiegel RM (1981) Percutaneous transluminal angioplasty. A comprehensive overview. Ariz Med 38: 680–686.

Spittell JA Jr (1981) Recognition and management of chronic atherosclerotic occlusive peripheral arterial disease. Mod Concepts Cardiovasc Dis 50: 19–23.

St. Louis EL, Provan JL, Gray RR, Grosman H, Ameli FM, Elliott DS (1982) Percutaneous transluminal angioplasty in peripheral vascular disease: a review. Can Fam Physician 28: 291–294.

Stanson AW (1983) A perspective of percutaneous transluminal angioplasty. Cardiovasc Clin 13: 245–259.

Stevens RK, Hyde GL, Loh FK (1982) Transluminal angioplasty (TLA) in occlusive vascular disease. J Ky Med Assoc 80: 278–282.

Stokes KR, Strunk HM, Campbell DR, Gibbons GW, Wheeler HG, Clouse ME (1990) Five-year results of iliac and femoropopliteal angioplasty in diabetic patients. Radiology 174: 977–982.

Stoney RJ, Wylie EJ (1966) Recognition and surgical management of visceral ischemic syndromes. Ann Surg 164: 714–721.

Sugrue ME, Lee M, Hederman WP, Legge D (1988) Percutaneous transluminal angioplasty in the treatment of lower limb ischaemia. Ir J Med Sci 157: 104–106.

Tegtmeyer C (1984) Peripheral and coronary angioplasty. Proc Annu Meet Med Sect Am Counc Life Insur: 23–31.

Tegtmeyer CJ (1987) Percutaneous transluminal angioplasty. Curr Probl Diagn Radiol 16: 75–139.

The SH, Wilson RA, Gussenhoven EJ, Pieterman H, Bom K, Roelandt JR, Van Urk H (1992) Extrinsic compression of the superficial femoral artery at the adductor canal: evaluation with intravascular sonography. AJR 159(1): 117–120.

The Second Meeting of the Cardiovascular and Interventional Radiological

Society of Europe (CIRSE) Porto Cervo, Sardinia, May 25–29, 1987. (1988) Proceedings. Ann Radiol (Paris) 31: 69–126.

Thomson KR (1987) Lower-limb angioplasty. Med J Aust 147: 342–344.

Thorvinger B, Norgren L, Albrechtsson U (1992) Patency after iliac and femoro-popliteal angioplasty. Difference between angiographic and clinical results. Acta Radiol 33(1): 29–30.

Tisnado J, Bezirdjian D, Cho SR (1987) An alternative method to identify location of catheter entrance (letter). AJR 148: 231.

Tisnado J, Cho SR, Beachley MC (1988) Percutaneous transluminal angioplasty following endarterectomy. REVIEW ARTICLE: 177 REFS. CRC Crit Rev Diagn Imaging 28: 213–293.

Tortolani EC, Tan AH, Butchart S (1984) Percutaneous transluminal angioplasty. An ineffective approach to the failing vascular access. Arch Surg 119: 221–223.

Train JS, Dan SJ, Mitty HA, Dikman SH, Harrington EB, Miller CM, Jacobson JH, 2d (1988) Occlusion during iliac angioplasty: a salvageable complication. Radiology 168: 131–135.

Turcotte JK, Lu CT, Zarins CK (1981) The role of transluminal angioplasty in limb salvage and claudication. J Surg Res 30: 428–434.

Turnbull IW, Bannister CM (1992) Can laser angioplasty replace carotid endarterectomy in the management of nonstenotic atheromatous disease of the carotid bifurcation? Surg Neurol 38(1): 73–76.

Valentine RJ, MacGillivray DC, DeNobile JW, Snyder DA, Rich NM (1990) Intermittent claudication caused by atherosclerosis in patients aged forty years and younger. Surgery 107: 560–565.

Valji K, Bookstein JJ (1988) Transluminal angioplasty in the treatment of arteriogenic impotence. Cardiovasc Intervent Radiol 11: 245–252.

Valji K, Bookstein JJ, Roberts AC, Davis GB (1991) Pharmacomechanical thrombolysis and angioplasty in the management of clotted hemodialysis grafts: early and late clinical results. Radiology 178: 243–247.

Vallance P (1989) EDRF and microvascular constriction after angioplasty [letter]. Lancet 1: 1139.

Van Andel GJ (1975) Transluminal angioplasty according to Dotter-Judkins. Radiol Clin 44: 228.

Van Andel GJ (1976) Percutaneous Transluminal Angioplasty. The Dotter Procedure: A Manual for the Radiologist. Amsterdam, Excerpta Medica.

Van Andel GJ (1976) Percutaneous Transluminal Angioplasty. The Dotter Procedure. New York, American Elsevier Publishing Company.

Van Andel GJ (1978) Review of the results of the Dotter procedure. In: Zeitler E et al. (eds) Percutaneous Vascular Recanalization. Berlin Heidelberg New York, Springer, chap 14, pp 91–95.

Veith FJ, Gupta SK, Wengerter KR, Rivers SP, Bakal CW (1991) Impact of nonoperative therapy on the clinical management of peripheral arterial disease. Circulation 83: I137–142.

Verstraete M, Vermylen J, Verhaeghe RH (1981) Peripheral arterial diseases. Clin Haematol 10: 669–689.

Vlietstra RE (1988) Angioplasty: long-term experience of the Mayo Clinic. Trans Assoc Life Insur Med Dir Am 71: 36–43.

Vujic I, Bradham GB, Gobien RP (1983) Percutaneous transluminal angioplasty (PTA) for treatment of claudication. J SC Med Assoc 79: 377–380.

Wakao F, Takayasu K, Muramatsu Y, Nawano S, Moriyama N (1990) MR evaluation of Budd-Chiari syndrome treated by percutaneous transluminal angioplasty [letter]. AJR Am J Roentgenol 154: 1350–1351.

Walker A, Plant G, Rees M (1990) New hope for claudicants. Practitioner 234: 328.

Wall CA, Murray RE, Myler RK (1980) Transluminal angioplasty: Adjunct or gimmick? Am J Surg 140: 228–230.

Wallace S (1976) Interventional Radiology. Cancer 37: 517–531.

Waller BF (1989) "Crackers, breakers, stretchers, drillers, scrapers, shavers, burners, welders and melters": the future treatment of atherosclerotic coronary artery disease? A clinical-morphologic assessment. JACC 13: 969–987.

Waters D, Cote G (1991) Angioplasty of bypass grafts and native arteries. Cardiovasc Clin 21: 241–256.

Weaver P (1987) Percutaneous transluminal angioplasty in the treatment of patients having angiography for ischaemic disease of the lower limb (letter). Clin Radiol 38: 659–660.

Welsh CL, Cumberland DC (1986) The role of percutaneous transluminal angioplasty for atherosclerotic disease of the lower extremities (letter). Ann R Coll Surg Engl 68: 54–55.

Wexler L (1989) Percutaneous transluminal angioplasty of peripheral vascular occlusions: a clinical perspective (editorial). J Am Coll Cardiol 13: 1555–1557.

White CJ, Ramee SR (1992) Options for percutaneous coronary and peripheral revascularization. Med Clin North Am 76(5): 1099–1124.

White GH (1988) Angioscopy and lasers in cardiovascular surgery: current applications and future prospects. REVIEW ARTICLE: 52 REFS. Aust N Z J Surg 58: 271–274.

White NW Jr, Yock PG (1989) Intravascular ultrasound: catheter-based Doppler and two-dimensional imaging. Cardiol Clin 7: 525–536.

White RA, White GH (1989) Laser thermal probe recanalization of occluded arteries. REVIEW ARTICLE: 31 REFS. J Vasc Surg 9: 598–608.

White RI (1981) Selected techniques in interventional radiology. JAMA 245: 741–744.

Wholey MH (1988) Advances in balloon technology and reperfusion devises for peripheral circulation. REVIEW ARTICLE: 25 REFS. Am J Cardiol 61: 87G-95G.

Wholey MH (1990) Controversies in perpheral vascular intervention. Radiology 174: 929–931.

Wierny LR, Plass R, Porstmannn W (1974) Long-term results in 100 consecutive patients treated by transluminal angioplasty. Radiology 112: 543–548.

Williams GM (1988) Who should blow up balloons in arteries? (editorial) Radiology 169: 857.

Wilson AR, Fuchs JC (1984) Percutaneous transluminal angioplasty. The radiologist's contribution to the treatment of vascular disease. Surg Clin North Am 64: 121–150.

Wilson SE, White GH, Wolf G, Cross AP (1990) Proximal percutaneous balloon angioplasty and distal bypass for multilevel arterial occlusion. Veterans Administration Cooperative Study No. 199. Ann Vasc Surg 4: 351–355.

Wollenweber J, Henne W, Kiefer H, Meves M, Schmarsow R (1986) Early and late results after percutaneous transluminal angioplasty in peripheral arterial occlusive disease. Vasa 15: 67–70.

Yamanashi WS, Patil AA, Hill DL, Lepage JR, Yassa NA, Valentine JL, Lester PD (1988) Precision surgery with an electromagnetically induced current convergence probe application in aneurysm treatment, angioplasty, and brain tumor resection in in vivo and in vitro models. Med Instrum 22: 205–216.

Yamanashi WS, Yassa NA, Hill DL, Lewis JE, Patil AA, Lester PD (1988) Electromagnetic field focusing probe (EFFP): a new angioplasty tool. Angiology 39: 1014–1021.

Yao JS, Flinn WR (1982) Comparison of long-term results after balloon dilatation to the results of arterial reconstructive surgery. Vasa 11: 340–343.

Zeevi B, Perry SB, Keane JF, Mandell VS, Lock JE (1988) Interventional cardiac procedures in neonates and infants: state of the art. Clin Perinatol 15: 633–658.

Zeitler E (1978) Appraisal of the techniques. In: Zeitler E et al. (eds) Percutaneous vascular recanalization. Berlin Heidelberg New York, Springer, pp 189–193.

Zeitler E (1980) Percutaneous transluminal angioplasty: cooperation among specialities. Cardiovasc Intervent Radiol 3: 221.

Zeitler E (1986) The beginning of cardiovascular intervention using roentgen rays and image intensifier-TV-fluoroscopy. Cardiovasc Intervent Radiol 9: 233–235.

Zeitler E (1986) Transluminal catheter dilatation. Indications, technical aspects, results. Int Angiol 5: 137–150.

Zeitler E, Grosse-Vorholt R, Richter EI, Saida Y (1981) Techniques of percutaneous transluminal angioplasty (PTA) and additional treatment of leg arteries. Ann Radiol (Paris) 24: 361–364.

Zeitler E, Gruentzig A, Schoop W (eds) (1978) Percutaneous vascular recanalization. Berlin Heidelberg New York, Springer.

Zeitler E, Richter EI, Roth FJ, Schoop W (1983) Results of percutaneous transluminal angioplasty. Radiology 146: 57–60.

Zeitler E, Schoop W, Zahnow W (1971) The treatment of occlusive arterial disease by transluminal catheter angioplasty. Radiology 99: 19–26.

Zollikofer CL, Cragg AH, Einzig S, et al (1983) Prostaglandins and angioplasty: an experimental study in canine arteries. Radiology 149: 681–685.

IV. Surgery and Its Interaction with PTA

Al-Salman M, Doyle DL, Hsiang YN, Fry PD, Fragoso M (1992) Intraoperative balloon angioplasty: a surgical approach. Can J Surg 35(3): 265–268.

AbuRahma AF, Boland JP, Robinson PA (1992) Adjunctive intraoperative linear extrusion (Fogarty-Chin) balloon angioplasty. Am J Surg 164(2): 109–113.

Ahn S, Rutherford RB (1992) A multicenter prospective randomized trial to determine the optimal treatment of patients with claudication and isolated superficial femoral artery occlusive disease: conservative versus endovascular versus surgical therapy. J Vasc Surg 15(5): 889–891.

Alpert JR, Ring EJ, Berkowitz HD, Freiman DB, Oleaga JA, Gordon R, Roberts B (1979) Treatment of vein graft stenosis by balloon catheter dilation. JAMA 242: 2769–2771.

Ammar AD, Hutchinson SA (1987) Management of acute infrainguinal arterial thrombosis: combined intraoperative balloon thrombectomy with balloon angioplasty: a preliminary report. Surgery 101: 176–180.

Angelini R, Salute L, Sardella L, Cichella G, Prosperi AD, Lalli T (1991) Surgical and radiological intervention in the treatment of peripheral arteriovenous fistulas [Ita]. Minerva Chir 46: 527–532.

Anonymous (1991) Donor limb vascular events following femoro-femoral bypass surgery. A Veterans Affairs Cooperative Study. Arch Surg 126: 681–685.

Arlart IP, Gerlach A, Grass HG (1991) Laser-assisted balloon angioplasty in complete femoropopliteal occlusions: preliminary results. Cardiovasc Intervent Radiol 14: 233–237.

Ashley S, Brooks SG, Gehani AA, Kester RC, Rees MR (1990) Experimental analysis of sapphire contact probes for Nd:YAG laser angioplasty. Angiology 41: 453–462.

Ashley S, Brooks SG, Gehani AA, Thorley P, Parkin A, Kester RC, Rees MR (1991) Isotope limb flow measurement in patients undergoing peripheral laser angioplasty. J Biomed Eng 13: 221–224.

Barnes RW (1989) Who took the "p" out of statistics? [editorial]. J Vasc Surg 10: 100–102.

Bauer R, Pokorny E, Muckenhuber P, Malekpour G, Werner H, Juptner J (1991) Is laser assisted angioplasty a real alternative to surgical treatment of occluded peripheral vessels? Eur J Vasc Surg 5(6): 637–640.

Becker GJ, Ferguson JG, Bakal CW, Kinnison ML, McLean GK, Pentecost MJ, Perler BA, et al. (1993) Angioplasty, bypass surgery, and amputation for lower extremity peripheral arterial disease in Maryland: a closer look [see comments]. Radiology 186(3): 635–638.

Becker GJ, Wenker JC, Rees CR, Reilly MK, Bendick PJ, Cockerill EM (1986) Percutaneous transluminal angioplasty and valvectomy in a failing in situ saphenous graft. Radiology 159: 431–433.

Belli AM, Cumberland DC, Procter AE, Welsh CL (1991) Total peripheral artery occlusions: conventional versus laser thermal recanalization with a hybrid probe in percutaneous angioplasty—results of a randomized trial [comments]. Radiology 181: 57–60.

Berkowitz HD, Fox AD, Deaton DH (1992) Reversed vein graft stenosis: early diagnosis and management. J Vasc Surg 15(1): 130–141; discussion 141–142.

Blair JM, Gewertz BL, Moosa H, Lu CT, Zarins CK (1989) Percutaneous transluminal angioplasty versus surgery for limb-threatening ischemia [see comments]. J Vasc Surg 9: 698–703.

Blankensteijn JD, van Vroonhoven TJ, Lampmann L (1986) Role of percutaneous transluminal angioplasty in aorto-iliac reconstruction. J Cardiovasc Surg (Torino) 27: 466–468.

Borio R, Chiocchini S, Lupattelli L, Barzi FM (1988) Personnel and patient doses during percutaneous transluminal angioplasty (PTA). Rays 13: 59–64.

Branchereau A, Espinoza H, Rudondy P, Magnan PE, Reboul J (1991) Descending thoracic aorta as an inflow source for late occlusive failures following aortoiliac reconstruction. Ann Vasc Surg 5: 8–15.

Bunt TJ (1986) Aortic reconstruction vs extra-anatomic bypass and angioplasty. Thoughts on evolving a protocol for selection. Arch Surg 121: 1166–1171.

Campbell WB, Higgins JR, Barker CS, von Eichstorff P, Fletcher EW (1988) Grading for angioplasty. Clin Radiol 39: 516–518.

Charlesworth D (1990) The benefits of proximal and distal vascular reconstruction as a one-stage procedure. Acta Chir Scand 555: 65–67.

Cheshire NJ, Wolfe JH (1992) ABC of vascular diseases. Critical leg ischaemia: amputation or reconstruction. BMJ 304(6822): 312–314.

Chin AK, Tawes RL Jr, Shannahan J, Zimmerman JJ, Shoor PM, Fogarty TJ (1989) Long-term results of intraoperative balloon dilatation. J Cardiovasc Surg (Torino) 30: 454–458.

Cikrit DF, O'Donnell DM, Dalsing MC, Sawchuk AP, Lalka SG (1991) Clinical implications of combined hypogastric and profunda femoral artery occlusion. Am J Surg 162: 137–140.

Creasy TS, McMillan PJ, Fletcher EW, Collin J, Morris PJ (1990) Is percutaneous transluminal angioplasty better than exercise for claudication? Preliminary results from a prospective randomised trial. Eur J Vasc Surg 4: 135–140.

Cull DL, Feinberg RL, Wheeler JR, Snyder SO Jr, Gregory RT, Gayle RG, Parent FN 3d (1991) Experience with laser-assisted angioplasty and a rotary angioplasty instrument: lessons learned. J Vasc Surg 14: 332–339.

Dalsing MC, Hoagland WP, Becker G, Holden RW, Cockerill E, Glover JL (1989) Limb salvage in high-risk patients with multisegmental disease. Indiana Med 82: 700–705.

Dardik H (1990) Maintaining an aggressive policy of graft surveillance to identify correctable lesions before graft occlusion [letter]. Ann Surg 212: 122.

Dewar ML, Blundell PE, Lidstone D, Herba MJ, Chiu RC (1985) Effects of abdominal aneurysmectomy, aortoiliac bypass grafting and angioplasty on male sexual potency: a prospective study. Can J Surg 28: 154–156, 159.

Diethrich EB (1989) Value of laser-assisted angioplasty in the community hospital [letter; comment]. Radiology 173: 877–878.

Do-dai-Do, Triller J, Walpoth BH, Stirnemann P, Mahler F (1992) A comparison study of self-expandable stents vs balloon angioplasty alone in femoropopliteal artery occlusions. Cardiovasc Intervent Radiol 15(5): 306–312.

Donaldson MC, Rosenberg JM (1986) Intraoperative arterial balloon angioplasty. Conn Med 50: 713–715.

Edwards RJ, Fulde GW, McGrath MA (1991) Successful limb salvage with prostaglandin infusion: a review of ergotamine toxicity. Med J Aust 155: 825–827.

Eidemiller ER, Porter JM, Rosch J, Dotter CT, Krippaehne WW (1974) Surgical treatment of bilateral iliac artery occlusive disease in high-risk patients. Am Surg 40: 511–517.

England WL, Roberts SD, Grim CE (1987) Surgery or angioplasty for cost-effective renal revascularization? Med Decis Making 7: 84–91.

Farina C, Mingoli A, Schultz RD, Castrucci M, Feldhaus RJ, Rossi P, Cavallaro A (1989) Percutaneous transluminal angioplasty versus surgery for subclavian artery occlusive disease. Am J Surg 158: 511–514.

Fletcher JP, Little JM, Kershaw LZ (1987) The changing pattern of vascular surgery: the effect of percutaneous transluminal angioplasty. Aust N Z J Surg 57: 221–224.

Fogarty TJ, Chin A, Shoor PM, Blair GL, Zimmerman JJ (1981) Adjunctive intraoperative arterial dilation: simplified instrumentation technique. Arch Surg 116: 1391–1398.

Fox RL, Kahn M, Adler J, Sussman B, Mendes D, Ibrahim IM, Dardik H (1985) Adventitial cystic disease of the popliteal artery: failure of percutaneous transluminal angioplasty as a therapeutic modality. J Vasc Surg 2: 464–467.

Francois F, Picard E, Nicaud P, Albat B, Thevenet A (1991) Femoro-femoral crossover bypass for noninfective complications of aortoiliac surgery. Ann Vasc Surg 5: 46–49.

Friedman SA (1990) The diagnosis and medical management of vascular ulcers. Clin Dermatol 8: 30–39.

Friedman SG (1989) Charles Dotter: interventional radiologist. Radiology 172: 921–924.

Gale SS (1989) Residual lesions and early recurrent stenosis after carotid endarterectomy [letter; comment]. J Vasc Surg 10: 705–707.

Gaylord GM, Pritchard WF, Chuang VP, Casarella WJ, Sprawls P (1988) The geometry of triple-balloon dilation. Radiology 166: 541–545.

Geschwind HJ (1988) Laser angioplasty: newer modalities. Ann Radiol (Paris) 31: 69–73.

Giessler R (1978) Surgical aspects of vascular reconstruction after PTR. In: Zeitler E, et al (eds) Percutaneous Vascular Recanalization. Berlin Heidelberg New York, Springer, chap. 27, pp 160–171.

Glover JL, Bendick PJ, Dilley RS, Becker GJ, Richmond BC, Yune HY, Holden RW (1983) Balloon catheter for limb salvage. Arch Surg 118: 557–560.

Greenstein SM, Verstandig A, McLean GK, DaFoe DC, Burke DR, Meranze SG, Naji A, Brayman KL, Grossman RA, Perloff LJ et al. (1987) Percutaneous transluminal angioplasty: the procedure of choice for renal allograft artery stenosis. Transplant Proc 19: 2194–2196.

Grim CE, Yune HY, Donahue JP, Weinberger MH, Dilley R, Klatte EC (1982) Unilateral renal vascular hypertension: surgery vs. dilation. Vasa 11: 367–368.

Gupta SK, Veith FJ, Kram HB, Wengerter KA (1990) Significance and management of inflow gradients unexpectedly generated after femoro-femoral, femoropopliteal, and femoroinfrapopliteal bypass grafting. J Vasc Surg 12: 278–283.

Harris RW, Dulawa LB, Andros G, Oblath RW, Salles-Cunha SX, Apyan RL (1991) Percutaneous transluminal angioplasty of the lower extremities by the vascular surgeon. Ann Vasc Surg 5: 345–353.

Hibberd AD (1983) Percutaneous transluminal angioplasty: a vascular surgeon's viewpoint. Australas Radiol 27: 303–304.

Holm J, Arfvidsson B, Jivegard L, Lundgren F, Lundholm K, Scherstoen T, Stenberg B, Tylen U, Zachrisson BF, Lindberg H, et al (1991) Chronic lower limb ischaemia. A prospective randomised controlled study comparing the 1-year results of vascular surgery and percutaneous transluminal angioplasty (PTA). Eur J Vasc Surg 5: 517–522.

Hopfner R, Wagner V (1978) Intraoperative transluminal angioplasty by Dotter's method. In: Zeitler E, et al (eds) Percutaneous Vascular Recanalization. Berlin Heidelberg New York, Springer, chap. 28, pp 172–174.

Humphries AL, Nesbit RR, Caruana RJ, Hutchins RS, Heimburger RA, Wray CH (1981) Thirty-six recommendations for vascular access operations. Am Surg 47: 145–151.

Jamieson C (1988) The management of intermittent claudication. Practitioner 232: 613–616.

Jeans WD (1989) Technical success, clinical success, and patency in laser angioplasty [letter]. Radiology 173: 572.

Johansen K, Anderson J, Morishima M (1983) Percutaneous transluminal angioplasty (PTA) as an adjunct in vascular trauma: case report. Angiology 34: 355–361.

Jorgensen B, Tonnesen KH, Holstein P (1991) Late hemodynamic failure following percutaneous transluminal angioplasty for long and multifocal femoropopliteal stenoses. Cardiovasc Intervent Radiol 14: 290–292.

Kadir S, Smith GW, White RI Jr, Kaufman SL, Barth KH, Williams GM, O'Mara CS, Burdick JF (1982) Percutaneous transluminal angioplasty as an adjunct to the surgical management of peripheral vascular disease. Ann Surg 195: 786–795.

Kantoch M, Ruzyllo W, Dabrowski M (1988) Transluminal dilation techniques in the management of congenital obstructive cardiovascular disease. Mater Med Pol 20: 103–113.

Kaufman JL (1989) Interventional procedures in peripheral atherosclerotic disease [letter; comment]. JAMA 262: 2387–2388.

Kaufman SL (1987) Intrathoracic interventional vascular techniques in congenital cardiovascular disease. J Thorac Imaging 2: 1–10.

Kram HB, Gupta SK, Veith FJ, Wengerter KR (1991) Unilateral aortofemoral bypass: a safe and effective option for the treatment of unilateral limb-threatening ischemia. Am J Surg 162: 155–158.

Krotovsky GS, Turpitko SA, Gerasimov VB, Zabelskaya TF, Mamedov DM, Klokov KI, Uchkin IG, Papandopulos E (1991) Surgical treatment and prevention of vasculopathic impotence in conjunction with revascularisation of the lower extremities in Leriche's syndrome. J Cardiovasc Surg 32: 340–343.

Kusel RD, Pereyra R (1986) Combined femorotibial bypass and distal intraoperative transluminal angioplasty. J Vasc Surg 4: 533–535.

Laissy JP, Peillon C, Clavier E, Pernes JM, Gaux JC, Watelet J, Testart J, Benozio M (1990) Transluminal angioplasty of failing infrainguinal arterial by-pass grafts: initial and long-term results in 13 patients. Cardiovasc Intervent Radiol 13: 14–17.

Lalka SG, Lash JM, Unthank JL, Lalka VK, Cikrit DF, Sawchuk AP, Dalsing MC (1991) Inadequacy of saphenous vein grafts for cross-femoral venous bypass. J Vasc Surg 13: 662–630.

Lewis JE (1989) Percutaneous transluminal angioplasty. Adjunctive treatment of ischemic ulcers. Int J Dermatol 28: 134–135.

Lorentzen JE, Jorgensen L, Johansen JJ (1990) The ideal operation for unilateral iliac occlusion. Should the asymptomatic iliac artery also be reconstructed? Acta Chir Scand 555: 69–71.

Lorenzi G, Domanin M, Constantini A (1991) PTA and laser assisted PTA combined with simultaneous surgical revascularization. J Cardiovasc Surg 32: 456–462.

Lowman BG, Queral LA, Holbrook WA, Estes JT, Bayly B (1981) The treatment of innominate artery stenosis by intraoperative transluminal angioplasty. Surgery 89: 565–568.

Lowman BG, Queral LA, Holbrook WA, Estes JT, Dagher FJ (1981) Transluminal angioplasty during vascular reconstructive procedures. Arch Surg 116: 829–832.

Lu C, Zarins CK, Yang C, Turcotte JK (1982) Percutaneous transluminal angioplasty for limb salvage. Radiology 142: 337–341.

Mandel SR, Jaques PF (1980) Salvage procedure of Thomas femoral shunts by balloon angioplasty. Surg Gynecol Obstet 151: 673–674.

McMillan PJ, Collin J, Fletcher EW (1988) Intraoperative transluminal balloon dilatation permits simpler safer reconstructive surgery. Clin Radiol 39: 91–93.

McShane MD, Birch S, Gazzard VM, Humphries KN, Chant AD (1988) Peroperative monitoring of distal transluminal dilatation. JCU 16: 659–662.

Meijenhorst GC, Linnebank F, Smit FW, van Elk PJ, Driessen LP (1986) Percutaneous transluminal angioplasty during operation. Diagn Imaging Clin Med 55: 266–269.

Menges HW, Jaschke W, Trede M (1988) Percutaneous transluminal angioplasty: the surgeon's role. World J Surg 12: 788–799.

Miller GA, Ford KK, Braun SD, Newman GE, Moore AV Jr, Malone R, Dunnick NR (1985) Percutaneous transluminal angioplasty vs. surgery for renovascular hypertension. AJR 144: 447–450.

Minich LL, Beekman RH 3d, Rocchini AP, Heidelberger K, Bove EL (1992) Surgical repair is safe and effective after unsuccessful balloon angioplasty of native coarctation of the aorta. J Am Coll Cardiol 19(2): 389–393.

Murie JA (1988) Percutaneous transluminal angioplasty and vascular surgery for lower limb ischaemia [editorial]. Br J Surg 75: 1051–1052.

Naylor AR, Ah-See AK, Engeset J (1990) Axillofemoral bypass as a limb salvage procedure in high risk patients with aortoiliac disease. Br J Surg 77: 659–661.

Newell DW, Eskridge J, Mayberg M, Grady MS, Lewis D, Winn HR (1992) Endovascular treatment of intracranial aneurysms and cerebral vasospasm. Clin Neurosurg 39: 348–360.

Norstein J, Brekke IB, Holdaas H, Vatne K (1990) Arterial stenoses in duct occluded segmental pancreatic grafts treated with percutaneous transluminal angioplasty. Transplant Proc 22: 599–601.

O'Byrne P, Blakeney C, Ham R, Murfitt J (1988) Transluminal balloon dilatation [letter]. Clin Radiol 39: 464–465.

Olbert F, Weidinger P, Schlegl A, Teiner G, Hagmuller GW, Denck H (1981) Combined transluminal percutaneous dilation and surgical reconstruction of the iliac, femoral and popliteal arteries. Ann Radiol (Paris) 24: 369–374.

Perler BA, Burdick JF, Williams GM (1991) Femoro-femoral or ilio-femoral bypass for unilateral inflow reconstruction? Am J Surg 161: 426–430.

Perler BA, Mitchell SE (1986) Percutaneous transluminal angioplasty and transaxillary first rib resection. A multidisciplinary approach to the thoracic outlet syndrome. Am Surg 52: 485–488.

Peterkin GA, Belkin M, Cantelmo NL, Guben J, Greenfield AJ, Johnson WC, Menzoian JO (1990) Combined transluminal angioplasty and infra-inguinal reconstruction in multilevel atherosclerotic disease. Am J Surg 160: 277–279.

Pfeiffer RB, String ST (1986) Adjunctive use of the balloon dilatation catheter during vascular reconstructive procedures. J Vasc Surg 3: 841–845.

Pilla TJ, Peterson GJ, Tantana S, Lang ER, Wolverson MK (1984) Percutaneous recanalization of iliac artery occlusions: an alternative to surgery in the high-risk patient. AJR 143: 313–316.

Pilla TJ, Tantana S, Smith KR (1988) Percutaneous transluminal angioplasty prior to carotid cavernous fistula embolization. AJNR 9: 789–790.

Porter JM, Eidemiller LA, Hood RW, Wesche EH, Dotter CT, Rosch J (1977) Transluminal angioplasty and distal arterial bypass. Am Surg 43: 695–701.

Porter JM, Eidemiller LR, Dotter CT, Rosch J, Vetto M (1973) Combined arterial dilatation and femorofemoral bypass for limb salvage. Surg Gynecol Obstet 137: 409–412.

Preter B, Gruentzig A, Greminge P (1978) (GE) Percutaneous transluminal recanalization after trauma. ROFO 129: 787–789.

Price BA (1990) Management of critical ischaemia by transluminal iliac angioplasty with distal bypass surgery [letter]. J R Coll Surg Edinb 35: 132.

Priest EM (1988) Treatment of shunt-produced edema [letter]. South Med J 81: 1204.

Ring EJ, Ehrenfeld WK (1988) Percutaneous transluminal angioplasty [letter]. J Vasc Surg 8: 92.

Roberts B, Gertner MH, Ring EJ (1981) Balloon-catheter dilation as an adjunct to arterial surgery. Arch Surg 116: 809–812.

Roberts L Jr, Wertman DA Jr, Mills SR, Moore AV Jr, Heaston DK (1983) Transluminal angioplasty of the superior mesenteric artery: an alternative to surgical revascularization. AJR 141: 1039–1042.

Rose BS, Van Aman ME, Simon DC, Sommer BG, Ferguson RM, Henry ML (1988) Transluminal balloon angioplasty of infrahepatic caval anastomotic stenosis following liver transplantation: case report. Cardiovasc Intervent Radiol 11: 79–81.

Rubay JE, Sluysmans T, Alexandrescu V, Khelif K, Moulin D, Vliers A, Jaumin P, Chalant CH (1992) Surgical repair of coarctation of the aorta in infants under one year of age. Long-term results in 146 patients comparing subclavian flap angioplasty and modified end-to-end anastomosis. J Cardiovasc Surg 33(2): 216–222.

Sacks D (1990) Percutaneous transluminal angioplasty versus surgery for limb-threatening ischemia [letter; comment]. J Vasc Surg 11: 358–359.

Sanchez LA, Gupta SK, Veith FJ, Goldsmith J, Lyon RT, Wengerter KR, Panetta TF, Marin ML, Cynamon J, Berdejo G, et al (1991) A ten-year experience with one hundred fifty failing or threatened vein and polytetrafluoroethylene arterial bypass grafts. J Vasc Surg 14: 729–736; discussion 736–738.

Savolainen HO (1992) Do thermal lasers increase the risk of distal embolism in angioplasties? An experimental study with cw Nd:YAG and excimer lasers. Vasa 21(4): 344–349.

Scobie TK (1986) Transluminal angioplasty: indications and overview. Can J Surg 29: 90–92.

Shaddy RE, Boucek MM, Sturtevant JE, Ruttenberg HD, Jaffe RB, Tani LY, Judd VE, et al. (1993) Comparison of angioplasty and surgery for unoperated coarctation of the aorta [see comments]. Circulation 87(3): 793–799.

Simonetti G, Urigo F, Guazzaroni M, Biglioli P, Dettori G, Bacciu PP (1986) Iliac artery lesions: a comparison between percutaneous transluminal angioplasty and surgery. Ann Radiol (Paris) 29: 127–129.

Skotnicki SH (1988) The vascular surgeon and transluminal angioplasty. Eur J Vasc Surg 2: 143–144.

Smith TP, Cragg AH, Castaneda F, Hunter DW (1989) Thrombosed polytetrafluoroethylene hemodialysis fistulas: salvage with combined thrombectomy and angioplasty. Radiology 171: 507–508.

Spoelstra H, Nevelsteen A, Wilms G, Suy R (1989) Balloon angioplasty combined with vascular surgery. Eur J Vasc Surg 3: 381–388.

Sprayregen S, Veith FJ (1983) Vein graft angioplasty with nonballoon catheters. Radiology 146: 224–225.

Sprayregen S, Veith FJ, Bakal CW (1988) Catheterization and angioplasty of the nonopacified peripheral autogenous vein bypass graft. Arch Surg 123: 1009–1012.

Stain SC, Weaver FA, Yellin AE (1991) Extra-anatomic bypass of failed traumatic arterial repairs. J Trauma 31: 575–578.

Stone J (1989) Balloon man. Ohio Med 85: 927–929.

Sundt TM Jr, Smith HC, Piepgras DG, Campbell LJK (1982) Bypass and transluminal dilatation procedures for advanced occlusive disease of the posterior circulation. Neurosurg Rev 5: 65–72.

Thompson JF, McShane MD, Chant AD (1989) Salvage of in situ femoropopliteal and femorotibial saphenous vein bypass with interventional radiology [letter]. J Vasc Surg 9: 178–179.

Thompson JF, McShane MD, Clifford PC, Gazzard V, Webster JH, Chant AB (1989) Intervention for graft stenoses: the role of surgery and transluminal angioplasty. Br J Surg 76: 1017.

Thompson JF, McShane MD, Gazzard V, Clifford PC, Chant AD (1989) Limitations of percutaneous transluminal angioplasty in the treatment of femoro-distal graft stenoses. Eur J Vasc Surg 3: 209–211.

Tisnado J, Vines FS, Barnes RW, Beachley MC, Cho SR (1984) Percutaneous transluminal angioplasty following endarterectomy. Radiology 152: 361–364.

Tortolani EC, Tan AH, Butchart S (1984) Percutaneous transluminal angioplasty. An ineffective approach to the failing vascular access. Arch Surg 119: 221–223.

Turcotte JK, Lu CT, Zarins CK (1981) The role of transluminal angioplasty in limb salvage and claudication. J Surg Res 30: 428–434.

Van Beers B, Roche A, Cauquil P (1988) Transluminal angioplasty of a stenotic surgical splenorenal shunt. Acta Radiol 29: 327–329.

Veith FJ, Perler BA, Bakal CW (1992) The use of angioplasty, bypass surgery, and amputation in the management of peripheral vascular disease (letter). N Engl J Med 326(6): 413–414; discussion 415–416.

Von Sommoggy S, Fraunhofer S, Wahba A, Blumel G, Maurer PC (1991) Coagulation in aortofemoral bifurication bypass grafting. Eur J Vasc Surg 5: 247–253.

Walker PJ, Harris JP, May J (1991) Combined percutaneous transluminal angioplasty and extra-anatomic bypass for symptomatic unilateral iliac artery occlusion with contralateral iliac artery stenosis. Ann Vasc Surg 5: 209–216.

Walker WJ, Giddings AE (1988) A protocol for the safe treatment of acute lower limb ischaemia with intra-arterial streptokinase and surgery [see comments]. Br J Surg 75: 1189–1192.

Weber G, Kiss T (1989) Intraoperative balloon angioplasty. Eur J Vasc Surg 3: 153–157.

Wehrmacher WH (1988) Angioplasty versus bypass surgery. Where do we stand today? Postgrad Med 84: 62–68.

Weibull H, Bergqvist D, Jendteg S, Lindgren B, Persson U, Jonsson K, Bergentz SE (1991) Clinical outcome and health care costs in renal revascularization—percutaneous transluminal renal angioplasty versus reconstructive surgery. Br J Surg 78: 620–624.

Weibull H, Bergqvist D, Jonsson K, Hulthen L, Mannhem P, Bergentz SE (1991) Long-term results after percutaneous transluminal angioplasty of atherosclerotic renal artery stenosis—the importance of intensive follow-up. Eur J Vasc Surg 5: 291–301.

Wexler L, Ginsburg R, Mitchell RS, Mehigan JT (1989) The vascular war of 1988. JAMA 261: 418–419.

Whittemore AD, Donaldson MC, Polak JF, Mannick JA (1991) Limitations of balloon angioplasty for vein graft stenosis. J Vasc Surg 14: 340–345.

Wilkins RA, Nunnerley HB, Allison DJ, Mason R, Kellett MJ, Cumberland DC, Sandin B (1989) The expansion of interventional radiology. Report of a survey conducted by the Royal College of Radiologists. Clin Radiol 40: 457–462.

Williams GM (1988) Who should blow up balloons in arteries? [editorial]. Radiology 169: 857.

Wilms G, Baert AL, Nevelsteen A, Suy R, Verbrugge H, Hauglustaine D, Michielsen P (1989) Balloon angioplasty of venous structures. J Belge Radiol 72: 273–277.

Wilson SE, White GH, Wolf G, Cross AP (1990) Proximal percutaneous balloon angioplasty and distal bypass for multilevel arterial occlusion. Veterans Administration Cooperative Study No. 199. Ann Vasc Surg 4: 351–355.

Wilson SE, Wolf GL, Cross AP (1989) Percutaneous transluminal angioplasty versus operation for peripheral arteriosclerosis. Report of a prospective randomized trial in a selected group of patients. J Vasc Surg 9: 1–9.

Wyffels PL, DeBord JR (1990) Increased limb salvage. Distal tibial/peroneal artery thrombectomy/embolectomy in acute lower extremity ischemia. Am Surg 56: 468–475.

Yao JS, Flinn WR (1982) Comparison of long-term results after balloon dilatation to the results of arterial reconstructive surgery. Vasa 11: 340–343.

Zarins CK (1989) The vascular war of 1988: the enemy is met. JAMA 261: 416–417.

Zarins CK, Lu CT, McDonnel AE, Whitehouse WM (1980) Limb salvage by percutaneous transluminal recanalization of the occluded superficial femoral artery. Surgery 87: 701–708.

Zeitler E, Raithel D, Gailer H, Nippold AV, Kasprcak P (1987) PTA combined with surgical vascular operations in iliac and femoral obstruction. Ann Radiol (Paris) 30: 142–144.

Section 3

Alternative or Complementary Devices

I. Adjunctive Devices

Berkowitz HD (1991) Plug technique for controlling lumbar and intercostal bleeding during aortic surgery. J Vasc Surg 13: 516–517.

Dick RJ, Popma JJ, Muller DW, Burek KA, Topol EJ (1991) In-hospital costs associated with new percutaneous coronary devices. Am J Cardiol 68: 879–885.

Goodkind J, Coombs V, Golobic RA (1993) Excimer laser angioplasty. Heart Lung 22(1): 26–35.

Greenberg MA, Menegus MA, Issenberg H, Spindola-Franco H (1990) Advances in interventional cardiology: coronary balloon angioplasty and alternative techniques. Curr Opin Radiol 2: 602–615.

Greenfield LJ, Cho KJ, Tauscher JR (1990) Limitations of percutaneous insertion of Greenfield filters. J Cardiovasc Surg 31: 344–350.

Gunther RW, Vorwerk D (1991) Minibasket for percutaneous embolectomy and filter protection against distal embolization: technical note. Cardiovasc Intervent Radiol 14: 195–198

Markowitz DM, Hughes SH, Shaw C, Denny DF Jr, Wilkinson LA, White RI Jr (1991) Transcatheter detachable balloon embolotherapy for catheter-induced pulmonary artery pseudoaneurysm. J Thorac Imaging 6: 75–78.

McFadden JT (1991) A new clip applier. Technical note. J Neurosurg 74: 304–305.

Nishida H, Grooters RK, Soltanzadeh H, Thiemen KC, Schneider RF (1991) Clinical alternative bypass conduits and methods for surgical coronary revascularization. Surg Gynecol Obstet 172: 161–174.

Pollak JS, Cooper SG, Denny DF Jr (1990) Use of the balloon on a guidewire as an adjunct to conventional angioplasty. AJR 155: 887–888.

Rosenschein U, Rozenszajn LA, Kraus L, Marboe CC, Watkins JF, Rose EA, David D, Cannon PJ, Weinstein JS (1991) Ultrasonic angioplasty in totally occluded peripheral arteries. Initial clinical, histological, and angiographic results. Circulation 83: 1976–1986.

Sawchuk AP, Flanigan DP, Tober JC, Eton D, Schwarcz TH, Eldrup-Jorgensen J, Meyer JP, Durham JR, Schuler JJ (1990) A rapid, accurate, noninvasive technique for diagnosing critical and subcritical stenoses in aortoiliac arteries. J Vasc Surg 12: 158–167.

Schmitz-Rode T, Gunther RW, Muller-Leisse C (1991) US-assisted aspiration thrombectomy: in vitro investigations. Radiology 178: 677–679.

Solomon RA, Fukushima T (1991) New aneurysm clip appliers for "keyhole" neurosurgery. Neurosurgery 28: 474–476.

Tani M, Mizuno K, Midorikawa H, Igari T, Egawa M, Niimura S, Fukuchi S, et al. (1993) Thermal laser-assisted angioplasty of renal artery stenosis for renovascular hypertension. Cardiovasc Intervent Radiol 16(1): 52–54.

Wholey MH (1988) Advances in balloon technology and reperfusion devices for peripheral circulation. REVIEW ARTICLE: 25 REFS. Am J Cardiol 61: 87G–95G.

Yamanashi WS, Yassa NA, Hill DL, Lewis JE, Patil AA, Lester PD (1988) Electromagnetic field focusing probe (EFFP)—a new angioplasty tool. Angiology 39: 1014–1021.

II. Angioscopy

Ahn SS, Auth D, Marcus DR, Moore WS (1988) Removal of focal atheromatous lesions by angioscopically guided high-speed rotary atherectomy. Preliminary experimental observations. J Vasc Surg 7: 292–300.

Ahn SS, Moore WS (1992) Endovascular surgery. Surg Annu 24: 107–142.

Bauriedel G, De Maio SJ Jr, Hofling B (1991) Role of angioscopy in the treatment of peripheral vascular disease with percutaneous atherectomy. Am J Cardiol 68: 226–231.

Bech A, Milic S, Spagnoli AM, Mundinger A, Blum U (1989) The clinical value of percutaneous transluminal angioscopy. Angioscopical findings in primary vascular diagnosis and in interventional radiology. Clin Ter 131: 93–105.

Beck A, Reinbold WD, Blum U, Nanko N, Milic S, Papacharalampous X (1988) Clinical application of percutaneous transluminal angioscopy. Comparison of findings in percutaneous transluminal angioplasty, thrombolysis, thrombus-extraction and stent-application. REVIEW ARTICLE: 44 REFS. Herz 13: 392–399.

Beyer-Enke SA, Zeitler E (1989) Angioplasty and angioscopy. Curr Opin Radiol 1: 183–185.

Diethrich EB, Hanafy HM, Santiago OJ, Bahadir I (1991) Angioscopy after coronary excimer laser angioplasty [letter]. J Am Coll Cardiol 18: 643–644.

Diethrich EB, Yoffe B, Kiessling JJ, Santiago O, Bahadir I, Stern LA, Lavine D (1992) Angioscopy in endovascular surgery: recent technical advances to enhance intervention selection and failure analysis. Angiology 43(1): 1–10.

Ennker J, Gross CM, Biamino G, Hetzer R (1992) First clinical experiences with a new angioscopic system for diagnosing peripheral vascular changes. Thorac Cardiovasc Surg 40(1): 33–37.

Franzen D, Hopp HW, Korsten J, Hilger HH (1992) A prospective study on percutaneous coronary angioscopy with different guiding techniques in patients with coronary heart disease. Eur Heart J 13(5): 655–660.

Halfman-Franey M, Coburn C (1990) Techniques in cardiac care: lasers, stents, and atherectomy devices. REVIEW ARTICLE: 128 REFS. AACN Clin Issues Crit Care Nurs 1: 87–109.

Konishi T, Inden M, Nakano T (1989) Clinical experience of percutaneous coronary angioscopy in cases with coronary artery disease. Angiology 40: 18–23.

Lai ST, Cheng KJ (1991) Results of angioscopy-assisted intraoperative transluminal angioplasty of the iliac and femoral artery. Chung Hua I Hsueh Tsa Chih 48: 25–30.

Nakamura F, Kvasnicka J, Uchida Y, Geschwind HJ (1992) Percutaneous angioscopic evaluation of luminal changes induced by excimer laser angioplasty. Am Heart J 124(6): 1467–1472.

Ramee SR, White CJ, Collins TJ, Mesa JE, Murgo JP (1991) Percutaneous angioscopy during coronary angioplasty using a steerable microangioscope. J Am Coll Cardiol 17: 100–105.

Stonebridge PA, Murie JA (1992) Angioscopy: a new light on peripheral vascular disease. Eur J Vasc Surg 6(4): 346–353.

Tatpati DA, Sensarma PK, Erskin JT (1988) Angioscopy as an adjunct to laser-assisted angioplasty in seven peripheral vascular cases. Kans Med 89: 305–307.

Tobis JM, Conroy R, Deutsch LS, Gordon I, Honye J, Andrews J, Profeta G, Chatzkel S, Berns M (1991) Laser-assisted versus mechanical recanalization of femoral arterial occlusions. Am J Cardiol 68: 1079–1086.

Uchida Y, Masuo M, Tomaru T, Kato A, Sugimoto T (1986) Fiberoptic observation of thrombosis and thrombolysis in isolated human coronary arteries. Am Heart J 112: 691–696.

White CJ, Ramee SR, Mesa JE, Collins TJ (1991) Percutaneous coronary angioscopy in patients with restenosis after coronary angioplasty. J Am Coll Cardiol 17: 46B–49B.

White GH, White RA, Colman PD, Kopchok GE (1989) Experimental and clinical applications of angioscopic guidance for laser angioplasty. Am J Surg 158: 495–500; discussion 500–501.

White RA (1990) Indications for fiberoptic angioscopy and intraluminal ultrasound. Compr Ther 16: 23–30.

III. Atherectomy

Ahn SS (1992) Status of peripheral atherectomy. Surg Clin North Am 72(4): 869–878.

Ahn SS, Auth D, Marcus DR, Moore WS (1988) Removal of focal atheromatous lesions by angioscopically guided high-speed rotary atherectomy. Preliminary experimental observations. J Vasc Surg 7: 292–300.

Ahn SS, Auth D, Marcus P, Moore W (1987) Removal of focal atheromatous lesions by angioscopically guided high speed rotary atherectomy. Forty-First Annual Meeting of the Society for Vascular Surgery. Abstract Book 1: 42, #13.

Ahn SS, Auth DC, Marcus D, Moore WS (1987) Removal of obstructing atheroma in human cadavers by angioscopically guided rotary atherectomy. Texas Heart Institute of Cardiology and Cardiovascular Surgery: Interventions, 1987 Annual Symposium, Abstract Book 50.

Ahn SS, Eton D, Yeatman LR, Deutsch LS, Moore WS (1992) Intraoperative peripheral rotary atherectomy: early and late clinical results. Ann Vasc Surg 6(3): 272–280.

Anderson MH, Ward DE (1991) Early experience with low speed rotational angioplasty. Br Heart J 66: 130–133.

Aretz HT, Martinelli MA, LeDet EG (1989) Intraluminal ultrasound guidance of transverse laser coronary atherectomy. Int J Card Imaging 4: 153–157.

Auth DC (1987) Micro-ablation catheters for removing cardiovascular obstructions. New Frontiers in Cardiovascular Therapy Conference (sponsored by Biomedical Business International), Newport Beach, California.

Barbano EF, Newman GE, McCann RL, Hackel DB, Stack RS, Palmos LE, Mikat EM (1989) Correlation of clinical history with quantitative histology of lower extremity atheroma biopsies obtained with the Simpson atherectomy catheter. Atherosclerosis 78: 183–196.

Bates ER, O'Neill WW, Topol EJ (1988) Percutaneous atherectomy catheters. REVIEW ARTICLE: 39 REFS. Cardiol Clin 6: 373–382.

Baumgart R, Steckmeier B, Pfeifer KJ, Thetter O, Schweiberer L (1988) Dynamic angioplasty: a milling catheter for transcutaneous and intraoperative treatment of vascular occlusive disease. Eur J Vasc Surg 2: 297–303.

Bauriedel G, Dartsch PC, Voisard R, Roth D, Simpson JB, Hofling B, Betz E (1989) Selective percutaneous "biopsy" of atheromatous plaque tissue for cell culture. Basic Res Cardiol 84: 326–331.

Bauriedel G, Windstetter U, DeMaio SJ Jr, Kandolf R, Hofling B (1992)

Migratory activity of human smooth muscle cells cultivated from coronary and peripheral primary and restenotic lesions removed by percutaneous atherectomy. Circulation 85(2): 554–564.

Belli AM, Cumberland DC (1989) Percutaneous atherectomy: early experience in Sheffield. Clin Radiol 40: 122–126.

Bertrand ME, Lablanche JM, Leroy F, Bauters C, De Jaegere P, Serruys PW, Meyer J, Dietz U, Erbel R (1992) Percutaneous transluminal coronary rotary ablation with Rotablator (European experience). Am J Cardiol 69(5): 470–474.

Bieler L (1988) Arterial catheter atherectomy. CARDIO, pp 67–70.

Blankenship J, Thomas W, Abrams G, Gallagher K, Pitt B, O'Neill WW (1987) Non-surgical percutaneous endarterectomy using a mechanical rotational catheter in normal canine coronary arteries in vivo. JACC 9: 188A.

Bowerman RE, Pinkerton CA, Kirk B, Waller BF (1991) Disruption of a coronary stent during atherectomy for restenosis. Cathet Cardiovasc Diagn 24(4): 248–251.

Bucay M, Zacca NM, Trakhtenbroit AD, Asimacopoulos PJ, Master H, Raizner AE (1992) Rotablator induced "shave" of intraluminal cap exposing intramural plaque crater. Cathet Cardiovasc Diagn 25(3): 209–212.

Castaneda F, Moradian G, Hunter D, Castaneda-Zuniga W, Amplatz K (1989) Percutaneous intravascular biopsy using a Simpson atherectomy catheter: technical note. Cardiovasc Intervent Radiol 12: 342–343.

Clugston RA, Eisenhauer AC, Matthews RV (1992) Atherectomy of the distal aorta using a "kissing-balloon" technique for the treatment of blue toe syndrome. AJR 159(1): 125–127.

Cohen AJ, Banks A, Cambier P, Edwards FH (1992) Post-atherectomy coronary artery aneurysm. Ann Thorac Surg 54(6): 1216–1218.

Coleman CC, Posalaky IP, Robinson JD, Payne WD, Vlodaver ZA, Amplatz K (1989) Atheroablation with the Kensey catheter: a pathologic study. Radiology 170: 391–394.

Culverwell M (1987) Blades and reamers move into balloon angioplasty turf. CARDIO, pp 22–25.

Dake MD (1990) Peripheral angiography, angioplasty, atherectomy, laser techniques, thrombolysis, and stents. Curr Opin Radiol 2: 239–249.

Dake MD, Zemel G, Dolmatch BL, Katzen BT (1990) The cause of superior vena cava syndrome: diagnosis with percutaneous atherectomy. Radiology 174: 957–959.

Dartsch PC, Bauriedel G, Schinko I, Weiss HD, Hofling B, Betz E (1989) Cell constitution and characteristics of human atherosclerotic plaques selectively removed by percutaneous atherectomy. Atherosclerosis 80: 149–157.

Dartsch PC, Voisard R, Bauriedel G, Hofling B, Betz E (1990) Growth characteristics and cytoskeletal organization of cultured smooth muscle cells from human primary stenosing and restenosing lesions. Arteriosclerosis 10: 62–75.

De Cesare NB, Popma JJ, Holmes DR Jr, Dick RJ, Whitlow PL, King SB, Pinkerton CA, Kereiakes DJ, Topol EJ, Haudenschild CC, et al (1992) Clinical angiographic and histologic correlates of ectasia after directional coronary atherectomy. Am J Cardiol 69(4): 314–319.

Dolmatch BL, Rholl KS, Moskowitz LB, Dake MD, van Breda A, Kaplan JO, Katzen BT (1989) Blue toe syndrome: treatment with percutaneous atherectomy. Radiology 173: 799–804.

Dorros G, Percutaneous rotational atherectomy (Rotablator®) in peripheral lesions. International Course on Peripheral Vascular Interventions, October 1990.

Dorros G, Iyer S, Lewin R, Zaitoun R, Mathiak L, Olson K (1991) Angiographic follow-up and clinical outcome of 126 patients after percutaneous directional atherectomy (Simpson AtheroCath) for occlusive peripheral vascular disease. Cathet Cardiovasc Diagn 22: 79–84.

Dorros G, Iyer S, Zaitoun R, Lewin R, Cooley R, Olson K (1991) Acute angiographic and clinical outcome of high speed percutaneous rotational atherectomy (Rotablator). Cathet Cardiovasc Diagn 22: 157–166.

Dorros G, Lewin RF, Sachdev N, Mathiak L (1989) Percutaneous atherectomy of occlusive peripheral vascular disease: stenoses and/or occlusions. Cathet Cardiovasc Diagn 18: 1–6.

Erbel R, Dietz U, Auth D, Haude M, Nixdorf U, Meyer J, III, (1989) Percutaneous transluminal coronary rotablation during heart catheterization. JACC 13: 228A.

Erbel R, Haude M, Iversen S, Nixdorff U, Dietz U, Oelert H, Dietz U, Meyer J 1991 High Frequency Rotational Angioplasty. In Fleck E, Frantz E (eds): Complications in PTCA. New York, Springer-Verlag.

Erbel R, O'Neill W, Auth D, Haude N, Nixdorf U, Rupprecht HJ, Dietz U, Meyer J (1989) High-frequency rotablation of occluded coronary artery during heart catheterization. Cathet Cardiovasc Diagn 17: 56–58.

Eton D, Ahn SS (1991) Trends in endovascular surgery. Crit Care Nurs Clin North Am 3: 535–549.

Fischell TA, Stadius ML (1991) New technologies for the treatment of obstructive arterial disease. Cathet Cardiovasc Diagn 22: 205–233.

Fourrier JL, Lefebvre JM, Henry M, Dorros G, Ginsburg R, Zacca NM, Walker CM. Rotational atherectomy in complex and long peripheral lesions—multicentric study. International Course on Peripheral Vascular Intervention, October 1990.

Garratt KN, Edwards WD, Kauffmann UP, Vlietstra RE, Holmes DR Jr (1991) Differential histopathology of primary atherosclerotic and restenotic lesions in coronary arteries and saphenous vein bypass grafts: analysis of tissue obtained from 73 patients by directional atherectomy. J Am Coll Cardiol 17: 442–448.

Garratt KN, Kaufmann UP, Edwards WD, Vlietstra RE, Holmes DR, Jr (1989) Safety of percutaneous coronary atherectomy with deep arterial resection. Am J Cardiol 64: 538–540.

Ginsburg R, Jenkins N, Wright A, Wexler L, McCowan L, Mehighan J (1988) Transluminal peripheral vessel angioplasty: clinical experience with new therapeutic devices. Circulation (Suppl II) 78: II-270.

Godlewski P, Nagurka M, Wholey M (1991) Engineering investigation of the Kensey dynamic angioplasty catheter. J Biomed Eng 13(5): 391–398.

Good LP, Gentzler RD (1991) Coronary atherectomy. An alternative to balloon angioplasty. Aorn J 53: 32–39.

Graor RA, Whitlow PL (1990) Transluminal atherectomy for occlusive peripheral vascular disease. J Am Coll Cardiol 15: 1551–1558.

Hall M, Hansen D, Intlekofer MJ, Auth D, Ritchie J (1988) PTCA vs rotational atherectomy (PTRA) in rabbit atherosclerosis: early and late effects. JACC 11: 173A.

Hansen DD, Auth D, Vracko R, Ritchie JL (1986) Rotating mechanical angioplasty in atherosclerotic iliac arteries in rabbits. JACC 7: 213A.

Hansen DD, Auth D, Vracko R, Ritchie JL (1986) Rotating mechanical angioplasty in atherosclerotic illiac (sic) vessels in rabbits. X World Congress of Cardiology, Abstract Book 1: 280, #1599.

Hansen DD, Auth DC, Hall M, Ritchie JL (1988) Rotational endarterectomy in normal canine coronary arteries: preliminary report. JACC 11: 1073–1077.

Hansen DD, Auth DC, Vracko R, Ritchie JL (1987) Mechanical thrombectomy: A comparison of two rotational devices and balloon angioplasty in subacute canine femoral thrombosis. Am Heart J: 1223–1231.

Hansen DD, Auth DC, Vracko R, Ritchie JL (1988) Rotational atherectomy in atherosclerotic rabbit iliac arteries. Am Heart J 115: 160–165.

Hansen DD, Auth DC, Vracko R, Ritchie JL (1988) Rotational thrombectomy in acute canine coronary thrombosis International Journal of Cardiology 22: 13–19.

Hansen DD, Hall M, Intlekofer MJ, Auth D, Ritchie JL (1986) In-vivo rotational angioplasty in atherosclerotic rabbits; comparison of angioscopy and angiography. Circulation (Suppl II) 74: II-362.

Hansen DD, Hall M, Intlekofer MJ, Auth D, Ritchie JL (1986) In-vivo rotational angioplasty in atherosclerotic rabbits: comparison of angioscopy and angiography. International Symposium on Interventional Cardiology, Abstract Book 1: 58.

Hansen DD, Intlekofer MJ, Hall M, Ritchie JL (1987) In-vivo rotational endarterectomy in canine coronary arteries. Lasers Surg Med 7: 82.

Hansen DD, Vracko R, Auth D, Ritchie JL, Intlekofer MJ (1986) In-vivo rotational angioplasty in canine coronary arteries. International Symposium Interventional Cardiology, Abstract Book 1: 106.

Hatfield S (1989) Research reporting preliminary success with Rotablator$_{TM}$. Advance 2: 1.

Hinohara T, Robertson GC, Selmon MR, Vetter JW, Rowe MH, Braden LJ, McAuley BJ, et al. (1992) Restenosis after directional coronary atherectomy. J Am Coll Cardiol 20(3): 623–632.

Hinohara T, Rowe MH, Robertson GC, Selmon MR, Braden L, Leggett JH, Vetter JW, Simpson JB (1991) Effect of lesion characteristics on outcome of directional coronary atherectomy. J Am Coll Cardiol 17: 1112–1120.

Hinohara T, Selmon MR, Robertson GC, Braden L, Simpson JS (1990) Directional atherectomy. New approaches for treatment of obstructive coronary and peripheral vascular disease. Circulation 81(Suppl 3): IV79–91.

Hofling B, Gonschior P, Simpson L, Bauriedel G, Nerlich A (1992) Efficacy of directional coronary atherectomy in cases unsuitable for percutaneous transluminal coronary angioplasty (PTCA) and after unsuccessful PTCA. Am Heart J 124(2): 341–348.

Hofling B, Simpson JB, Remberger K, Lauterjung L, Backa D (1987) Percutaneous atherectomy in iliac, femoral and popliteal arteries. Klin Wochenschr 65: 528.

Isner JM, Rosenfield K, Losordo DW, Kelly S, Palefski P, Langevin RE, Razvi S, Pastore JO, Kosowsky BD (1990) Percutaneous intravascular US as adjunct to catheter-based interventions: preliminary experience in patients with peripheral vascular disease. Radiology 175: 61–70.

Isner JM, Rosenfield K, White CJ, Rame S, Kearney M, Pieczek A, Langevin RE Jr, Razvi S (1992) In vivo assessment of vascular pathology resulting from laser irradiation. Analysis of 23 patients studied by directional atherectomy immediately after laser angioplasty. Circulation 85(6): 2185–2196.

Jenkins RD, Sinclair IN, Anand R, Kalil AG, Hr, Schoen FJ, Spears JR (1988) Laser balloon angioplasty: effect of tissue temperature on weld strength of human postmortem intima-media separations. Lasers Surg Med 8: 30–39.

Johnson DE (1990) Directional peripheral atherectomy: histopathologic aspects of a new interventional technique. J Vasc Intervent Radiol 1(1): 29–33.

Johnson DE, Braden L, Simpson JB (1990) Mechanism of directed transluminal atherectomy. Am J Cardiol 65: 389–391.

Johnson DE, Hinohara T, Selmon MR, Braden LJ, Simpson JB (1990) Primary peripheral arterial stenoses and restenoses excised by transluminal atherectomy: a histopathologic study (see comments). Comment in: J Am Coll Cardiol 15: 426–428. J Am Coll Cardiol 15: 419–425.

Kahn JK, Hartzler GO (1990) Retrieval of vein graft suture fragments with directional coronary atherectomy: a note of caution. Am Heart J 120: 692–696.

Karsch KR, Haase KK, Mauser M, Voelker W (1989) Initial angiographic results in ablation of atherosclerotic plaque by percutaneous coronary excimer laser angioplasty without subsequent balloon dilatation. Am J Cardiol 64: 1253–1257.

Kaufmann UP, Garratt KN, Vlietstra RE, Holmes DR, Jr (1990) Transluminal atherectomy of saphenous vein aortocoronary bypass grafts. Am J Cardiol 65: 1430–1433.

Kim D, Gianturco LE, Porter DH, Orron DE, Kuntz RE, Kent KC, Siegel JB, Schlam BW, Skillman JJ (1992) Peripheral directional atherectomy: 4-year experience. Radiology 183(3): 773–778.

Kim D, Porter DH, Siegel JB, Mowschenson PM, Steer ML (1990) Common bile duct biopsy with the Simpson atherectomy catheter. AJR Am J Roentgenol 154: 1213–1215.

Kimball BP, Bui S, Carere RG, Cohen EA, Adelman AG (1992) Acute outcome of directional coronary atherectomy vs standard balloon angioplasty in de novo left anterior descending stenoses. Chest 102(6): 1676–1682.

Kimball BP, Bui S, Cohen EA, Carere RG, Adelman AG (1992) Comparison of acute elastic recoil after directional coronary atherectomy versus standard balloon angioplasty. Am Heart J 124(6): 1459–1466.

Kirn TF (1989) Atheroma curettage: an idea whose time may come as several devices begin trials (news). JAMA 261: 498–499.

Krolick MA, Bugni WJ, Walsh JW (1992) Coronary artery aneurysm formation following directional coronary atherectomy. Cathet Cardiovasc Diagn 27(2): 117–121.

Kuhn FP, Kutkuhn B, Torsello G, Modder U (1991) Renal artery stenosis: preliminary results of treatment with the Strecker stent. Radiology 180: 367–372.

Kuntz RE, Gibson CM, Nobuyoshi M, Baim DS (1993) Generalized model of restenosis after conventional balloon angioplasty, stenting and directional atherectomy. J Am Coll Cardiol 21(1): 15–25.

Kuntz RE, Hinohara T, Robertson GC, Safian RD, Simpson JB, Baim DS (1992) Influence of vessel selection on the observed restenosis rate after endoluminal stenting or directional atherectomy. Am J Cardiol 70(13): 1101–1108.

Kuntz RE, Hinohara T, Safian RD, Selmon MR, Simpson JB, Baim DS

(1992) Restenosis after directional coronary atherectomy. Effects of luminal diameter and deep wall excision. Circulation 86(5): 1394–1399.

Kuntz RE, Piana R, Schnitt SJ, Johnson RG, Safian RD, Baim DS (1991) Early ostial vein graft stenosis: management by atherectomy. Cathet Cardiovasc Diagn 24: 41–44.

Kuntz RE, Safian RD, Carrozza JP, Fishman RF, Mansour M, Baim DS (1992) The importance of acute luminal diameter in determining restenosis after coronary atherectomy or stenting. Circulation 86(6): 1827–1835.

Kusnick CA, Wright AM, Ginsburg R, Thorpe PE, Jenkins N, Wexler L (1988) High speed rotary atherectomy in the lower extremities: early results with Rotablator$_{TM}$. Radiology 169P: (Suppl) 306.

Lai P, O'Neill WW, Auth D, Abrams GD, Glass H, Long R, Pitt B (1985) Nonsurgical human coronary endarterectomy: Use of a mechanical rotary catheter. Circulation (Part II) 72: 4, III-371.

Langes K, Schofer J, Bleifeld W, Mathey DG (1989) Catheter atherectomy: functional results in peripheral arterial disease. Angiology 40: 830–834.

Leclerc G, Isner JM, Kearney M, Simons M, Safian RD, Baim DS, Weir L (1992) Evidence implicating nonmuscle myosin in restenosis. Use of in situ hybridization to analyze human vascular lesions obtained by directional atherectomy (see comments). Circulation 85(2): 543–553.

Lee G, Morelli R, Long JB, Shea W, Lopez AC, Cunningham TM, Mason DT (1989) Combined laser-thermal and atherectomy treatment of peripheral arterial occlusion: documentation by angioscopy and angiography. Am Heart J 118: 1324–1327.

Lee TC, Hartzler GO, Rutherford BD, McConahay DR (1990) Removal of an occlusive coronary dissection flap by using an atherectomy catheter. Cathet Cardiovasc Diagn 20: 185–188.

Lukes P, Wihed A, Tidebrant G, Risberg B, Ortenwall P, Seeman T (1992) Combined angioplasty with the Kensey catheter and balloon angioplasty in occlusive arterial disease. A preliminary report. Acta Radiol 33(3): 230–233.

Maynar M, Reyes R, Cabrera V, Roman M, Pulido JM, Castaneda F, Letourneau JG, Castaneda-Zuniga WR (1989) Percutaneous atherectomy as an alternative treatment for postangioplasty obstructive intimal flaps. Radiology 170: 1029–1031.

Miller BV, Sharp WJ, Shamma AR, Kresowik TF, Petrone S, Corson JD (1991) Surveillance for recurrent stenosis after endovascular procedures. A prospective study. Arch Surg 126: 867–871.

Miller MJ, Kuntz RE, Friedrich SP, Leidig GA, Fishman RF, Schnitt SJ, Baim DS, et al. (1993) Frequency and consequences of intimal hyperplasia in specimens retrieved by directional atherectomy of native primary coronary artery stenoses and subsequent restenoses. Am J Cardiol 71(8): 652–658.

Mintz GS, Potkin BN, Keren G, Satler LF, Pichard AD, Kent KM, Popma JJ, et al. (1992) Intravascular ultrasound evaluation of the effect of rotational atherectomy in obstructive atherosclerotic coronary artery disease. Circulation 86(5): 1383–1393.

Naftilan AJ (1991) Chemical atherectomy. A novel approach to restenosis [editorial; comment]. Circulation 84: 945–947.

Nakagawa N, Cragg AH, Smith TP, Landas SK, De Jong SC (1990) Peripheral atherectomy: experimental results with a new device. J Vasc Intervent Radiol 1(1): 127–132.

Newman GE, Miner DG, Sussman SK, Phillips HR, Mikat EM, McCann RL (1988) Peripheral artery atherectomy: description of technique and report of initial results. Radiology 169: 677–680.

O'Neill WW (1992) Mechanical rotational atherectomy. Am J Cardiol 69(15): 12F–18F.

O'Neill WW, Bates RE, Kirsh M, Bassett J, Sakwa M, Elliott M, Doppke D (1989) Mechanical transluminal coronary endarterectomy: initial clinical experience with the Auth mechanical rotary catheter. JACC 13: 227A.

O'Neill WW, Friedman HZ, Cragg D, Strzelecki MR, Gangadharan V, Levine AB, Ramos RG (1989) Initial clinical experience and early follow-up of patients undergoing mechanical rotary endarterectomy. Circulation (Suppl II) 80: 4.

Overmeyer K, Genetos BC, Kaminsky ME, Mirro MJ (1989) Percutaneous atherectomy of the popliteal artery. Indiana Med 82: 362–365.

Parker BC, Morano JU, Huckabee RE (1990) Radiological seminar CCXLV: Use of the Simpson atherectomy catheter in a lesion resistant to percutaneous transluminal angioplasty. J Miss State Med Assoc 31: 71–74.

Payne JS (1992) Alternatives for revascularization: peripheral atherectomy devices. J Vasc Nursing 10(1): 2–8.

Penny WF, Schmidt DA, Safian RD, Erny RE, Baim DS (1991) Insights into the mechanism of luminal improvement after directional coronary atherectomy. Am J Cardiol 67: 435–437.

Pomerantz RM, Kuntz RE, Carrozza JP, Fishman RF, Mansour M, Schnitt SJ, Safian RD, Baim DS (1992) Acute and long-term outcome of narrowed saphenous venous grafts treated by endoluminal stenting and directional atherectomy. Am J Cardiol 70(2): 161–167.

Popma JJ, De Cesare NB, Pinkerton CA, Kereiakes DJ, Whitlow P, King SB 3d, Topol EJ, et al. (1993) Quantitative analysis of factors influencing late lumen loss and restenosis after directional coronary atherectomy. Am J Cardiol 71(7): 552–557.

Porter DH, Kim D, Siegel JB, Storella JM, Silverstone DZ (1991) Atherectomy facilitated by long vascular sheaths. AJR 156: 173–175.

Prevosti LG, Cook JA, Unger EF, Sheffield CD, Almajor Y, Bartorelli AL, Leon MB (1988) Particulate debris from rotational atherectomy: size distribution and physiologic effect. Circulation (Suppl II) 78: II-83.

Rees M, Gehani AA, Richens D (1988) Percutaneous dynamic removal of atheroma [letter] Lancet 1: 174.

Reid JD, Hsiang YN, Doyle DL, Sladen JG, Fry PD, Machan LS, Chipperfield P, Marsh JI, Harrison PB (1992) Atherectomy. Early use of three differenct methods. Can J Surg 35(3): 242–245.

Ritchie JL, Hansen DD, Intlekofer MJ, Hall M, Auth DC (1987) Rotational approaches to atherectomy and thrombectomy. Zeitschrift fur Kardiologie (Suppl 6) 76: 59–65.

Ritchie JL, Hansen DD, Intlekofer MJ, Vracko R, Auth D (1986) Thrombolysis: a new rotational thrombectomy catheter and evaluation by angioscopy. International Symposium on Interventional Cardiology, Abstract Book 1: 61.

Rosenblum J, Stertzer SH, Schechtmann NS, Hidalgo B, Baciewicz PA, Myler RK (1991) Brachial rotational atherectomy. Cathet Cardiovasc Diagn 24: 32–36.

Rowe MH, Hinohara T, White NW, Robertson GC, Selmon MR, Simpson JB (1990) Comparison of dissection rates and angiographic results following directional coronary atherectomy and coronary angioplasty. Am J Cardiol 66: 49–53.

Sabri MN, Johnson D, Warner M, Cowley MJ (1992) Intracoronary thrombolysis followed by directional atherectomy: a combined approach for thrombotic vein graft lesions considered unsuitable for angioplasty. Cathet Cardiovasc Diagn 26(1): 15–18.

Safian RD, Gelbfish JS, Erny RE, Schnitt SJ, Schmidt DA, Baim DS (1990) Coronary atherectomy. Clinical, angiographic, and histological findings and observations regarding potential mechanisms [see comments]. Comment in: Circulation 82: 305–307. Circulation 82: 69–79.

Sanborn TA (1990) Percutaneous peripheral atherectomy: what are its indications? [editorial; comment] Comment on: J Am Coll Cardiol 15: 682–688. J Am Coll Cardiol 15: 689–690.

Schnitt SJ, Safian RD, Kuntz RE, Schmidt DA, Baim DS (1992) Histologic findings in specimens obtained by percutaneous directional coronary atherectomy. Hum Pathol 23(4): 415–420.

Serruys PW, Umans VA, Strauss BH, van Suylen RJ, van den Brand M, Suryapranata H, de Feyter PJ, Roelandt J (1991) Quantitative angiography after directional coronary atherectomy. Br Heart J 66: 122–129.

Simons M, Leclerc G, Safian RD, Isner JM, Weir L, Baim DS (1993) Relation between activated smooth-muscle cells in coronary-artery lesions and restenosis after atherectomy. N Engl J Med 328(9): 608–613.

Simpson JB, Selmon MR, Robertson GC, Cipriano PR, Hayden WG, Johnson DE, Fogarty TJ (1988) Transluminal atherectomy for occlusive peripheral vascular disease. Am J Cardiol 61: 96G–101G.

Smalling RW, Cassidy DB, Schmidt WA, Barrett R, Fulford S, Kirkeeide RL (1991) Effects of rotational atherectomy in normal canine coronary and diseased human cadaveric arteries: potential for plaque removal from distal, tortuous, and diffusely diseased vessels. Cathet Cardiovasc Diagn 24(4): 300–307.

Snyder SO Jr, Wheeler JR, Gregory RT, Gayle RG, Mariner DR (1988) The Kensey catheter: preliminary results with a transluminal atherectomy tool. J Vasc Surg 8: 541–543.

Stack RS (1989) New interventional technologies in cardiology. (1989) Mayo Clin Proc 64: 867–870.

Steenkiste AR, Baim DS, Sipperly ME, Desvigne-Nickens P, Robertson T, Detre K (1991) The NACI Registry: an instrument for the evaluation of new approaches to coronary intervention. The NACI Investigators. Cathet Cardiovasc Diagn 23: 270–281.

Stokes KR, Strunk HM, Campbell DR, Gibbons GW, Wheeler HG, Clouse ME (1990) Five-year results of iliac and femoropopliteal angioplasty in diabetic patients. Radiology 174: 977–982.

Strauss BH, Umans VA, van Suylen RJ, de Feyter PJ, Marco J, Robertson GC, Renkin J, et al. (1992) Directional atherectomy for treatment of restenosis within coronary stents: clinical, angiographic and histologic results. J Am Coll Cardiol 20(7): 1465–1473.

Thorpe PE, Ginsburg R, Wright AM, Kusnick CA, Baxter R, Wittich GR, Jenkins N, Wexler L (1988) Evolution of lower extremity angioplasty: Stanford experience comparing the use of Laser, Kensey Catheter, Rotablator$_{TM}$, and Atherectomy Catheter as adjuncts to balloon angioplasty for vascular occlusions. Radiology 169P: (Suppl) 306.

Triller J, Do DD, Maddern G, Mahler F (1992) Femoropopliteal artery occlusion: clinical experience with the Kensey catheter. Radiology 182: 257–261.

Umans V, Haine E, Renkin J, de Feyter P, Wijns W, Serruys PW (1992) One hundred and thirteen attempts at directional coronary atherectomy: the early and combined experience of two European centres using quantitative angiography to assess their results. Eur Heart J 13(7): 918–924.

Umans VA, Beatt KJ, Rensing BJ, Hermans WR, de Feyter PJ, Serruys PW (1991) Comparative quantitative angiographic analysis of directional coronary atherectomy and balloon coronary angioplasty. Am J Cardiol 68: 1556–1563.

Umans VA, Strauss BH, de Feyter PJ, Serruys PW (1991) Edge detection versus videodensitometry for quantitative angiographic assessment of directional coronary atherectomy. Am J Cardiol 68: 534–539.

Umans VA, Strauss BH, Rensing BJ, de Jaegere P, de Feyter PJ, Serruys PW (1991) Comparative angiographic quantitative analysis of the immediate efficacy of coronary atherectomy with balloon angioplasty, stenting, and rotational ablation. Am Heart J 122: 836–843.

Vallbracht C, Liermann D, Prignitz I, Beinborn W, Landgraf H, Paasch C, Roth FJ, Kollath J, Schoop W, Bamberg W, et al (1988) Results of low speed rotational angioplasty for chronic peripheral occlusions. Am J Cardiol 62: 935–940.

Vallbracht C, Liermann DD, Prignitz I, Beinborn W, Roth FJ, Kollath J, Landgraf H, Kaltenbach M (1989) Low-speed rotational angioplasty in chronic peripheral artery occlusions: experience in 83 patients. Work in progress. Radiology 172: 327–330.

Von Polnitz A, Hofling B (1989) Percutaneous atherectomy of a recurrent renal transplant artery stenosis. Transplantation 48: 880–883.

Von Polnitz A, Nerlich A, Berger H, Hofling B (1990) Percutaneous peripheral atherectomy: angiographic and clinical follow-up of 60 patients [see comments]. Comment in: J Am Coll Cardiol 1: 689–690. J Am Coll Cardiol 1: 682–688.

Vorwerk D, Guenther RW (1990) Removal of intimal hyperplasia in vascular endoprostheses by atherectomy and balloon dilatation. AJR Am J Roentgenol 154: 617–619.

Vroegindeweij D, Kemper FJ, Tielbeek AV, Buth J, Landman G (1992) Recurrence of stenoses following balloon angioplasty and Simpson atherectomy of the femoro-popliteal segment. A randomised comparative 1-year follow-up study using colour flow duplex. Eur J Vasc Surg 6(2): 164–171.

Webb JG, Dodek AA, Allard M, Carere R, Marsh I (1992) 'Salvage atherectomy' for discrete arterial dissections resulting from balloon angioplasty. Can J Cardiol 8(5): 481–486.

Weibull H, Lundqvist B, Falt K, Spangen L, Feith F, Bergqvist D (1991) Peroperative arterial recanalization with Kensey dynamic angioplasty. Histopathologic studies. Eur J Surg 157: 385–387.

Wholey MH, Jarmolowski CR (1989) New reperfusion devices: The Kensey catheter, the atherolytic reperfusion wire device, and the transluminal extraction catheter. Radiology 172: 947–952.

Wholey MH, Smith JA, Godlewski P, Nagurka M (1989) Recanalization of total arterial occlusions with the Kensey dynamic angioplasty catheter. Radiology 172: 95–98.

Widlus DM, Osterman FA Jr (1989) Evaluation and percutaneous management of atherosclerotic peripheral vascular disease. JAMA 261: 3148–3154.

Willekens FG, Wever J, Nevelsteen A, Boeckxstaens C, Suy R, Cuesta M, Bengoechea E, Doblas M (1987) Extensive disobliteration of the aorto-iliac and common femoral arteries using the LeVeen plaque cracker. Eur J Vasc Surg 1: 391.

Wilms G, Pauwels P, Peene P, Baert AL, Vermylen J, Nevelsteen A, Suy R (1990) Percutaneous transluminal atherectomy: preliminary results. Cardiovasc Intervent Radiol 13: 18–21.

Wilms G, Peene P, Baert AL, Vermylen J, Suy R, Nevelsteen A, Pauwels P (1990) Preliminary results of percutaneous transluminal atherectomy. J Belge Radiol 73: 107–111.

Yock PG, Linker DT, White NW, Rowe MH, Selmon MR, Robertson GC, Hinohara T, Simpson JB (1989) Clinical applications of intravascular ultrasound imaging in atherectomy. Int J Card Imaging 4: 117–125.

Zacca N, Raizner A, Short D, Noon G, Wilbeacher D, Roehm J, Gotto A, Jr, Roberts R (1987) First in-vivo human experience with a recently developed rotational atherectomy device. Circulation (Suppl IV) 76: IV-46.

Zacca NM, Kleiman NS, Rodriguez AR, Heibig J, Warth D, Harris S, Minor ST, Raizner AE (1992) Rotational ablation of coronary artery lesions using single, large burrs. Cathet Cardiovasc Diagn 26(2): 92–97.

Zacca NM, Raizner AE, Noon GP, Short D, III, Weilbaecher D, Gotto A Jr, Roberts R (1989) Treatment of symptomatic peripheral atherosclerotic disease with a rotational atherectomy device. Am J Cardiol 63: 77–80.

Zacca NM, Raizner AE, Noon GP, Short DH III, Weilbaecher DG, Gotto AM Jr, Roberts R (1988) Short term follow up of patients treated with a recently developed rotational atherectomy device and in-vivo assessment of the particles generated. JACC 11: 109A.

Zacca NM, Raizner AE, Short HD III, Noon GP, Weilbaecher DG, Roehm JOJ Jr, Gotto AM Jr, Roberts R (1987) First in-vivo human experience with a recently developed rotational atherectomy device. Texas Heart Institute Cardiology and Cardiovascular Surgery: Interventions, 1987 Annual Symposium, Abstract Book 32.

Zacca NM, Short HD III, Edwards T, Rosborough J, Raizner AE, Noon GP, Weilbaecher DG, Bolli R (1987) In-vivo assessment of particles generated by rotational atherectomy of human atheroma. Texas Heart Institute of Cardiology and Cardiovascular Surgery: Interventions, 1987 Annual Symposium, Abstract Book 158.

Zaitoun R, Dorros G, Iyer SS, Lewin RF (1990) Percutaneous high-speed rotational atherectomy (Rotablator) of a restenosed ostial renal artery: a case report. Cathet Cardiovasc Diagn 20: 254–256.

Zeitler E, Kensey K (1988) First own results with dynamic angioplasty with the Kensey-catheter. Ann Radiol 31: 77–81.

Zemel G, Katzen BT, Dake MD, Benenati JF, Lempert TE, Moskowitz L (1990) Directional atherectomy in the treatment of stenotic dialysis access fistulas. J Vasc Intervent Radiol 1(1): 35–38.

Zotz RJ, Erbel R, Philipp A, Judt A, Wagner H, Lauterborn W, Meyer J (1992) High-speed rotational angioplasty-induced echo contrast in vivo and in vitro optical analysis. Cathet Cardiovasc Diagn 26(2): 98–109.

IV. Catheters, Guide Wires, and Angiography

Abele JE (1980) Balloon catheters and transluminal dilatation: technical considerations. AJR 135: 901–906.

Abele JE (1983) Technical considerations: physical properties of balloon catheters, inflation devices, and pressure measurement devices. In: Castaneda WR (ed) Transluminal Angioplasty. New York, Thieme-Stratton, pp 20–27.

Abrams HL (ed) (1983) Abrams angiography: vascular and interventional radiology, third edition. Boston, Little, Brown and Company.

Amplatz K, Formanek G, Stanger P, Wilson W (1967) Mechanics of Selective Coronary Artery Catheterization via Femoral Approach. Radiology 89: 1040–1047.

Angelini P (1989) Use of mechanical injectors during percutaneous transluminal coronary angioplasty (PTCA). Cathet Cardiovasc Diagn 16: 193–194.

Au PK (1991) Nonionic contrast media and intracatheter clot formation during use of a perfusion balloon catheter [letter]. Cathet Cardiovasc Diagn 22: 235–236.

Bakal CW, Friedland RJ, Sprayregen S, Calligaro KD, Cynamon J, Veith FJ (1991) Translumbar arch aortography: a retrospective controlled study of usefulness, technique, and safety. Radiology 178: 225–228.

Bakal CW, Sprayregen S (1986) Determining arterial entry side for catheter (letter). AJR 147: 438.

Banka VS, Baker HA 3d, Vemuri DN, Voci G, Maniet AR (1992) Effectiveness of decremental diameter balloon catheters (tapered balloon). Am J Cardiol 69(3): 188–193.

Bauriedel G, DeMaio SJ Jr, Hofling B (1992) Sheath introducer technique for recanalizing total occlusions of the superficial femoral artery. Cathet Cardiovasc Diagn 25(1): 66–70.

Bell MR, Berger PB, Menke KK, Holmes DR Jr (1992) Balloon angioplasty of chronic total coronary artery occlusions: what does it cost in radiation exposure, time, and materials? Cathet Cardiovasc Diagn 25(1): 10–15.

Berman HL, Katz SG, Tihansky DP (1986) Guided direct antegrade puncture of the superficial femoral artery. AJR 147: 632–634.

Berman HL, Martin MB (1982) A simplified method for antegrade sheath introduction into the common femoral artery. AJR 138: 973.

Bertrand ME, Lablanche JM, Bauters C, Leroy F, Mac Fadden E (1993) Discordant results of visual and quantitative estimates of stenosis severity before and after coronary angioplasty. Cathet Cardiovasc Diagn 28(1): 1–6.

Bishop AF, Berkman WA, Palagallo GL (1985) Antegrade selective catheterization of the superficial femoral artery using a movable-core guide wire. Radiology 157: 548.

Bogart DB, Brown B, Mortko P, Miller JT (1989) Use of exchange wires in coronary angioplasty. Cathet Cardiovasc Diagn 16: 139–140.

Bowser MA, Lozner EC, Johnson LW (1989) Simplified two-wire technique for bifurcation lesions during coronary angioplasty. Cathet Cardiovasc Diagn 16: 136–138.

Campbell DR, Mason WF, Flemming BK, Fraser DB (1983) Digital subtraction arteriography (DSA) in re-evaluation of angioplasties. J Can Assoc Radiol 34: 258–260.

Cardella JF, Kotula F, Hunter DW, Young AT, Castaneda-Zuniga WR, Amplatz K (1985) Very stiff guide wire with a floppy tip. Radiology 156: 837.

Castellanos A, Pereiras R (1980) Counter-current aortography. Rev Cubana Cardiol 2: 187.

Cho KJ (1982) Renal angiography in renovascular hypertension. Urol Radiol 3: 213–218.

Chopra PS, Grassi CJ (1992) Superior mesenteric artery angioplasty with the TEGwire: usefulness and technical difficulties. J Vasc Intervent Radiol 3(3): 523–526.

Chuang V (1981) Basic rule in catheter selection for visceral angiography. AJR, 136: 432–433.

Chuang V, Soo C, Wallace S (1983) Superselective Catheterization Technique in Hepatic Angiography. AJR 141: 803–811.

Clermont A, Gourdol Y, Valette PJ, Pinet F (1985) Cine-angiography during percutaneous transluminal angioplasty of the lower limbs. Int Angiol 4: 99–100.

Coons HG (1985) A floppy-tipped wire guide for interventional procedures. AJR 144: 254.

Cope C (1983) Stiff fine-needle guide wire for catheterizations and drainage. Radiology 147: 264.

Corcos T, Favereau X, Poirot G, Souffrant G (1990) Orion, an improved balloon on a wire system: initial experience. Cathet Cardiovasc Diagn 20: 103–107.

De Muinck ED, van Dijk RB, den Heijer P, Meeder JG, Lie KI (1992) Autoperfusion balloon catheter for complicated coronary angioplasty: a prospective study with retrospective controls. Int J Cardiol 37(3): 317–327.

Dorros G, Lewin RF (1989) The Probe exchange catheter. Cathet Cardiovasc Diagn 16: 263–266.

Dorros G, Lewin RF, Mathiak L (1988) Probe, a balloon wire: initial experience. Cathet Cardiovasc Diagn 14: 286–288.

Dotter CT (1968) Therapeutic catheter systems. Proceedings of the Fifth Annual Rocky Mountain Bioengineering Symposium, May 6–7, 1968. IEEE Trans Biomed Eng 102–104.

Dotter CT (1983) Vascular catheterization using a rigid guide. Radiology 148: 305.

Dotter CT, Rosch J, Robinson M (1978) Fluoroscopically aided femoral artery puncture: technical note. Radiology 127: 266–267.

Duda SH, Wehrmann M, Haase KK, Huppert PE, Karsch KR, Claussen CD (1992) Holmium:YAG laser angioplasty. Experimental ablation of vascular tissue via flexible ring catheters. Acta Radiologica 33(6): 538–541.

Dwyer ML, Colombo A, Bozzi G (1989) Retrieval technique of a PTCA guidewire. G Ital Cardiol 19: 170–172.

Esplugas E, Cequier AR, Sabate X, Jara F (1990) False coronary dissection with the new Monorail angioplasty balloon catheter. Cathet Cardiovasc Diagn 19: 30–33.

Favaloro RG (1990) Computerized tabulation of cine coronary angiograms. Its implication for results of randomized trials. Circulation 81: 1991–2003.

Fields WS, Lemak NA (1972) Joint study of extracranial arterial occlusion VII subclavian steal: a review of 168 cases. JAMA 222: 1139–1143.

Fink U, Heywang SH, Hilbertz T, Fischer K, Jenner E, Buchsteiner W (1991) Peripheral DSA with automated stepping. Eur J Radiol 13: 50–54.

Fogarty TJ, Chin A, Shoor PM, Blair GL, Zimmerman JJ (1981) Adjunctive intraoperative arterial dilation: simplified instrumentation technique. Arch Surg 116: 1391–1398.

Fogarty TJ, Kinney TB, Finn JC (1984) Current status of dilatation catheters and guiding systems. Am J Cardiol 53: 97C-101C.

Frainas PL (1941) A new technique for arteriographic examination of the abdominal aorta and its branches. Am J Roentgenol 46: 641–645.

Frink NC, Paolella LP, Dorfman GS (1990) Angioplasty sites: assessment with the dual-access technique. Radiology 174: 264.

Gaines PA, Cumberland DC (1988) Wire-loop technique for angioplasty of total iliac artery occlusions. Radiology 168: 275–276.

Gaylord GM, Pritchard WF, Chuang VP, Casarella WJ, Sprawls P (1988) The geometry of triple-balloon dilation. Radiology 166: 541–545.

Gerlock AJ, Regen DM, Shaff MI (1982) An examination of the physical characteristics leading to angioplasty balloon rupture. Radiology 144: 421–422.

Ginsburg R, Thorpe P, Bowles CR, Wright AM, Wexler L (1989) Pull-through approach to percutaneous angioplasty of totally occluded common iliac arteries. Radiology 172: 111–113.

Ginsburg R, Wexler L (1989) Hydrophilic guide wire for laser-assisted angioplasty [letter]. J Vasc Surg 9: 507–508.

Goudreau E, Vetrovec GW (1992) A technique to access severely diseased arteries. Cathet Cardiovasc Diagn 26(1): 53–54.

Grable GS, Smith DC (1980) The use of the Simmons "sidewinder" catheter in percutaneous transluminal angioplasty of the renal arteries. Radiology 137: 541–543.

Grollman JH, Rennar JW (1981) Transfemoral pulmonary angiography: update on technique. AJR 136: 624–626.

Gruentzig A, Kumpe DA (1979) Technique of percutaneous transluminal angioplasty with the Gruentzig balloon catheter. AJR 132: 547–552.

Gruentzig AR, Meier B (1984) Current status of dilatation catheters and guiding systems. Am J Cardiol 53: 92C-93C.

Gunther RW, Vorwerk D (1991) Minibasket for percutaneous embolectomy and filter protection against distal embolization: technical note. Cardiovasc Intervent Radiol 14: 195–198.

Gurley JC, Booth DC, Hixson C, Smith MD (1990) Removal of retained intracoronary percutaneous transluminal coronary angioplasty equipment by a percutaneous twin guidewire method. Cathet Cardiovasc Diagn 19: 251–255.

Halden WJ Jr., White RI, Jr., Bright J, Mitchell SE, Chang R (1986) Vessel measurement using digital subtraction arteriography. Radiology 161: 556–557.

Hamada Y, Matsuda Y, Takashiba K, Ohno H, Fujii B, Ebihara H, Hyakuna E (1989) Difficult deflation of Probe balloon due to twisting the system. Cathet Cardiovasc Diagn 18: 12–14.

Hawkins IF (1972) A deflector catheter approach to the abdominal aorta. AJR 116: 196–198.

Hawkins IF, Hawkins MC (1983) New coaxial exchange guide wire with a variable-length tip. Radiology 148: 303–304.

Henson JH, Jeans WD, Newham FJ, Paice C, Blakeborough A (1988) Assessment of angioplasty balloon catheters: preliminary studies. Br J Radiol 61: 1026–1031.

Hibbard MD, Holmes DR, Jr (1992) The Tracker catheter: a new vascular access system. Cathet & Cardiovasc Diagn 27(4): 309–316.

Horvath L, Illes I (1979) The use of Gruentzig balloon catheter in obstructive arterial disease. Intervention radiology. Proceedings of the First International Symposium on Intervention Radiology, Algarve, Portugal.

Jorgensen B, Skovgaard N, Norgard J, Karle A, Holstein P, Percutaneous transluminal angioplasty in 226 iliac artery stenoses: role of the superficial femoral artery for clinical success. Vasa 21(4): 382–386.

Jorgensen RA, Dobrin PB (1983) Balloon embolectomy catheters in small arteries: IV. Correlation of shear forces with histologic injury. Surgery 93: 798–808.

Kadir S (1980) Loop catheter technique: a simple, rapid method for left adrenal vein catheterization. AJR 134: 31–33.

Kadir S (1981) Loop catheter technique. Med Radiogr Photogr (Kodak) 57: 22–30.

Katritsis D, Webb-Peploe MM (1990) Cardiac phase-related variability of border detection or densitometric quantitation of postangioplasty lumens. Am Heart J 120: 537–543.

Katzen BT, Chang J (1979) Percutaneous transluminal angioplasty with the Gruentzig balloon catheter. Radiology 130: 623–626.

Kaufman SL (1980) Femoral puncture using Doppler ultrasound guidance: aid to transluminal angioplasty and other applications. AJR 134: 402.

Kerber, CW, Newton TH (1972) The long tapered catheter. J Neuroradiol 3: 182–183.

Kinnison ML, Steinberg EP, Powe NR, Anderson GF (1988) Reducing the cost of using contrast media: a look at discarded volumes. Radiology 166: 367–370.

Korogi Y, Takahashi M (1993) A double-guide-wire technique in renal angioplasty. A modified approach. Acta Radiol 34(2): 196–197.

Kumar K, Kaul U, Dev V, Rajani M, Sharma S (1991) Probe angioplasty through an intracoronary probing catheter in lesions which are difficult to cross. Int J Cardiol 30: 157–162.

Kumpe D, Gruentzig A (1979) Technique of percutaneous transluminal angioplasty with the Gruentzig balloon catheter. AJR 132: 547–552.

Lee DW, Garnic JD (1988) Application of tapered teflon dilator to PTCA. Angiology 39: 381–384.

Levin DC (1983) Catheters for selective arteriography: additional configuration alternatives. Radiology 146: 553–554.

Levin DC, Harrington DP, Bettmann MA, Garnic JD, Torman H, Murray P, Boxt LM, Geller SC (1984) Equipment choices, technical aspects and pitfalls of percutaneous transluminal angioplasty. Cardiovasc Intervent Radiol 7: 1–10.

Link DP, Foerster JM, Lantz Bo MT, Holcroft JW (1981) Assessment of peripheral blood flow in man by video dilution technique: a preliminary report. Invest Radiol 16: 298–304.

Link DP, Lantz BM, Meinke WB, Foerster JM, Holcroft JW (1982) Vasodilator response in the lower extremity induced by contrast medium. III.

Before and after percutaneous transluminal angioplasty. Acta Radiol (Diagn) (Stockh) 23: 381–387.

Ludwig JW; Engels PH (1983) Overtoom TT Application of digital vascular imaging in interventional radiology. Ann Radiol (Paris) 26: 585–588.

Lukes P, Wihed A, Tidebrant G, Risberg B, Ortenwall P, Seeman T (1992) Combined angioplasty with the Kensey catheter and balloon angioplasty in occlusive arterial disease. A preliminary report. Acta Radiol 33(3): 230–233.

Lurie PR, Armer RM, Klatte EC (1963) Percutaneous guide wire catheterization: diagnosis and therapy. Am J Dis Child 106: 189–196.

Maat L, van Herwerden LA, van den Brand M, Bos E (1991) An unusual problem during surgical removal of a broken guidewire. Ann Thorac Surg 51: 829–830.

Mani RL (1970) A new double-curve catheter for selective femorocerebral angiography. Radiology 94: 607–611.

Mantoni MY, Holstein P (1990) Aorto-femoral digital subtraction angiography in old patients with symptoms of peripheral arterial disease. Findings, efficacy, and consequences. Dan Med Bull 37: 192–193.

Marache P, Asseman P, Jabinet JL, Prat A, Bauchart JJ, Aisenfarb JC, Lesenne M, et al. (1993) Percutaneous transluminal venous angioplasty in occlusive iliac vein thrombosis resistant to thrombolysis. Am Heart J 125(2 Pt 1): 362–366.

Markowitz DM, Hughes SH, Shaw C, Denny DF Jr, Wilkinson LA, White RI Jr (1991) Transcatheter detachable balloon embolotherapy for catheter-induced pulmonary artery pseudoaneurysm. J Thorac Imaging 6: 75–78.

Martinelli MJ, Deutsch E, Ferraro A, Bove AA (1992) Comparison of angiographic center and local site analysis of PTCA results in a multicenter angioplasty-restenosis trial. The M Heart Group. Cathet Cardiovasc Diagn 27(1): 8–13.

Mayer JH, Wills PJ (1982) A localization grid for percutaneous transluminal angioplasty. Radiology 144: 649–650.

McDermott JC, Babel SG, Crummy AB, Wojtowycz M, Starck E (1989) Review of the uses of digital "road map" techniques in interventional radiology. Ann Radiol 32: 11–13.

McDermott JC, Starck E, Crummy AB (1986) Road map application to the pulseless common femoral artery. Cardiovasc Intervent Radiol 9: 109–110.

McFadden JT (1991) A new clip applier. Technical note. J Neurosurg 74: 304–305.

McIvor ME, Kaufman SL, Satre R, Porterfield JK, Brinker JA (1989) Search and retrieval of a radiolucent foreign object. Cathet Cardiovasc Diagn 16: 19–23.

McLean GK, Burke DR, Marinelli DL (1989) Comment on the clinical appropriateness of an emerging technology (editorial). Radiology 172: 941–942.

Meier B, Carlier M, Finci L, Nukta E, Urban P, Niederhauser W, Favre J (1989) Magnum wire for balloon recanalization of chronic total coronary occlusions. Am J Cardiol 64: 148–154.

Mitchell SE, White RI Jr, Kan J, Tolkoff J (1984) Improved balloon catheters for large-vessel and valvular angioplasty. AJR 142: 571–572.

Mullan S, Duda EE, Patronas NJ (1980) Some examples of balloon technology in neurosurgery. J Neurosurg 52: 321–329.

Murray A, Wood RF, Mitchell DC, Edwards DH, Grasty M, Basu R (1989) Peripheral laser angioplasty with pulsed dye laser and ball-tipped optical fibres. Lancet 2: 1471–1474.

Myler RK, McConahay DR, Stertzer SH, Johnson W, Cumberland DC, Boucher RA, Hidalgo B (1989) Coronary bifurcation stenoses: the kissing balloon Probe technique via a single guiding catheter. Cathet Cardiovasc Diagn 16: 267–278.

Myler RK, Mooney MR, Stertzer SH, Clark DA, Hidalgo BO, Fishman J (1988) The balloon on a wire device: a new ultra-low-profile coronary angioplasty system/concept. Cathet Cardiovasc Diagn 14: 135–140.

Nakhjavan FK (1988) Use of angioplasty guidewire for technically difficult angiography. Cathet Cardiovasc Diagn 14: 213.

Nakhjavan FK, Najmi M (1990) Exit block: a new technique for difficult side branch angioplasty. Cathet Cardiovasc Diagn 20: 43–45.

Nath A, Vetrovec GW, Cowley MJ, Newton M, DiSciascio G, Mukharji J, Lewis SA (1988) Double-wire angioplasty of the right coronary artery bifurcational stenosis. Cathet Cardiovasc Diagn 14: 37–40.

Newton CM, Lewis SA, Vetrovec GW (1988) Technique for guiding catheter exchange during coronary angioplasty while maintaining guidewire access across a coronary stenosis. Cathet Cardiovasc Diagn 15: 173–175.

Nichols AB, Smith R, Berke AD, Shlofmitz RA, Powers ER (1989) Importance of balloon size in coronary angioplasty. J Am Coll Cardiol 13: 1094–1100.

O'Connor HE, Browne KF, Bourne G, Brenner AS (1992) Sitting up post angioplasty: a new sheath technology. Cathet Cardiovasc Diagn 25(1): 76–78.

Ofili EO, Kern MJ, Labovitz AJ, St. Vrain JA, Segal J, Aguirre FV, Castello R (1993) Analysis of coronary blood flow velocity dynamics in angiographically normal and stenosed arteries before and after endolumen enlargement by angioplasty. J Am Coll Cardiol 21(2): 308–316.

O'Keefe JH Jr, Holmes DR Jr, Reeder GS, Bresnahan DR (1989) A new approach for dilation of bifurcation stenoses: the dual probe technique. Mayo Clin Proc 64: 277–281.

Olbert F, Hanecka L (1978) Transluminal vascular dilation with a modified dilatation catheter. In: Zeitler E, et al (eds) Percutaneous Vascular Recanalization. Berlin, Heidelberg, New York, Springer, chap. 6, pp 32–38.

Olbert F, Kasprzak P, Muzika N, Schlegl A (1984) Percutaneous transluminal dilatation and recanalization: long-term results and report on experience with a new catheter system. Ann Radiol (Paris) 27: 349–356.

Pan M, Medina A, Romero M, Suarez de Lezo J, Hernandez E, Pavlovic D, Melian F, et al (1992) Peripheral stent recovery after failed intracoronary delivery. Cathet Cardiovasc Diagn 27(3): 230–233.

Pande AK, Meier B, Urban P, de la Serna F, Villavicencio R, Dorsaz PA, Favre J (1992) Magnum/Magnarail versus conventional systems for recanalization of chronic total coronary occlusions: a randomized comparison. Am Heart J 123(5): 1182–1186.

Park JH, Han MC, Kim SH, Oh BH, Park YB, Seo JD (1989) Takayasu's arteritis: angiographic findings and results of angioplasty. AJR Am J Roentgenol 153: 1069–1074.

Patel YD (1990) Catheter for conversion of retrograde to antegrade femoral artery catheterization. AJR Am J Roentgenol 154: 179–180.

Patel YD (1991) Ipsilateral antegrade femoral arteriography (letter). AJR 157: 199.

Picus D (1990) Angiography in the 1990s: diagnosis and therapy [editorial; comment]. Comment on: Radiology 1990 175: 71–74. Radiology 175: 33.

Pijls NH, Aengevaeren WR, Uijen GJ, Hoevelaken A, Pijnenburg T, van Leeuwen K, van der Werf T (1991) Concept of maximal flow ratio for immediate evaluation of percutaneous transluminal coronary angioplasty result by videodensitometry. Circulation 83: 854–865.

Pollak JS, Cooper SG, Denny DF Jr (1990) Use of the balloon on a guidewire as an adjunct to conventional angioplasty. AJR 155: 887–888.

Porter BA, Link DP (1985) Interventional and angiographic uses of the Bentson guide wire. Cardiovasc Intervent Radiol 8: 204–205.

Powills S (1989) Cardiology. Heart conscious. Hospitals 63: 69, 71.

Price J, Hands LJ, Fletcher EW (1989) Removal of a nondeflating balloon angioplasty catheter after percutaneous aspiration [letter]. AJR Am J Roentgenol 152: 1347.

Proctor MS, Koch LV (1988) Surgical removal of guidewire fragment following transluminal coronary angioplasty. Ann Thorac Surg 45: 678–679.

Quigley PJ, Hinohara T, Phillips HR, Peter RH, Behar VS, Kong Y, Simonton CA, Perez JA, Stack RS (1988) Myocardial protection during coronary angioplasty with an autoperfusion balloon catheter in humans. Circulation 78: 1128–1134.

Radner S (1948) Thoracal aortography by catheterization from the radial artery. Acta Radiol (Diagn) (Stockh) 29: 178–180.

Rao KJ, Blake H, Theodossi A (1990) Use of a modified angioplasty balloon catheter in the dilatation of tight biliary strictures. Gut 31: 565–567.

Rees M, Gehani AA, Richens D (1988) Percutaneous dynamic removal of atheroma [letter]. Lancet 1: 174.

Ring EJ, Alpert JR, Freiman DB, Oleaga JA, Berkowitz H, Roberts B (1980) Early experience with percutaneous transluminal angioplasty using a vinyl balloon catheter. Ann Surg 192: 438–442.

Rizzo TF, Ciccone J, Werres R (1989) Dilating guide wire: use of a new ultra-low-profile percutaneous transluminal coronary angioplasty system. Cathet Cardiovasc Diagn 16: 258–262.

Rogers WF, Kraft MA (1990) Outpatient angioplasty. Radiology 174: 735–755.

Rosch J, Grollman JII Jr (1969) Superselective arteriography in the diagnosis of abdominal pathology: technical considerations. Radiology 92: 1008–1013.

Rosen RJ, McLean GK, Oleaga JA, Freiman DB, Ring EJ (1981) A new exchange guide wire for transluminal angioplasty. Radiology 140: 242–243.

Rozenbaum EA, Topaz O, Wysham DG (1993) Balloon catheter systems for PTCA: the importance of the catheter length. Cathet Cardiovasc Diagn 28(3): 252–255.

Saddekni S, Srur M, Cohn DJ, Rozenblit G, Wetter EB, Sos TA (1985) Antegrade catheterization of the superficial femoral artery. Radiology 157: 531–532.

Saibil EA, Maggisano R (1988) Combined antegrade-retrograde catheterization of the occluded common iliac artery prior to angioplasty. J Can Assoc Radiol 39: 228–229.

Savas V, Schreiber T, O'Neill W (1991) Percutaneous extraction of fractured guidewire from distal right coronary artery. Cathet Cardiovasc Diagn 22: 124–126.

Schwarten DE (1986) Extracardiac uses for the "steerable" coronary balloon angioplasty systems. Ann Radiol (Paris) 29: 120–126

Seggewiss H, Gleichmann U, Fassbender D, Vogt J, Mannebach H, Minami K (1992) Therapy for acute vascular complications in percutaneous transluminal coronary angioplasty with the autoperfusion balloon catheter. Euro H J 13(12): 1649–1657.

Seifert PE, Auer JE (1989) Removal of guidewire fragment (letter). Ann Thorac Surg 47: 638.

Selby JB Jr, Tegtmeyer CJ (1990) New balloon-through-balloon angioplasty technique for the treatment of segmental lesions. Radiology 177: 276–277.

Seldinger SI (1953) Catheter replacement of the needle in percutaneous arteriography. Acta Radiol (Diagn) (Stockh) 39: 368–376.

Seldinger SI (1984) Catheter replacement of needle in percutaneous arteriography: new technique, Acta Radiologica, 39 (1953), 368–376. Reproduced: The Seldinger Technique. AJR 142: 5–7.

Serota H, Deligonul U, Lew B, Kern MJ, Aguirre F, Vandormael M (1989) Improved method for transcatheter retrieval of intracoronary detached angioplasty guidewire segments. Cathet Cardiovasc Diagn 17: 248–251.

Serruys PW, Juilliere Y, Bertrand ME, Peul J, Rickards AP, Sigwart U (1988) Additional improvement of stenosis geometry in human coronary arteries by stenting after balloon dilatation. Am J Cardiol 61: 71G-76G.

Shaver RW, Soong J (1982) Angioplasty through aortofemoral graft: use of catheter-introducer sheath. AJR 138: 168–169.

Sheikh KH, Davidson CJ, Newman GE, Kisslo KB, Schwab SJ (1991) Intravascular ultrasound assessment of the renal artery. Ann Int Med 115: 22–25.

Simmons KC (1985) Crossing femoral artery occlusions and stenoses with stiffening cannula and Van Andel catheter. Cardiovasc Intervent Radiol 8: 115–6.

Simpson JB, Selmon MR, Robertson GC, Cipriano PR, Hayden WG, Johnson DE, Fogarty TJ (1988) Transluminal atherectomy for occlusive peripheral vascular disease. Am J Cardiol 61: 96G-101G.

Smith DC, Durkos JL (1982) An improved ruptured-balloon retrieval set. Radiology 144: 430–431.

Smith LD, Katritsis D, Webb-Peploe MM (1989) Use of a hollow wire to facilitate angioplasty of occluded vessels. Br Heart J 61: 326–330.

Smith TP, Darcy MD, Hunter DW, Castaneda-Zuniga WR, Amplatz K (1986) New super-stiff guide wire. Radiology 161: 551–552.

Smith TP, Derauf BJ, Darcy MD, Hunter DW, Castaneda-Zuniga WR, Amplatz K (1986) Movable core guide wire: evaluation of improved model. Radiology 159: 552–553.

Sniderman KW, Bodner L, Saddekni S, Srur M, Sos TA (1984) Percutaneous embolectomy by transcatheter aspiration. Work in progress. Radiology 150: 357–361.

Sniderman KW, Kalman PG, Shewchun J, Goldberg RE (1989) Lower-extremity in situ saphenous vein grafts: angiographic interventions. Radiology 170: 1023–1027.

Solomon RA, Fukushima T (1991) New aneurysm clip appliers for "keyhole" neurosurgery. Neurosurgery 28: 474–476.

Sos TA, Sniderman KW, Beinart C (1981) Gruentzig catheter with a 10-cm-long balloon. Radiology 141: 825–826.

Stack RS (1989) New interventional technologies in cardiology. Mayo Clin Proc 64: 867–870.

Stack RS, Quigley PJ, Collins G, Phillips HR 3rd (1988) Perfusion balloon catheter. Am J Cardiol 61: 77G-80G.

Staple TW (1968) Modified catheter for percutaneous transluminal treatment of arteriosclerotic obstructions. Radiology 91:1041–1043.

Stein MA, Winter J, Grollman JH Jr (1975) The value of the pulmonary-artery-seeking catheter in percutaneous selective pulmonary arteriography. Radiology 114: 299–304.

Stokes KR, Strunk HM, Campbell DR, Gibbons GW, Wheeler HG, Clouse ME (1990) Five-year results of iliac and femoropopliteal angioplasty in diabetic patients. Radiology 174: 977–982.

Strauss AL, Schaberle W, Rieger H, Roth FJ (1991) Use of duplex scanning in the diagnosis of arteria profunda femoris stenosis. J Vasc Surg 13: 698–704.

Tegtmeyer CJ (1988) Guide wire angioplasty balloon catheter: preliminary report. Radiology 169: 253–254.

Teitelbaum GP, Joseph GJ, Matsumoto AH, Barth KH (1989) Double-guide-wire access through a single 6-F vascular sheath. Radiology 173: 871–873.

Tenaglia AN, Quigley PJ, Kereiakes DJ, Abbottsmith CW, Phillips HR, Tcheng JE, Rendall D, et al (1992) Coronary angioplasty performed with gradual and prolonged inflation using a perfusion balloon catheter: procedural success and restenosis rate. Am Heart J 124(3): 585–589.

Thompson KR, Goldin AR (1979) Angiographic techniques in interventional radiology. Radiol Clin North Am 17: 375–391.

Tonkin IL, Stapleton FB, Roy S 3d (1988) Digital subtraction angiography in the evaluation of renal vascular hypertension in children. Pediatrics 81: 150–158.

Train JS, Mitty HA, Efremidis SC, Rabinowitz JG (1982) Visualization of a fine periluminal vascular network following transluminal angioplasty: possible demonstration of the vasa vasorum. Radiology 143: 399–403.

Van Andel GJ (1978) Transluminal dilatation with separate teflon catheters. In: Zeitler E, et al (eds) Percutaneous Vascular Recanalization. Berlin, Heidelberg, New York, Springer, chap. 3, pp 13–16.

Van Leeuwen K, Blans W, Pijls NH, Van Der Werf T (1989) Kissing balloon angioplasty of a circumflesx artery bifurcation lesion. A new approach utilizing two balloon-on-wire probes and a single guiding catheter. Chest 95: 1144–1145.

Vassanelli C, Turri M, Morando G, Menegatti G, Zardini P (1989) Open-ended guidewire: new technique for balloon angioplasty of chronically occluded coronary arteries. Cathet Cardiovasc Diagn 17: 224–227.

Violini R (1989) Guidewire technique [letter]. Cathet Cardiovasc Diagn 16: 80.

Voda J (1993) Long-tip guiding catheter: successful and safe for left coronary artery angioplasty. Cathet Cardiovasc Diagn 27(3): 234–242.

Walter JF, Bookstein JJ, Kramer RA, Cannon WB, Trollope MD, Jamplis RW (1978) Therapeutic angiography. Arch Surg 113: 432–439.

Waltman AC, Courey WR, Athanasoulis C, Baum S (1973) Technique for left gastric artery catheterization. Radiology 109: 732–734.

Weaver FA, Pentecost MJ, Yellin AE, Davis S, Finck E, Bitelbaum G (1991) Clinical applications of carbon dioxide/digital subtraction arteriography. J Vasc Surg 13: 266–272.

White RI Jr, Frech RS, Amplatz K (1971) An improved technique for right coronary artery catheterization. AJR 113: 562–566.

Wholey MH (1987) The design and clinical application of a new #5 French angioplasty catheter. Cathet Cardiovasc Diagn 13: 347–351.

Wholey MH (1988) A newly designed angioplasty catheter: "the Gemini balloon". Cardiovasc Intervent Radiol 11: 42–44.

Wikholm G (1983) Use of a modified lunderquist guide wire for percutaneous transluminal renal angioplasty. AJR 141: 605–606.

Wilson WJ, Lee GB, Amplatz K (1967) Biplane selective coronary arteriography via percutaneous transfemoral approach. AJR 100: 332–340.

Yazdanfar S, Ledley GS, Alfieri A, Strauss C, Kotler MN (1993) Parallel angioplasty dilatation catheter and guide wire: a new technique for the dilatation of calcified coronary arteries. Cathet Cardiovasc Diagn 28(1): 72–75.

Zaitoun R, Dorros G, Iyer SS, Lewin RF (1990) Percutaneous high-speed rotational atherectomy (Rotablator) of a restenosed ostial renal artery: a case report. Cathet Cardiovasc Diagn 20: 254–256.

V. Intravascular Ultrasound (Intravascular, Doppler)

Alfonso F, Macaya C, Goicolea J, Iniguez A, Hernandez R, Banuelos C, Castillo JA, et al. (1993) Angiographic changes induced by intracoronary ultrasound imaging before and after coronary angioplasty. Am Heart J 125(3): 877–880.

Amendt K, Schomig A, Wilhelm C, Hsu E, Weiss T, Diehm C, Kubler W (1992) Intravascular ultrasound (IVUS) in patients with peripheral arterial occlusive disease (PAOD). Vasa 21(1): 27–38.

Angelsen BA, et al (1990) Comparison between phased array and mechanical scanning for cross-sectional intraluminal ultrasound imaging. ASE.

Anonymous (1989) Intravascular ultrasound techniques, developments, clinical perspectives. Int J Card Imaging 4: 79–216.

Aretz HT, Gregory KW, Martinelli MA, Gregg RE, LeDet EG, Hatch GF, Sedlacek T, Haase WC (1991) Ultrasound guidance of laser atherectomy. Int J Card Imaging 6: 231–237.

Aretz HT, Martinelli MA, LeDet EG (1989) Intraluminal ultrasound guidance of transverse laser coronary atherectomy. Int J Card Imaging 4: 153–157.

Bartorelli AL, et al (1989) Intravascular ultrasound imaging of atherosclerotic coronary arteries: an in vitro validation study. J Am Coll Cardiol 13: 4A.

Bartorelli AL, Neville RF, Keren G, et al (1992) In vitro and in vivo intravascular ultrasound imaging. Eur Heart J 13: 102–108.

Barzilai BS, Saffitz JE, Miller JG, Sobel BE (1987) Quantitative ultrasonic characterization of the nature of atherosclerotic plaques in human aorta. Circ Res 60: 459–463.

Basile RM, Waters BD, Curletti EL (1990) Image-directed Doppler ultrasonography in the management of failing infrainguinal bypass grafts. JCU 18: 132–137.

Becker AE (1989) Ultrasound imaging and atherogenesis. Int J Card Imaging 4: 99–104.

Becker GJ, Lee BI, Waller BF, Barry KJ, Kaplan J, Connolly R, Dreesen RG, Nardella P (1988) Radiofrequency balloon angioplasty. Rationale and proof of principle. Invest Radiol 23: 810–817.

Bergeron P, Rudondy P, Poyen V, Pinot JJ, Alessandri C, Martelet JP (1991) Long-term peripheral stent evaluation using angioscopy. Int Angiol 10(3): 182–186.

Bom N, Slager CJ, van Egmond FC, Lancee CT, Serruys PW (1988) Intra-arterial ultrasonic imaging for recanalization by spark erosion. Ultrasound Med Biol 14: 257–261.

Bom N, Ten Hoff H, Lancee CT, Gussenhoven WJ, Bosch JG (1989) Early and recent intraluminal ultrasound devices. Int J Card Imaging 4: 79–88.

Borst C, Rienks R, Mali WP, Van Erven L (1989) Laser ablation and the need for intraarterial imaging. Int J Card Imaging 4: 127–133.

Borst C, Savalle LH, Smits PC, Post MJ, Gussenhoven WJ, Bom N (1991) Imaging of post-mortem coronary arteries by 30 MHz intravascular ultrasound. Int J Card Imaging 6: 239–246.

Buller CE, Davidson CJ, Virmani, et al (1992) Real-time assessment of experimental arterial angioplasty with transvenous intravascular ultrasound. J Am Coll Cardiol 19: 217–222.

Cacchione JG, Reddy K, Richards F, Sheehan H, Hodgson JM (1991) Combined intravascular ultrasound/angioplasty balloon catheter: initial use during PTCA. Cathet Cardiovasc Diagn 24: 99–101.

Cavaye DM, French WJ, White RA, Lerman RD, Mehringer CM, Tabbara MR, Kopchok GE (1991) Intravascular ultrasound imaging of an acute dissecting aortic aneurysm: a case report. J Vasc Surg 13: 510–512.

Cavaye DM, Tabbara MR, Kopchok GE, Laas TE, White RA (1991) Three dimensional vascular ultrasound imaging. Am Surg 57: 751–755.

Cavaye DM, Tabbara MR, Kopchok GE, Termin P, White RA (1991) Intraluminal ultrasound assessment of vascular stent deployment. Ann Vasc Surg 5: 241–246.

Cavaye DM, White RA, Lerman RD, et al (1992) Usefulness of intravascular ultrasound imaging for detecting experimentally induced aortic dissection in dogs and for determining the effectiveness of endoluminal stenting. Am J Cardiol 69: 705–707.

Collier P, Wilcox G, Brooks D, Laffey S, Dalton T (1990) Improved patient selection for angioplasty utilizing color Doppler imaging. Am J Surg 160: 171–174.

Coy KM, Maurer G, Siegel RJ (1991) Intravascular ultrasound imaging: a current perspective. J Am Coll Cardiol 18: 1811–1823.

Coy KM, Park JC, Sheffer A, Smith A, Ariani M, Chae JS, Siegel RJ (1991) Spontaneous echo contrast effect as an indicator of flow-limiting coronary stenosis. Am J Cardiol 68: 276–277.

Crowley RJ, Hamm MA, Joshi SH, Lennox CD, Roberts GT (1991) Ultrasound guided therapeutic catheters: recent developments and clinical results. Int J Card Imaging 6: 145–156.

Crowley RJ, Von Behren PL, Couvillon LA Jr, Mai DE, Abele JE (1989) Optimized ultrasound imaging catheters for use in the vascular system. Int J Card Imaging 4: 145–151.

Dake MD (1991) Intravascular ultrasound. Curr Opin Radiol 3: 181–187.

Davidson CJ, Newman GE, Sheikh KH, Kisslo K, Stack RS, Schwab SJ (1991) Mechanisms of angioplasty in hemodialysis fistula stenoses evaluated by intravascular ultrasound. Kidney Int 40: 91–95.

Davidson CJ, Sheikh KH, Harrison JK, Himmelstein SI, Leithe ME, Kisslo KB, Bashore TM (1990) Intravascular ultrasonography versus digital subtraction angiography: a human in vivo comparison of vessel size and morphology. J Am Coll Cardiol 16: 633–636.

Davidson CJ, Sheikh KH, Kisslo KB, Phillips HR, Peter RH, Behar VS, Kong YH, Krucoff M, Ohman EM, Tcheng JE, et al (1991) Intracoronary ultrasound evaluation of interventional technologies. Am J Cardiol 68: 1305–1309.

Demer LL, Ariani M, Siegel RJ (1991) High intensity ultrasound increases distensibility of calcific atherosclerotic arteries. J Am Coll Cardiol 18: 1259–1262.

DeSouza NM, King DH, Pilgrim P, Bates P, Reidy JF, Gosling RG (1991) Quickscan: Doppler ultrasound emulation of angiography—its value prior to arteriography in peripheral vascular disease. Br J Radiol 64: 479–484.

DiMario C, The SH, Madretsma S, et al (1992) Detection and characterization of vascular lesions by intravascular ultrasound: an in vitro study correlated with histology. J Am Soc Echocardiogr 5: 135–146.

Duber C, Klose KJ, Erbel R, Schmiedt W, Thelen M (1991) Intravascular sonography: initial clinical results [Ger]. Rofo: Fortschritte Auf Dem Gebiete Der Rontgenstrahlen Und Der Nuklearmedizin 154: 164–171.

Edwards JM, Coldwell DM, Goldman ML, Strandness DE Jr (1991) The role of duplex scanning in the selection of patients for transluminal angioplasty. J Vasc Surg 13: 69–74.

Edwards JM, Zaccardi MJ, Strandness DE Jr (1992) A preliminary study of the role of duplex scanning in defining the adequacy of treatment of patients with renal artery fibromuscular dysplasia. J Vasc Surg 15(4): 604–609; discussion 609–611.

Ehrlich S, Honye J, Mahon D, Bernstein R, Tobis J (1991) Unrecognized stenosis by angiography documented by intravascular ultrasound imaging. Cathet Cardiovasc Diagn 23: 198–201.

Ellis R, et al (1988) Ultrasonic imaging catheter. SPIE 904: 127–130.

Engeler CE, Yedlicka JW, Letourneau JG, Castaneda-Zuniga WR, Hunter DW, Amplatz K (1991) 1990 ARRS Executive Council Award. Intravascular sonography in the detection of arteriosclerosis and evaluation of vascular interventional procedures. AJR 156: 1087–1090.

Fitzgerald PJ, et al (1989) Catheter-tipped ultrasonic intravascular imaging. Perspect Vascular Surg 2: 113–125.

Fitzgerald PJ, et al (1987) Two-dimensional ultrasonic tissue characterization: backscatter power, endocardial wall motion, and their phase relationship for normal, ischemic and infarcted myocardium. Circulation 4: 850–859.

Fitzgerald PJ, Ports TA, Yock PG (1992) Contribution of localized calcium deposits to dissection after angioplasty. An observational study using intravascular ultrasound (see comments). Circulation 86(1): 64–70.

Fitzgerald PJ, St. Goar FG, Connolly AJ, et al (1992) Intravascular ultrasound imaging of coronary arteries. Circulation 86: 154–158.

Garrand TJ, Mintz GS, Popma JJ, Lewis SA, Vaughn NA, Leon MB (1993) Intravascular ultrasound diagnosis of a coronary artery pseudoaneurysm following percutaneous transluminal coronary angioplasty. Am Heart J 125(3): 880–882.

Gerber TC, Erbel R, Gorge G, Ge J, Rupprecht HJ, Meyer J (1992) Classification of morphologic effects of percutaneous transluminal coronary angioplasty assessed by intravascular ultrasound. Am J Cardiol 70(20): 1546–1554.

Giller CA, Mathews D, Purdy P, Kopitnik TA, Batjer HH, Samson DS (1992) The transcranial Doppler appearance of acute carotid artery occlusion. Ann Neurol 31(1): 101–103.

Goldberg BB, et al (1990) Endoluminal US: experiments with nonvascular uses in animals. Radiology 175: 39–43.

Gorge G, Erbel R, Schuster S, Ge J, Meyer J (1991) Intravascular ultrasound in diagnosis of acute pulmonary embolism (letter). Lancet 337: 623–624.

Grayburn PA, Willard JE, Brickner ME, Eichhorn EJ (1991) In vivo thrombus formation on a guidewire during intravascular ultrasound imaging: evidence for inadequate heparinization. Cathet Cardiovasc Diagn 23: 141–143.

Grayburn PA, Willard JE, Haagen DR, Brickner ME, Alvarez LG, Eichhorn EJ (1992) Measurement of coronary flow using high-frequency intravascular ultrasound imaging and pulsed Doppler velocimetry: in vitro feasibility studies. J Am Soc Echocardiogr 5: 5–12.

Gussenhoven EJ, Essed CE, Frietman P, Mastik F, Lancee C, Slager C, Serruys P, Gerritsen P, Pieterman H, Bom N (1989) Intravascular echographic assessment of vessel wall characteristics: a correlation with histology. Int J Card Imaging 4: 105–116.

Gussenhoven EJ, Essed CE, Frietman P, Van Egmond F, Lancee CT, Van Kappellen WH, Roelandt J, Serruys PW, Gerritsen GP, Van Urk H, et al (1989) Intravascular ultrasonic imaging: histologic and echographic correlation. Eur J Vasc Surg 3: 571–576.

Gussenhoven EJ, Essed CE, Lancee CT, et al (1989) Arterial wall characteristics determined by intravascular ultrasound imaging: an in vitro study. J Am Coll Cardiol 14: 947–952.

Gussenhoven EJ, Frietman PA, The SH, Van Suylen RJ, Van Egmond FC, Lancee CT, Van Urk H, Roelandt JR, Stijnen T, Bom N (1991) Assessment of medial thinning in atherosclerosis by intravascular ultrasound. Am J Cardiol 68: 1625–1632.

Harrison JK, et al (1990) Balloon angioplasty of coarctation of the aorta evaluated with intravascular ultrasound imaging. J Am Coll Cardiol 65: 1392–1396.

Harrison JK, Sheikh KH, Davidson CJ, Kisslo KB, Leithe ME, Himmelstein SI, Kanter RJ, Bashore TM (1990) Balloon angioplasty of coarctation of the aorta evaluated with intravascular ultrasound imaging. J Am Coll Cardiol 15: 906–909.

Hodgson JM, Graham SP, Savakus AD, Dame SG, Stephens DN, Dhillon PS, Brands D, Sheehan H, Eberle MJ (1989) Clinical percutaneous imaging of coronary anatomy using an over-the-wire ultrasound catheter system. Int J Card Imaging 4: 187–193.

Hodgson JM, Reddy KG, Suneja R, Nair RN, Lesnefsky EJ, Sheehan HM (1993) Intracoronary ultrasound imaging: correlation of plaque morphology with angiography, clinical syndrome and procedural results in patients undergoing coronary angioplasty. J Am Coll Cardiol 21(1): 35–44.

Honye J, Mahon DJ, Jain A, White CJ, Ramee SR, Wallis JB, Al-Zarka A, Tobis JM (1992) Morphological effects of coronary balloon angioplasty in vivo assessed by intravascular ultrasound imaging. Circulation 85(3): 1012–1025.

Hunt AC, Chow SC, Escaned J, Perry RA, Seth A, Shiu MF (1991) Changes in Doppler indices of cardiac function during and after percutaneous transluminal coronary angioplasty. Br Heart J 66: 346–350.

Hurst RW, Schnee C, Raps EC, Farber R, Flamm ES (1993) Role of transcranial Doppler in neuroradiological treatment of intracranial vasospasm. Stroke 24(2): 299–303.

Isner JM, et al (1990) Catheter-based intravascular ultrasound discriminates bicuspid from tricuspid valves in adults with calcific aortic stenosis. J Am Coll Cardiol 15: 1575–1585.

Isner JM, Losordo DW, Rosenfield K, et al (1990) Catheter-based intravascular ultrasound discriminates bicuspid from tricuspid valves in adults with calcific aortic stenosis. J Am Coll Cardiol 15: 310–317.

Isner JM, Rosenfield K, (1992) Enough with the fantastic voyage: will IVUS pay in Peoria? Cathet Cardiovasc Diag 26: 192–199.

Isner JM, Rosenfield K, Losordo DW, Kelly S, Palefski P, Langevin RE, Razvi S, Pastore JO, Kosowsky BD (1990) Percutaneous intravascular US as adjunct to catheter-based interventions: preliminary experience in patients with peripheral vascular disease. Radiology 175: 61–70.

Isner JM, Rosenfield K, Losordo DW, Rose L, Langevin RE Jr, Razvi S, Kosowsky BD (1991) Combination balloon ultrasound imaging catheter for percutaneous transluminal angioplasty. Validation of imaging, analysis of recoil, and identification of plaque fracture. Circulation 84: 739–754.

Iwai T, Sakurazawa K, Sato S, Muraoka Y, Inoue Y, Endo M (1991) Intraoperative monitoring of the pelvic circulation using a transanal Doppler probe. Eur J Vasc Surg 5: 71–74.

Jackman JD, Hermiller JB, Sketch MH, et al (1992) Combined rotational and directional atherectomy guided by intravascular ultrasound in an occluded vein graft. Am Heart J 124: 214–216.

Jain A, Ramee SR, Culpepper WR, Mesa JE, Murgo JP, White CJ (1992) Intravascular ultrasound-assisted percutaneous angioplasty of aortic coarctation. Am Heart J 123(2): 514–515.

Jain A, Ramee SR, Mesa J, Collins TJ, White CJ (1992) Intracoronary thrombus: chronic infusion and evaluation with intravascular ultrasound. Cathet Cardiovasc Diagn 26: 212–214.

Jain SP, Roubin GS, Nanda NC, Dean LS, Agrawal SK, Pinheiro L (1992) Intravascular ultrasound imaging of saphenous vein graft stenosis. Am J Cardiol 69(1): 133–136.

Jorgensen JJ, Stranden E, Gilbers T (1987) Hemodynamic effect of percutaneous transluminal angioplasty for lower limb atherosclerosis. A study based on pulsed Doppler ultrasound flowmetry. Acta Radiol 28: 761–766.

Karnik R, Winkler WB, Valentin A, Urban M, Slany J (1992) Intravascular ultrasound imaging of Guenther vena caval filters. Am J Cardiol 69: 1504–1505.

Keren G, Douek P, Oblon C, Bonner RF, Pichard AD, Leon MB (1992) Atherosclerotic saphenous vein grafts treated with different interventional procedures assessed by intravascular ultrasound. Am Heart J 124(1): 198–206.

Keren G, Leon MB (1991) Characterization of atherosclerotic lesions by intravascular ultrasound: possible role in unstable coronary syndromes and in interventional therapeutic procedures. Am J Cardiol 68: 85B–91B.

Keren G, Pichard AD, Kent KM, Satler LF, Leon MB (1992) Failure or success of complex catheter-based interventional procedures assessed by intravascular ultrasound. Am Heart J 123(1): 200–208.

Kitney RI, Moura L, Straughan K (1989) 3-D visualization of arterial structures using ultrasound and Voxel modelling. Int J Card Imaging 4: 135–143.

Klein HM, Gunther RW, Verlande M, et al (1992) 3-D surface reconstruction of intravascular ultrasound images using personal computer hardware and motorized catheter control. Cardiovasc Intervent Radiol 15: 97–101.

Kopchok GE, et al (1990) Intravasculasr ultrasound: a new potential modality for angioplasty guidance. Angiology 41: 785–792.

Laissy JP, Thiebot J, Peillon C, Watelet J, Testart J, Benozio M (1987) Axillo-femoral bypass failure secondary to axillary stenosis: ultrasound-guided percutaneous transluminal and angioplasty. Bildgebung 56: 185–186.

Landini L, Sarnelli R, Picano E, Salvadori M (1986) Evaluation of frequency dependence of backscatter coefficient in normal and atherosclerotic aortic walls. Ultrasound Med Biol 12: 397–401.

Lee RT, Loree HM, Cheng GC, Lieberman EH, Jaramillo N, Schoen FJ (1993) Computational structural analysis based on intravascular ultrasound imaging before in vitro angioplasty: prediction of plaque fracture locations. J Am Coll Cardiol 21(3): 777–782.

Lee RT, Richardson SG, Loree HM, et al (1992) Prediction of mechanical properties of human athersclerotic tissue by high-frequency intravascular ultrasound imaging: an in vitro study. Arterioscler Thromb 12: 1–5.

Lehner K, et al (1990) Intravascular ultrasound. Methods and diagnostic significance. Rontgenpraxis 43: 413–419.

Liebson PR, Klein LW (1992) Intravascular ultrasound in coronary atherosclerosis: a new approach to clinical assessment. Am Heart J 123: 1643–1660.

Linker DT, Kleven A, Gronningsaether A, Yock PG, Angelsen BA (1991) Tissue characterization with intra-arterial ultrasound: special promise and problems. Int J Card Imaging 6: 255–263.

Linker DT, Yock PG, Gronningsaether A, Johansen E, Angelsen BA (1989) Analysis of backscattered ultrasound from normal and diseased arterial wall. Int J Card Imaging 4: 177–185.

Lockwood GR, Ryan LK, Gotlieb AI, et al (1992) In vitro high resolution intravascular imaging in muscular and elastic arteries. J Am Coll Cardiol 20: 153–160.

Ludwig M, et al (1990) Experiences with the use of an intravascular 6 French endosonography catheter in vivo. Klin Wochenschr 68: 570–575.

Mallery JA, Gregory K, Morcos NC (1987) Evaluation of an ultrasound balloon dilation imaging catheter. Circulation 76: IV–371.

Mallery JA, Tobis JM, Griffith J, Gessert J, McRae M, Moussabeck O, Bessen M, Moriuchi M, Henry WL (1990) Assessment of normal and atherosclerotic arterial wall thickness with an intravascular ultrasound imaging catheter. Am Heart J 119: 1392–1400.

Mandelbrot L, Daffos F, Forestier F, MacAleese J, Descombey D (1988) Assessment of fetal blood volume for computer-assisted management of in utero transfusion. Fetal Ther 3: 60–66.

Martin RW, Johnson CC (1989) Design characteristics for intravascular ultrasonic catheters. REVIEW ARTICLE: 23 REFS. Int J Card Imaging 4: 201–216.

Martin RW, Silverstein FE, Kimmey MB (1989) A 20-MHz ultrasound system for imaging the intestinal wall. Ultrasound Med Biol 15: 273–280.

Marx MV, Tauscher JR, Williams DM, Greenfield LJ (1991) Evaluation of the inferior vena cava with intravascular US after Greenfield filter placement. J Vasc Intervent Radiol 2: 261–268.

McCowan TC, et al (1990) Inferior vena caval filter thrombi: evaluation with intravascular US. Radiology 177: 783–788.

Meier B (1992) Recanalization of chronically occluded coronary arteries. Herz 17(1): 27–39.

Mewissen MW, Kinney EV, Bandyk DF, Reifsnyder T, Seabrook GR, Lipchik EO, Towne JB (1992) The role of duplex scanning versus angiography is predicting outcome after balloon angioplasty in the femoropopliteal artery. J Vasc Surg 15(5): 860–865; discussion 865–866.

Meyer CR, Chiang EH, Fechner KP, Fitting DW, Williams DM, Buda AJ (1988) Feasibility of high resolution intravascular ultrasonic imaging catheters. Radiology 168: 113–116.

Milunski MR, Mohr GA, Pérez JE, et al (1989) Ultrasonic tissue characterization with integrated backscatter. Circulation 80: 491–503.

Mintz GS, Potkin BN, Cooke RH, et al (1992) Intravascular ultrasound imaging in a patient with unstable angina. Am Heart J 123: 1692–1694.

Mintz GS, Potkin BN, Keren G, Satler LF, Pichard AD, Kent KM, Popma JJ, et al. (1992) Intravascular ultrasound evaluation of the effect of rotational atherectomy in obstructive atherosclerotic coronary artery disease. Circulation 86(5): 1383–1393.

Moneta GL, Schneider E, Jager K, Brulisauer M, Thuring-Vollenweider U, Bollinger A (1988) Laser Doppler flux and vasomotion in patients before and after transluminal angioplasty for limb salvage. Vasa 17: 26–31.

Moriuchi M, Saito S, Hoyne, et al (1992) Intravascular ultrasound imaging in human peripheral and coronary arteries in vivo. Jpn Circ J 56: 578–585.

Moriuchi M, Tobis JM, Mahon D, et al (1990) The reproducibility of intravascular ultrasound imaging in vitro. J Am Soc Echocardiogr 3:444–450

Neville RF, Bartorelli AL, Sidawy AN, et al (1989) An in vivo feasibility study of intravascular ultrasound imaging. Am J Surg 158: 142–145.

Neville RF, Hobson RW, Jamil Z, et al (1991) Intravascular ultrasonography: validation studies and preliminary intraoperative observations. J Vasc Surg 13: 274–283.

Neville RF, Padberg FT, DeFouw D, Hernanadez J, Duran W, Hobson RW (1992) The arterial wall response to intimal injury in an experimental model. Ann Vasc Surg 6: 50–54.

Neville RF Jr, Hobson RW 2d, Watanabe B, Yasuhara H, Padberg FT Jr, Duran W, Franco CD (1991) A prospective evaluation of arterial intimal injuries in an experimental model. J Trauma 31: 669–674.

Neville RF Jr, Yasuhara H, Watanabe BI, Canady J, Duran W, Hobson RW 2d (1991) Endovascular management of arterial intimal defects: an experimental comparison by arteriography, angioscopy, and intravascular ultrasonography. J Vasc Surg 13: 496–502.

Nishimura RA, Edwards WD, Warnes CA, Reeder GS, Holmes DR Jr, Tajik AJ, Yock PG (1990) Intravascular ultrasound imaging: in vitro validation and pathologic correlation. J Am Coll Cardiol 16: 145–154.

Nishimura RA, Reeder GS (1992) Intravascular ultrasound: research technique or clinical tool? Circulation 86: 322–324.

Nishimura RA, Welch TJ, Stanson AW, Sheedy PF 2d, Holmes DR Jr (1990) Intravascular US of the distal aorta and iliac vessels: initial feasibility studies. Radiology 176: 523–525.

Nissen SE, et al (1990) Assessment of vascular disease by intravascular ultrasound. Cardiology 77: 398–410.

Nissen SE, Grines CL, Gurley JC, et al (1990) Application of a new phased-array ultrasound imaging catheter in the assessment of vascular dimensions: in vivo comparison to cineangiography. Circulation 81: 660–666.

Nissen SE, Gurley JC (1991) Application of intravascular ultrasound for detection and quantitation of coronary atherosclerosis. Int J Card Imaging 6: 165–177.

Nissen SE, Gurley JC, Grines CL, Booth DC, McClure R, Berk M, Fischer C, DeMaria AN (1991) Intravascular ultrasound assessment of lumen size and wall morphology in normal subjects and patients with coronary artery disease. Circulation 84: 1087–1099.

Pande A, Meier B, Fleisch M, Kammerlander R, Simonet F, Lerch R (1991) Intravascular ultrasound for diagnosis of aortic dissection. Am J Cardiol 67: 662–663.

Pandian NG (1989) Intravascular and intracardiac ultrasound imaging: an old concept, now on the road to reality. Circulation 80: 1091–1094.

Pandian NG, et al (1989) Ultrasound angioscopy: feasibility and potential. Echocardiography 4: 1–7.

Pandian NG, Hsu TL (1992) Intravascular ultrasound of the coronary arteries: current applications and future directions. Am J Cardiol 69: 18H–29H.

Pandian NG, Kreis A, Brockway B, et al (1988) Ultrasound angioscopy: real-time, two-dimensional, intraluminal ultrasound imaging of blood vessels. Am J Cardiol 62: 493–494.

Pandian NG, Kreis A, Brockway B, Sacharoff A, Boleza E, Caro R (1990) Detection of intrarterial thrombus by high frequency two-dimensional ultrasound imaging in vivo studies. Am J Cardiol 65: 1280–1283.

Pandian NG, Kreis A, Brockway B, Sacharoff A, Boleza E, Caro RE (1990) Intravascular high frequency two-dimensional ultrasound detection of arterial dissection and intimal flaps. Am J Cardiol 65: 1278–1280.

Pandian NG, Kreis A, O'Donnell T (1989) Intravascular ultrasound estimation of arterial stenosis. J Am Soc Echocardiogr 2:390–397.

Pandian NG, Kreis A, O'Donnell T, Sacharoff A, Boleza E, Caro R (1989) Intraluminal two-dimensional ultrasound angioscopic quantitation of arterial stenosis: comparison with external high-frequency ultrasound imaging and anatomy. J Am Coll Cardiol 13: 5A.

Pandian NG, Kreis A, Weintraub A (1990) Real-time intravascular ultrasound imaging in humans. Am J Cardiol 65: 1392–1396.

Pandian NG, Kumar R, Katz SE, et al (1991) Real-time, intracardiac, two-dimensional echocardiography. Echocardiography: Am J CV Ultrasound and Allied Tech 8: 407–421.

Pandian NG, Weintraub A, Kreis A, Schwartz SL, Konstam MA, Salem DN (1990) Intracardiac, intravascular, two-dimensional, high-frequency ultrasound imaging of pulmonary artery and its branches in humans and animals. Circulation 81: 2007–2012.

Peene P, Wilms G, Marchal G, Baert AL (1991) Intravascular ultrasonography, a new alternative for the assessment of vascular lesions. Eur J Radiol 12: 141–146.

Pellerito JS, Taylor KJ (1992) Doppler color imaging. Peripheral arteries. Clin Ultrasound 27: 97–112.

Picano E, et al (1988) Ultrasonic tissue characterization of atherosclerosis: state of the art of 1988. J Nucl Med Allied Sci 32: 174–185.

Picano E, Pelosi G, Marzilli M (1990) In vivo quantitative ultrasonic evaluation of myocardial fibrosis in humans. Circulation 81: 58–64.

Pignoli P, et al (1986) Intimal plus medial thickness of the anterial wall: a direct measurement with ultrasound imaging. Circulation 74: 1399–1406.

Pinto FJ, St. Goar FG, Fischell TA, et al (1992) Nitroglycerin-induced coronary vasodilation in cardiac transplant recipients: evaluation with in vivo intracoronary ultrasound. Circulation 85: 69–77.

Potkin BN, Bartorelli AL, Gessert JM, et al (1990) Coronary artery imaging with intravascular high-frequency ultrasound. Circulation 81: 1575–1585.

Ricou F, Ludomirsky A, Weintraub RG, Sahn DJ (1991) Applications of intravascular scanning and transesophageal echocardiography in congenital heart disease: tradeoffs and the merging of technologies. Int J Card Imaging 6: 221–230.

Ricou F, Nicod PH, Moser KM, Peterson KL (1991) Catheter-based intravascular ultrasound imaging of chronic thromboembolic pulmonary disease. Am J Cardiol 67: 749–752.

Roelandt J, Serruys PW (1989) Intraluminal real-time ultrasonic imaging: clinical perspectives. Int J Card Imaging 4: 89–97.

Rosenfield K, Kaufman J, Pieczek A, Langevin RE Jr, Razvi S, Isner JM (1992) Real-time three-dimensional reconstruction of intravascular ultrasound images of iliac arteries. Am J Cardiol 70(3): 412–415.

Rosenfield K, Losordo DW, Ramaswamy K, Pastore JO, Langevin RE, Razvi S, Kosowsky BD, Isner JM (1991) Three-dimensional reconstruction of human coronary and peripheral arteries from images recorded during two-dimensional intravascular ultrasound examination (see comments). Circulation 84: 1938–1956.

Rosenschein U, Rozenszajn LA, Kraus L, Marboe CC, Watkins JF, Rose EA, David D, Cannon PJ, Weinstein JS (1991) Ultrasonic angioplasty in totally occluded peripheral arteries. Initial clinical, histological, and angiographic results. Circulation 83: 1976–1986.

Rothman A, Ricou F, Weintraub RG, et al (1992) Intraluminal ultrasound imaging through a balloon dilation catheter in an animal model of coarctation of the aorta. Circulation 85: 2291–2295.

Sacks D, Robinson ML, Marinelli DL, Perlmutter GS (1990) Evaluation of the peripheral arteries with duplex US after angioplasty. Radiology 176: 39–44.

Salo JO (1987) Intravesical ultrasound for staging bladder tumors. Scand J Urol Nephrol 21: 203–207.

Schmitz-Rode T, Gunther RW, Muller-Leisse C (1991) US-assisted aspiration thrombectomy: in vitro investigations. Radiology 178: 677–679.

Schryver TE, Popma JJ, Kent KM, Leon MB, Eldredge S, Mintz GS (1992) Use of intracoronary ultrasound to identify the "true" coronary lumen in chronic coronary dissection treated with intracoronary stenting. Am J Cardiol 69(12): 1107–1108.

Schwartz RA, Kerns DB, Mitchell DG (1991) Color Doppler ultrasound imaging in iatrogenic arterial injuries. Am J Surg 162: 4–8.

Sheikh KH, Adams DB, McCann R, Lyerly HK, Sabiston DC, Kisslo J (1989) Utility of Doppler color flow imaging for identification of femoral arterial complications of cardiac catheterization. Am Heart J 117: 623–628.

Sheikh KH, Davidson CJ, Kisslo KB, Harrison JK, Himmelstein SI, Kisslo J, Bashore TM (1991) Comparison of intravascular ultrasound, external ultrasound and digital angiography for evaluation of peripheral artery dimensions and morphology. Am J Cardiol 67: 817–822.

Sheikh KH, Davidson CJ, Newman GE, Kisslo KB, Schwab SJ (1991) Intravascular ultrasound assessment of the renal artery. Ann Intern Med 115: 222–225.

Sheikh KH, Harrison JK, Harding MB, et al (1991) Detection of angiographically silent coronary atherosclerosis by intracoronary ultrasonography. Am Heart J 121: 1803–1807.

Siegel RJ, Ariani M, Fishbein MC, Chae JS, Park JC, Maurer G, Forrester JS (1991) Histopathologic validation of angioscopy and intravascular ultrasound. Circulation 84: 109–117.

Siegel RJ, Chae JS, Forrester JS, Ruiz CE (1990) Angiography, angioscopy, and ultrasound imaging before and after percutaneous balloon angioplasty. Am Heart J 120: 1086–1090.

Siegel RJ, Cumberland DC, Crew JR (1992) Ultrasound recanalization of diseased arteries. From experimental studies to clinical application. Surg Clin North Am 72(4): 879–897.

Siegel RJ, Cumberland DC, Myler RK, DonMichael TA (1989) Percutaneous ultrasonic angioplasty: initial clinical experience. Lancet 2: 772–774.

Siegel RJ, et al (1989) Intravascular ultrasound imaging: clinical—pathological correlation. SPIE 1068: 119–126.

Slepian MJ (1991) Application of intraluminal ultrasound imaging to vascular stenting. Int J Card Imaging 6: 285–311.

Slordahl SA, Piene H, Linker DT, Vik A (1991) Segmental aortic wall stiffness from intravascular ultrasound at normal and subnormal aortic pressure in pigs. Acta Physiol Scand 143: 227–232.

St. Goar FG, Pinto FJ, Alderman EL, et al (1992) Intracoronary ultrasound in cardiac transplant recipients: in vivo evidence of "angiographically silent" intimal thickening. Circulation 85: 979–987.

St. Goar FG, Pinto FJ, Alderman EL, Fitzgerald PJ, Stadius ML, Popp RL (1991) Intravascular ultrasound imaging of angiographically normal coronary arteries: an in vivo comparison with quantitative angiography. J Am Coll Cardiol 18: 952–958.

Struass AL, Roth FJ, Rieger H (1993) Noninvasive assessment of pressure gradients across iliac artery stenoses: duplex and catheter correlative study. J Ultrasound Med 12(1): 17–22.

Strauss AL, Schaberle W, Rieger H, Roth FJ (1991) Use of duplex scanning in the diagnosis of arteria profunda femoris stenosis. J Vasc Surg 13: 698–704.

Stumper O, et al (1991) Role of intraoperative ultrasound examination in patients undergoing a Fontan-type procedure. Br Heart J 65: 204–210.

Sudhir K, Fitzgerald PJ, MacGregor JS, DeMarco T, Ports TA, Chatterjee K, Yock PG (1991) Transvenous coronary ultrasound imaging. A novel approach to visualization of the coronary arteries. Circulation 84: 1957–1961.

Tabbara M, Kopchok G, White RA (1990) In vitro and in vivo evaluation of intraluminal ultrasound in normal and atherosclerotic arteries. Am J Surg 160: 556–560.

Tabbara M, White R, Cavaye D, Kopchok G (1991) In vivo human comparison of intravascular ultrasonography and angiography. J Vasc Surg 14: 496–502; discussion 502–504.

Tabbara MR, Mehringer CM, Cavaye DM, Schwartz M, Kopchok GE, Maselly M, White RA (1992) Sequential intraluminal ultrasound evaluation of balloon angioplasty of an iliac artery lesion. Ann Vasc Surg 6(2): 179–184.

Tapson VF, Davidson CJ, Gurbel PA, Sheikh KH, Kisslo KB, Stack RS (1991) Rapid and accurate diagnosis of pulmonary emboli in a canine model using intravascular ultrasound imaging. Chest 100: 1410–1413.

Taylor KJ, et al (1989) Tissue characterization. Ultrasound Med Biol 15: 421–428.

Tegeler CH, Downes TR (1991) Thrombosis and the heart. Semin Neurol 11: 339–352.

Tenaglia AN, Buller CE, Kisslo KB, Phillips HR, Stack RS, Davidson CJ (1992) Intracoronary ultrasound predictors of adverse outcomes after coronary artery interventions. J Am Coll Cardiol 20(6): 1385–1390.

Ten Hoff H, Korbijn A, Smith TH, Klinkhamer JF, Bom N (1989) Imaging artifacts in mechanically driven ultrasound catheters. Int J Card Imaging 4: 195–199.

The SH, Gussenhoven EJ, Du Bois NA, Pieterman H, Roelandt JR, Wilson RA, Van Urk H (1991) Femoro-popliteal vein bypass grafts studied by intravascular ultrasound. Eur J Vasc Surg 5: 523–526.

The SH, Gussenhoven EJ, Zhong Y, Li W, Van Egmond F, Pieterman H, Van Urk H, Gerritsen GP, Borst C, Wilson RA, et al (1992) Effect of balloon angioplasty on femoral artery evaluated with intravascular ultrasound imaging. Circulation 86(2): 483–493.

The SH, Wilson RA, Gussenhoven EJ, Pieterman H, Bom K, Roelandt JR, Van Urk H (1992) Extrinsic compression of the superficial femoral artery at the adductor canal: evaluation with intravascular sonography. AJR 159(1): 117–120.

Tobis JM (1991) Intravascular ultrasound. A fantastic voyage (editorial; comment). Circulation 84: 2190–2192.

Tobis JM, Mahon DJ, Moriuchi M, Honye J, McRae M (1991) Intravascular ultrasound imaging following balloon angioplasty. Int J Card Imaging 6: 191–205.

Tobis JM, Mallery JA, Gessert J, Griffith J, Mahon D, Bessen M, Moriuchi M, McLeay L, McRae M, Henry WL (1989) Intravascular ultrasound cross-sectional arterial imaging before and after balloon angioplasty in vitro. Circulation 80: 873–882.

Tobis JM, Mallery J, Mahon D, Lehmann K, Zalesky P, Griffith J, Gessert J, Moriuchi M, McRae M, Dwyer ML, et al (1991) Intravascular ultrasound imaging of human coronary arteries in vivo. Analysis of tissue characterizations with comparison to in vitro histological specimens. Circulation 83: 913–926.

Valantine H, Pinto FJ, Frederick G, et al (1992) Intracoronary ultrasound imaging in heart transplant recipients: the Stanford experience. J Heart Lung Transplant 11: S60–64.

Valdes-Cruz LM, et al (1991) Transvascular intracardiac applications of a miniaturized phased-array ultrasonic endoscope: initial experience with intracardiac imaging in piglets. Circulation 83: 1023–1027.

Van der Heijden FH, Legemate DA, van Leeuwen MS, Mali WP, Eikelboom BC (1993) Value of Duplex scanning in the selection of patients for percutaneous transluminal angioplasty. Europ J Vasc Surg 7(1): 71–76.

Van Urk H, Gussenhoven WJ, Gerritsen GP, Pieterman H, The SH, Van Egmond F, Lancee CT, Bom N (1991) Assessment of arterial disease and arterial reconstructions by intravascular ultrasound. Int J Card Imaging 6: 157–164.

Ventura HO, Ramee SR, Jain A, et al (1992) Coronary artery imaging with intravascular ultrasound in patients following cardiac transplantation. Transplantation 53: 216–219.

Violaris AG, Linnemeier TJ, Campbell S, Rothbaum DA, Cumberland DC (1992) Intravascular ultrasound imaging combined with coronary angioplasty. Lancet 339(8809): 1571–1572.

Vroegindeweij D, Kemper FJ, Tielbeek AV, Buth J, Landman G (1992) Recurrence of stenoses following balloon angioplasty and Simpson atherectomy of the femoro-popliteal segment. A randomised comparative 1-year follow-up study using colour flow duplex. Eur J Vasc Surg 6(2): 164–171.

Waller BF (1989) Anatomy, histology, and pathology of the major epicardial coronary arteries relevant to echocardiographic imaging techniques. J Am Soc Echocardiogr 2: 232–252.

Waller BF, Orr CM, Slack JD, Pinkerton CA, Van Tassel J, Peters T (1992) Anatomy, histology, and pathology of coronary arteries: a review relevant to new interventional and imaging techniques—Part I. Clin Cardiol 15(6): 451–457.

Waller BF, Orr CM, Slack JD, Pinkerton CA, Van Tassel J, Peters T (1992) Anatomy, histology, and pathology of coronary arteries: a review relevant to new interventional and imaging techniques—Part II. Clin Cardiol 15(7): 535–540.

Waller BF, Orr CM, Slack JD, Pinkerton CA, Van Tassel JV, Peters T (1992) Anatomy, histology, and pathology of coronary arteries: a review relevant to new interventional and imaging techniques—Part III. Clin Cardiol 15(8): 607–615.

Waller BF, Pinkerton CA, Slack JD (1992) Intravascular ultrasound: a histological study of vessels during life. The new 'gold standard' for vascular imaging. Circulation 85(6): 2305–2310.

Wenguang L, Gussenhoven WJ, Zhong Y, The SH, Di Mario C, Madretsma S, Van Egmond F, De Feyter P, Pieterman H, Van Urk H, et al (1991)

Validation of quantitative analysis of intravascular ultrasound images. Int J Card Imaging 6: 247–253.

Werner GS, Corovic D, Buchwald A, et al (1990) Intravascular ultrasonic diagnosis. In vivo findings before and after angioplasty in peripheral arterial occlusive disease. Dtsch Med Wochenschr 115: 1259–1265.

Werner GS, et al (1991) Intravascular ultrasound imaging of human coronary arteries after percutaneous transluminal angioplasty: morphologic and quantitative assessment. Am Heart J 122: 212–220.

Werner GS, Sold G, Buchwald A, Kreuzer H, Wiegand V (1991) Intravascular sonography of the coronary vessels following percutaneous transluminal angioplasty [Ger]. Dtsch Med Wochenschr 116: 81–86.

Werner GS, Sold G, Buchwald A, Kreuzer H, Wiegand V (1991) Intravascular ultrasound imaging of human coronary arteries after percutaneous transluminal angioplasty: morphologic and quantitative assessment. Am Heart J 122: 212–220.

White CJ, Rameo SR, Collins TJ, Jain A, Mesa JE (1992) Ambiguous coronary angiography: clinical utility of intravascular ultrasound. Cathet Cardiovasc Diagn 26: 200–203.

White NW Jr, Yock PG (1989) Intravascular ultrasound: catheter-based Doppler and two-dimensional imaging. REVIEW ARTICLE: 39 REFS. Cardiol Clin 7: 525–536.

White RA (1990) Indications for fiberoptic angioscopy and intraluminal ultrasound. Compr Ther 16: 23–30.

Whyman MR, Gillespie I, Ruckley CV, Allan PL, Fowkes FG (1992) Screening patients with claudication from femoropopliteal disease before angioplasty using Doppler colour flow imaging. Br J Surg 79(9): 907–909.

Wickline SA, Barzilai B, Thomas LJ, Saffitz JE (1990) Quantitative of intimal and medial thickness of human coronary arteries by acoustic microscopy. Coronary Artery Dis 1: 375–381.

Willard JE, Netto D, Demian SE, et al (1992) Intravascular ultrasound imaging of saphenous veins grafts in vitro: comparison and histologic and quantitative angiographic findings. J Am Coll Cardiol 19: 759–764.

Williams DM, Simon HJ, Marx MV, Starkey TD (1992) Acute traumatic aortic rupture: intravascular US findings. Radiology 182: 247–249.

Wilson MW, Webb RC, Marx MV, Meyer CR, Gallagher MA, Haarer SL, Buda AJ, Williams DM (1991) Intravascular ultrasound imaging of vascular responsiveness in isolated perfused canine arteries. Invest Radiol 26: 248–253.

Windeck P, Labs KH, Jaeger KA (1992) How useful are acceleration- and deceleration-based Doppler indices? A trial on patients with percutaneous transluminal angioplasty. Ultrasound Med Biol 18(6-7): 525–534.

Yock PG, et al (1989) Intravascular two-dimensional ultrasound: clinical studies in the periphery. Society of Photo-Optical Instrumentation Engineers Catheter-Based Sensing and Imaging Technology 1068: 151–156.

Yock PG, et al (1990) Intravascular ultrasound: looking below the surface of vascular disease. Circulation 81: 1715–1718.

Yock PG, Fitzgerald PJ, Linker DT, Angelsen BA (1991) Intravascular ultrasound guidance for catheter-based coronary interventions. J Am Coll Cardiol 17: 39B–45B.

Yock PG, Fitzgerald PJ, Sudhir K, Linker DT, White W, Ports A (1991) Intravascular ultrasound imaging for guidance of atherectomy and other plaque removal techniques. Int J Card Imaging 6: 179–189.

Yock PG, Johnson EL, Linker DT (1988) Intravascular ultrasound: development and clinical potential. Am J Card Imaging 2: 185–193.

Yock PG, Linker DT (1990) Intravascular ultrasound: looking below the surface of vascular disease (comment). Circulation 1990;8: 1715–1718. Journal comment on circulation. Circulation 81: 1575–1585.

Yock PG, Linker DT, Angelsen BAJ, Tech DR (1989) Two-dimensional intravascular ultrasound: technical development and initial clinical experience. J Am Soc Echocardiogr 2: 296–304.

Yock PG, Linker DT, White NW, Rowe MH, Selmon MR, Robertson GC, Hinohara T, Simpson JB (1989) Clinical applications of intravascular ultrasound imaging in atherectomy. Int J Card Imaging 4: 117–125.

Yoshida K, Yoshikawa J, Akasaka T, et al (1992) Intravascular ultrasound imaging in vitro and vivo validation. Jpn Circ J 56: 572–577.

Yuan YW, et al (1988) Ultrasonic backscatter from flowing whole blood: II dependence on frequency and fibrinogen concentration. J Acoust J Am 84: 1195–1200.

VI. Lasers

A. Peripheral

AbuRahma AF, Kennard W (1990) Yag laser-assisted thermal balloon angioplasty. Our early experience at Charleston Area Medical Center. W V Med J 86: 242–245.

AbuRahma AF, Robinson PA, Kennard W, Boland JP (1990) Intraoperative peripheral Nd:YAG laser-assisted thermal balloon angioplasty: short-term and intermediate-term follow-up. J Vasc Surg 12: 566–572.

Akchurin RS, Beliaev AA, Savchenko AP, Pomerantsev EV (1989) Transcutaneous laser angioplasty of fine coronary and renal arteries (the first clinical experience). Kardiologiia 29: 100–103.

Allen B, Loflin TG, Embry BM, Gaskin TA, Isobe JH, Martin RG (1990) Occluded peripheral arteries: clinical utility of argon laser recanalization. Radiology 176: 543–547.

Apfelberg DB, Smith T, Maser MR, Lash H, White DN (1987) Study of three lasers systems for treatment of superficial varicosities of the lower extremity. Lasers Surg Med 7: 219–223.

Arai T, Mizuno K, Fujikawa A, Nakagawa M, Kikuchi M (1990) Infrared absorption spectra ranging from 2.5 to 10 microns at various layers of human normal abdominal aorta and fibrofatty atheroma in vitro. Lasers Surg Med 10: 357–362.

Arlart IP, Gerlach A, Grass HG (1991) Laser-assisted balloon angioplasty in complete femoropopliteal occlusions: preliminary results. Cardiovasc Intervent Radiol 14: 233–237.

Ashley S, Brooks SG, Gehani AA, Thorley P, Parkin A, Kester RC, Rees MR (1991) Isotope limb blood flow measurement in patients undergoing peripheral laser angioplasty. J Biomed Eng 13: 221–224.

Barbeau GR, Abela GS, Seeger JM, Friedl SE, Tomaru T, Giacomino PP (1990) Temperature monitoring during peripheral thermo-optical laser recanalization in humans [comments]. Clin Cardiol 13: 690–697.

Bauer R, Pokorny E, Muckenhuber P, Malekpour G, Werner H, Juptner J (1991) Is laser assisted angioplasty a real alternative to surgical treatment of occluded peripheral vessels? Eur J Vasc Surg 5(6): 637–640.

Belli AM, Cumberland DC, Myler RK, Crew JR, Stertzer SH (1990) Peripheral arterial occlusions: initial results from percutaneous angioplasty with a hybrid laser probe. Radiology 174: 447–449.

Belli AM, Cumberland DC, Procter AE, Welsh CL (1991) Follow-up of conventional angioplasty versus laser thermal angioplasty for total femoropopliteal artery occlusions: results of a randomized trial. J Vasc Intervent Radiol 2(4): 485–488.

Belli AM, Cumberland DC, Procter AE, Welsh CL (1991) Total peripheral artery occlusions: conventional versus laser thermal recanalization with a hybrid probe in percutaneous angioplasty—results of a randomized trial [comments]. Radiology 181: 57–60.

Belli AM, Proctor AE, Cumberland DC (1990) Peripheral vascular occlusions: mechanical recanalization with a metal laser probe after guidewire dissection. Radiology 176: 539–541.

Berengoltz-Zlochin SN, Westerhof PW, Mali WP, Rienks R, Smits PC, Verdaasdonk RM, Van der Tweel I, Robles de Medina EO, Borst C (1992) Nd:YAG laser-assisted angioplasty in femoropopliteal artery occlusions: "hot" versus "cold" recanalization with transparent contact probe. Radiology 182(2): 409–414.

Blebea J, Ouriel K, Green RM, Fiore WM, Welch EL, Svoboda JJ, Balaji MR (1991) Laser angioplasty in peripheral vascular disease symptomatic versus hemodynamic results. J Vasc Surg 13: 222–228.

Bonn J (1991) Clinical utility of laser recanalization in occluded peripheral arteries [editorial]. Radiology 178: 323–325.

Bonnier JJ, van Gemert MJ, Stassen EG, Verdaasdonk RM, Schets GA, Lahaye C (1986) Thermal and optical properties of human blood, vessel wall and plaque using different lasers. Ann Radiol (Paris) 29: 211–214.

Borst C, Rienks R, Mali WP, van Erven L (1989) Laser ablation and the need for intra-arterial imaging. Int J Card Imaging 4: 127–133.

Cheong WF, Spears JR, Welch AJ (1991) Laser balloon angioplasty. Crit Rev Biomed Eng 19(2-3): 113–146.

Choy DS, Ascher P, Lammer J, Rothman L, Snowdon J (1986) Percutaneous laser catheter recanalization of carotid arteries in seven cadavers and one patient. AJNJ 7: 1050–1052.

Cikrit DF, Becker GJ, Dalsing MC, Ehrman KO, Lalka SG, Sawchuk AP (1991) Early experience with the Palmaz expandable intraluminal stent in iliac artery stenosis. Ann Vasc Surg 5: 150–155.

Cox JL, Jacobs CP (1987) Laser-assisted angioplasty. Treating peripheral vascular disease. AORN J 46: 835–846.

Cragg AH, Gardiner GA Jr, Smith TP (1989) Vascular applications of laser. Radiology 172: 925–935.

Creamer-Bauer C, Webber (1990) Patient teaching strategies for peripheral laser procedures. Prog Cardiovasc Nurs 5: 50–58.

Criado FJ, Queral LA, Patten P, Rudolphi D (1990) Laser angioplasty in the lower extremities: an early surgical experience. J Vasc Surg 11: 532–535.

Cull DL, Feinberg RL, Wheeler JR, Snyder SO Jr, Gregory RT, Gayle RG,

Parent FN 3d (1991) Experience with laser-assisted balloon angioplasty and a rotary angioplasty instrument: lessons learned. J Vasc Surg 14: 332–339.

Cumberland DC, Sanborn TA, Tayler DI, Moore DJ, Welsh CL, Greenfield AJ, Guben JK, Ryan TJ (1986) Percutaneous laser thermal angioplasty: initial clinical results with a laser probe in total peripheral artery occlusions. Lancet 1: 1457–1459.

Cumberland DC, Tayler DI, Procter AE (1986) Laser-assisted percutaneous angioplasty: initial clinical experience in peripheral arteries. Clin Radiol 37: 423–428.

Cumberland DC, Tayler DI, Procter AE (1986) Percutaneous laser angioplasty. Initial clinical experience. Ann Radiol (Paris) 29: 215–218.

Deckelbaum LI (1989) Laser-assisted angioplasty of inferior vena caval obstructions: what's good for the artery is good for the vein. Hepatology 9: 338–339.

De Scheerder IK, Strauss BH, De Feyter PJ, Beatt KJ, Baur LH, Wijns W, Heyndrix GR, Suryapranata H, Van den Brand M, Buis B, et al (1992) Stenting of venous bypass grafts: a new treatment modality for patients who are poor candidates for reintervention. Am Heart J 123(4 Pt 1): 1046–1054.

Diethrich EB, Santiago O, Bahadir I (1991) Laser-assisted angioplasty in the treatment of prosthetic graft stenosis. Angiology 42: 576–580.

Diethrich EB, Timbadia E, Bahadir I (1989) Applications and limitations of laser-assisted angioplasty. Eur J Vasc Surg 3: 61–70.

Dixon JA (1988) Current laser applications in general surgery. REVIEW ARTICLE: 105 REFS. Ann Surg 207: 355–372.

Douek PC, Leon MB, Geschwind H, Cook PS, Selzer P, Miller DL, Bonner RF (1990) Occlusive peripheral vascular disease: a multicenter trial of fluorescence-guided, pulsed dye laser-assisted balloon angioplasty. Radiology 180: 127–133.

Doyle JE (1986) Treatment modalities in peripheral vascular disease. REVIEW ARTICLE: 29 REFS. Nurs Clin North Am 21: 241–253.

Duda SH, Huppert PE, Arndt V, Wehrmann M, Haase KK, Claussen CD (1992) In vitro and clinical feasibility and study with an over-the-wire delivery system for pulsed dye laser angioplasty. J Vasc Intervent Radiol 3(1): 59–65.

Duda SH, Wehrmann M, Haase KK, Huppert PE, Karsch KR, Claussen CD (1992) Holmium:YAG laser angioplasty. Experimental ablation of vascular tissue via flexible ring catheters. Acta Radiol 33(6): 538–541.

Dutta AL, Panja M (1989) Laser angioplasty (editorial) (published erratum appears in J Indian Med Assoc 1989 Nov;87(11): 258). J Indian Med Assoc 87: 225–226.

Enge IP, Schilvold A (1988) Recanalization of occluded peripheral vessels by laser assisted PTA. Ann Radiol (Paris) 31: 74–76.

Farrell EM, Higginson LA, Nip WS, Walley VM, Keon WJ (1986) Pulsed excimer laser angioplasty of human cadaveric arteries. J Vasc Surg 3: 284–287.

Feinberg RL, Wheeler JR, Gregory RT, Snyder SO Jr, Gayle RG, Parent FN 3d (1990) Initial results and subsequent outcome of laser thermal-assisted balloon angioplasty of 56 consecutive femoropopliteal lesions. Am J Surg 160: 166–169; discussion 169–170.

Fleisher HL 3rd, Thompson BW, McCowan TC, Ferris EJ, Reifsteck JE, Barnes RW (1987) Human percutaneous laser angioplasty. Patient selection criteria and early results. Am J Surg 154: 666–670.

Fletcher JP, Hazelton S, Wong KP, Carr P, Kenny J, Taylor A, Avramovic JR, Fisher P, Moylan D (1992) Laser angioplasty for superficial femoral and proximal popliteal artery occlusion. J Cardiovasc Surg 33(1): 75–78.

Fletcher JP, Wong KP (1989) Early experiences with laser-assisted thermal angioplasty for peripheral vascular disease. Med J Aust 151: 372, 375, 378–379.

Fuller TA (1983) Surgical application of lasers. In Fundamentals of Laser Surgery and Medicine. (Dixon J A, Ed). Chicago, Year Book.

Furui S, Yamauchi T, Ohtomo K, Tsuchiya K, Makita K, Takenaka E (1988) Hepatic inferior vena cava obstructions: clinical results of treatment with percutaneous transluminal laser-assisted angioplasty. Radiology 166: 673–677.

Garcia AT (1992) Laser-assisted angioplasty: an intervention and backup system for catheterization laboratories conducting angioplasty. Tex Med 88(4): 70–71.

Gaylord GM (1991) Vascular interventional radiologists, the development of new technologies, marketing, and the auk [editorial; comment]. Radiology 181: 15–16.

Geschwind H, Fabre M, Chaitman Br, Lefebvre-Villardebo M, Ladouch A, Boussignac G, Blair JD, Kennedy HL (1986) Histopathology after Nd-YAG laser percutaneous transluminal angioplasty of peripheral arteries. J Am Coll Cardiol 8: 1089–1095.

Geschwind HJ (1986) Destructive lasers in arterial disease. Life Support Syst 4: 95–97.

Geschwind HJ (1988) Laser angioplasty: newer modalities. Ann Radiol (Paris) 31: 69–73.

Gindi GR, Darken CJ, O'Brien KM, Stetz ML, Deckelbaum LI (1991) Neural network and conventional classifiers for fluorescence-guided laser angioplasty. Ieee Trans Biomed Eng 38: 246–252.

Ginsburg R (1988) Percutaneous laser angioplasty in the treatment of peripheral vascular disease. REVIEW ARTICLE: 0 REFS. Thorac Cardiovasc Surg (Suppl 2): 142–145.

Ginsburg R, Kim DS, Cuthener D, Toth J, Mitchell RS (1984) Salvage of an ischemic limb by laser and angioplasty: description of a new technique. Clin Cardiol 7: 54–58.

Ginsburg R, Wexler L (1989) Hydrophilic guide wire for laser-assisted angioplasty (letter). J Vasc Surg 9: 507–508.

Ginsburg R, Wexler L, Mitchell RS, Profitt D (1985) Percutaneous transluminal laser angioplasty for the treatment of peripheral vascular disease: clinical experience in sixteen patients. Radiology 156: 619–624.

Goldsmith MF (1987) More light shed on structure and destruction of plaque as laser angioplasty research heats up (news). JAMA 257: 288.

Grundfest WS, Litvack F, Hickey A, Doyle L, Glick D, Lee M, Chaux A, Treiman R, Cohen L, Foran R, et al (1987) The current status of angioscopy and laser angioplasty. J Vasc Surg 5: 667–673.

Gunby P (1987) Laser may provide better channel, smoother lumen in future coronary arterial occlusions: full potential awaits improved technology (news). JAMA 257: 1283.

Haase KK, Baumbach A, Wehrmann M, Duda S, Cerullo G, Ruckle B, Steiger E, Karsch KR (1991) Potential use of holmium lasers for angioplasty: evaluation of a new solid-state laser for ablation of atherosclerotic plaque. Lasers Surg Med 11: 232–237.

Hallett JW Jr (1986) Trends in revascularization of the lower extremity. Mayo Clin Proc 61: 369–376.

Harrington ME, Schwartz ME, Sanborn TA, Mitty HA, Miller CA, McGinnis K, Harrington EB (1990) Expanded indications for laser-assisted balloon angioplasty in peripheral arterial disease. J Vasc Surg 11: 146–154; discussion 154–155.

Huppert PE, Duda SH, Helber U, Karsch KR, Claussen CD (1992) Comparison of pulsed laser-assisted angioplasty and balloon angioplasty in femoropopliteal artery occlusions. Radiology 184(2): 363–367.

Huppert PE, Duda SH, Seboldt H, Claussen CD (1991) Dye laser-assisted angioplasty with multifiber catheters: short-term results in the treatment of 29 peripheral arterial occlusions. AJR 157: 1253–1257.

Huppert PE, Seboldt H, Duda SH, Seiter H, Claussen CD, Hoffmeister HE (1991) Laser angioplasty of peripheral arterial occlusive disease. Thorac Cardiovasc Surg 39(Suppl 3): 248–251.

Isner JM (1988) Excimer laser angioplasty: Pygmalion makes it to the ball. Lasers Surg Med 8: 447–449.

Isner JM, Lucas AR, Fields CD (1988) Laser therapy in the treatment of cardiovascular disease. Br J Hosp Med 40: 172–178.

Isner JM, Pickering JG, Mosseri M (1992) Laser-induced dissections: pathogenesis and implications for therapy (editorial; comment). J Am Coll Cardiol 19(7): 1619–1621.

Isner JM, Rosenfield K, Losordo DW (1990) Excimer laser atherectomy. The greening of Sisyphus (comment). REVIEW ARTICLE: 32 REFS. Comment on: Circulation 81: 1849–1859. Circulation 81: 2018–2021.

Isner JM, Rosenfield K, White CJ, Ramee S, Kearney M, Pieczek A, Langevin RE Jr, Razvi S (1992) In vivo assessment of vascular pathology resulting from laser irradiation. Analysis of 23 patients studied by directional atherectomy immediately after laser angioplasty. Circulation 85(6): 2185–2196.

Jeans WD, Murphy P, Hughes AO, Horrocks M, Baird RN (1990) Randomized trial of laser-assisted passage through occluded femoro-popliteal arteries. Br J Radiol 63: 19–21.

Jenkins RD, Sinclair IN, Anand R, Kalil AG Jr, Schoen FJ, Spears JR (1988) Laser balloon angioplasty: effect of tissue temperature on weld strength of human postmortem intima-medial separations. Lasers Surg Med 8: 30–39.

Jenkins RD, Sinclair IN, Anand RK, James LM, Spears JR (1988) Laser balloon angioplasty: effect of exposure duration on shear strength of welded layers of postmortem human aorta. Lasers Surg Med 8: 392–396.

Kaminow IP, Wiesenfeld JM, Choy, DSJ (1984) Argon laser disintegration of thrombus and atherosclerotic plaque. Appl Optics 23: 1,301.

Kelly PJ, Kall BA, Goerss S, Earnest F 4th (1986) Computer-assisted stereotaxic laser resection of intra-axial brain neoplasms. J Neurosurg 64: 427–439.

Kipshidze N, Petrosyan J (1990) New trends in laser application: atherolysis. Int Angiol 9: 111–116.

Kjellstrom BT, Cothren RM, Kramer JR (1987) The use of lasers in vascular and cardiac surgery. Clinical review. Acta Chir Scand 153: 493–499.

Koga N, Sato T, Baba T, Ueda O, Okazaki H, Kohchi K, Norita H, Maw PR, Moriyama A (1989) Angioscopy in transluminal balloon and laser angioplasty in the management of chronic hemodialysis fistulae. ASAIO Trans 35: 193–196.

Kvasnicka J, Boudik F, Stanek F, Kubecek V, Krivanek J, Keclik R, Prochazkova H, Hamal K (1991) Percutaneous laser angioplasty with a pulsed Nd:YAG laser. Initial clinical experience and early follow-up. Int Angiol 10: 29–33.

Labs JD, Merillat JC, Williams GM (1988) Analysis of solid phase debris from laser angioplasty: potential risks of atheroembolism. J Vasc Surg 7: 326–335.

Labs JD, White RI Jr, Anderson JH, Williams GM (1987) Thermodynamic correlates of hot tip laser angioplasty. Invest Radiol 22: 954–959.

Lai ST, Cheng KJ (1991) Results of angioscopy-assisted intraoperative transluminal angioplasty of the iliac and femoral artery. Chin Med J 48: 25–30.

Lammer J, Karnel F (1988) Percutaneous transluminal laser angioplasty with contact probes. Radiology 168: 733–737.

Lammer J, Kleinert R, Pilger E, Schmidt-Kloiber H, Reichel E (1989) Contact probes for intravascular laser recanalization. Experimental evaluation. Invest Radiol 24: 190–195.

Lammer J, Pilger E, Decrinis M, Quehenberger F, Klein GE, Stark G (1992) Pulsed excimer laser versus continuous-wave Nd:YAG laser versus conventional angioplasty of peripheral arterial occlusions: prospective, controlled, randomised trial. Lancet 340(8829): 1183–1188.

Lammer J, Pilger E, Karnel F, Schurawitzki H, Horvath W, Riedl M, Umek H, Klein GE, Schreyer H, Kretschmer G, et al. (1991) Laser angioplasty: results of a prospective, multicenter study at 3-year follow-up. Radiology 178: 335–337.

LaMuraglia GM, Murray S, Anderson RR, Prince MR (1988) Effect of pulse duration on selective ablation of atherosclerotic plaque by 480- to 490-nanometer laser radiation. Lasers Surg Med 8: 18–21.

Leachman DR, Avedissian MG, Krajcer Z, Angelini P (1989) Transluminal laser angioplasty of the femoropopliteal circulation by use of a percutaneous popliteal approach. Am J Cardiol 64: 106–108.

Lee BI, Becker GJ, Waller BF, Barry KJ, Connolly RJ, Kaplan J, Shapiro AR, Nardella PC (1989) Thermal compression and molding of atherosclerotic vascular tissue with use of radiofrequency energy: implications for radiofrequency balloon angioplasty. J Am Coll Cardiol 13: 1167–1175.

Lee G, Ikeda RM, Stobbe D, et al (1984) Intraoperative use of dual fiberoptic catheter for simultaneous in vivo visualization and laser vaporization of peripheral atherosclerotic obstructive disease. Cath Cardiovasc Diag 10: 11–16.

Lee G, Masden R, Weiss JA, Falk RL, Temes GD, Pool GE, Argenal A, Wixson D, Mason DT (1988) Percutaneous peripheral laser angioplasty: demonstration of the clinical safety and efficacy of a new coaxial-guided laser-heated cap system. Am Heart J 116: 1640–1641.

Lee G, Morelli R, Long JB, Shea W, Lopez AC, Cunningham TM, Mason DT (1989) Combined laser-thermal and atherectomy treatment of peripheral arterial occlusion: documentation by angioscopy and angiography. Am Heart J 118: 1324–1327.

Lee G, Reis RL, Boggan MD, Chan MC, Lee MH, Low RI, Hannah H 3rd, Mason DT (1987) Laser recanalization in severe end-stage peripheral vascular disease. Am J Cardiol 59: 386–387.

Leon MB, Almagor Y, Bartorelli AL, Prevosti LG, Teirstein PS, Chang R, Miller DL, Smith PD, Bonner RF (1990) Fluorescence-guided laser-assisted balloon angioplasty in patients with femoropopliteal occlusions. Circulation 81: 143–155.

Levy JM, Hessel SJ, Horsley WW, Cook GC, Dickey JE (1989) Value of laser-assisted angioplasty in the community hospital. Radiology 170: 1017–1018.

Lindgren I, Raekallio J (1966) Accumulation of tetracycline in atherosclerotic lesions of human aorta. Acta Pathol Microbiol Scand 66: 323.

Litvack F, Grundfest W, Beeder C, Forrester JS (1986) Laser angioplasty: status and prospects. Semin Intervent Radiol 3: 75.

Litvack F, Grundfest WS, Adler L, Hickey AE, Segalowitz J, Hestrin LB, Mohr FW, Goldenberg T, Laudenslager JS, Forrester JS (1989) Percutaneous excimer-laser and excimer-laser-assisted angioplasty of the lower extremities: results of initial clinical trial. Radiology 172: 331–335.

Litvack F, Grundfest WS, Goldenberg T, Laudenslager J, Forrester JS (1989) Percutaneous excimer laser angioplasty of aortocoronary saphenous vein grafts. JACC 14: 803–808.

Litvack F, Grundfest WS, Lee ME, Carroll RM, Foran R, Chaux A, Berci G, Rose HB, Matloff JM, Forrester JS (1985) Angioscopic visualization of blood vessel interior in animals and humans. Clin Cardiol 8: 65–70.

Litvack F, Grundfest WS, Papaioannou T, Mohr FW, Jakubowski AT, Forrester JS (1988) Role of laser and thermal ablation devices in the treatment of vascular diseases. REVIEW ARTICLE: 53 REFS. Am J Cardiol 61: 81G-86G.

Lothian CL (1992) Laser angioplasty. Nursing 22(1): 62–64.

Masotti M, Riambau V, Crexells C, Oriol A (1992) Two-year follow-up after laser thermal balloon angioplasty (LTBA) in lower extremities: initial experience. Clin Cardiol 15(5): 336–342.

Matsumoto T, Koyanagi N, Yang Y, DuPree J, Naide D (1988) Argon laser arterial recanalization. Pa Med 91: 27–28, 30.

Matsumoto T, Okamura T, Yang Y, Rajyaguru V, Morris RJ (1989) Laser-assisted reconstructive vascular surgery. Circulation 80: III49–53.

May J, White GH, Waugh RC, Walker PJ, Harris JP (1991) Laser angioplasty of the iliac arteries. Aust N Z J Surg 61: 267–270.

McAlpin GM, Rama K, Berg RA (1991) Thermal laser assisted balloon angioplasty in lower extremity occlusive disease. Am Surg 57: 558–565; discussion 565–566.

McCarthy WJ, Vogelzang RL, Nemcek AA Jr, Joseph A, Pearce WH, Flinn WR, Yao JS (1991) Excimer laser-assisted femoral angioplasty: early results. J Vasc Surg 13: 607–614.

McCowan TC, Ferris EJ, Baker ML, Robbins KV, Reifsteck JE, Fleisher HL, Barnes RW (1986) Human percutaneous laser angioplasty. J Arkansas Med Soc 82: 594–596.

McCowan TC, Ferris EJ, Barnes RW, Baker ML (1988) Laser thermal angioplasty for the treatment of obstruction of the distal superficial femoral or popliteal arteries. AJR 150: 1169–1173.

Michaels JA, Cross FW, Shaw P, Raphael M, Bowker TJ, Brown SG, Adiseshiah M, Marston A (1989) Laser angioplasty with a pulsed NdYAG laser: early clinical experience. Br J Surg 76: 921–924.

Mitchell DC, Murray A, Wood RF, Grasty M, Smith RE, Dacie JE, Walters TK, Cotton G (1992) Laser-assisted angioplasty for arterial occlusion of the lower limb: initial results and follow-up. Br J Surg 79(1): 81–85.

Mitty HA, Sanborn TA, Train JS, Dan SJ (1989) Laser catheter thermal angioplasty: technique and early results in 34 patients. AJR 153: 617–621.

Mohan SR, Hawker RJ, Wolinski AP, Dunham JA, Grimley RP, Downing R, (1992) Platelet accumulation after laser angioplasty—a scintigraphic assessment. Angiology 43(1): 11–21.

Moneta GL, Schneider E, Jager K, Brulisauer M, Thuring-Vollenweider U, Bollinger A (1988) Laser Doppler flux and vasomotion in patients before and after transluminal angioplasty for limb salvage. Vasa 17: 26–31.

Morcos NC, Berns M, Henry WL (1988) Phycocyanin: laser activation, cytotoxic effects, and uptake in human atherosclerotic plaque. Lasers Surg Med 8: 10–17.

Murray A, Crocker PR, Wood RF (1988) The pulsed dye laser and atherosclerotic vascular disease. Br J Surg 75: 349–351.

Murray A, Wood RF (1989) Peripheral laser angioplasty with the pulsed dye laser and ball-tipped optical fibres (letter). Lancet 1: 324–325.

Nordstrom LA, Castaneda-Zuniga AR, Grewe DD, Schoster JV (1986) Laser enhanced transluminal angioplasty: the role of coaxial fiber placement. Semin Intervent Radiol 3: 47–52.

Nordstrom LA, Castaneda-Zuniga WR, Lindeka CC, Rasmussen TM, Burnside DK (1988) Laser angioplasty: controlled delivery of argon laser energy. Radiology 167: 463–465.

Nordstrom LA, Castaneda-Zuniga WR, Von Seggern KB (1991) Peripheral arterial obstructions: analysis of patency 1 year after laser-assisted transluminal angioplasty. Radiology 181: 515–520.

Nordstrom LA, Castaneda-Zuniga WR, Young EG, Von Seggern KB (1988) Direct argon laser exposure for recanalization of peripheral arteries: early results. Radiology 168: 359–364.

O'Brien KM, Gmitro AF, Gindi GR, Stetz ML, Cutruzzola FW, Laifer LI, Deckelbaum LI (1989) Development and evaluation of spectral classification algorithms for fluorescence guided laser angioplasty. IEEE Trans Biomed Eng 36: 424–431.

Odink HF, de Valois HC, Eikelboom BC (1991) Femoropopliteal arterial occlusions: laser-assisted versus conventional percutaneous transluminal angioplasty. Radiology 181: 61–66.

Okadome K, Muto Y, Onohara T, Yamamura S, Sugimachi K (1991) Laser thermal angioplasty for early repair of anastomotic stenosis after lower extemity arterial reconstruction: initial experience. Eur J Vasc Surg 5: 303–309.

Pia HW (1986) The future role of neurosurgery in the case of vascular diseases of the central nervous system. Neurosurg Rev 9: 51–68.

Pilger E, Lammer J, Bertuch H, Stark G, Decrinis M, Pfeiffer KP, Krejs GJ (1991) Nd:YAG laser with sapphire tip combined with balloon angioplasty in peripheral arterial occlusions. Long-term results [comments]. Circulation 83: 141–147.

Pilger E, Lammer J, Kleinert R, Ascher W, Bertuch H (1988) Laser angioplasty with a contact probe for the treatment of peripheral vascular disease. Cardiovasc Res 22: 149–153.

Polla LL, Tan OT, Garden JM, Parrish JA (1987) Tunable pulsed dye laser for the treatment of benign cutaneous vascular ectasia. Dermatologica 174: 11–17.

Poulain M (1985) The paths ahead for fluoride fibres. Photon Spectra 19: 68–70.

Prince MR (1988) Laser angioplasty in peripheral vascular disease (letter). Cardiovasc Res 22: 446.

Prince MR, Athanasoulis CA (1992) Fluorescence-guided pulsed dye laser-assisted angioplasty (letter; comment). Radiology 182(3): 896–897.

Rajyaguru V, Okamura T, Matsumoto T (1989) YAG laser angioplasty in lower extremity: sole therapy as well as adjunct to balloon dilatation. J Indian Med Assoc 87: 227–229.

Redd DC, Yue KT, Martin LG, Kaufman SL (1991) Young Investigator Award. Raman spectroscopy of human atherosclerotic plaque: implications for laser angioplasty. J Vasc Intervent Radiol 2(2): 247–252.

Rienks R, Verdaasdonk RM, Borst C, Smits PC, Jambroes G, van Gemert MJ, Robles de Medina EO, Hitchcock JF (1988) Nd-YAG laser energy distribution in an artificial obstruction: influence of lasing parameters in a model of laser angioplasty. Lasers Surg Med 8: 90–94.

Rosenthal D, Pesa FA, Gottsegen WL, Crew JR, Moss CA, Walsky R, Pallos LL (1991) Thermal laser-assisted balloon angioplasty of the superficial femoral artery: a multicenter review of 602 cases. J Vasc Surg 14: 152–159.

Rosenthal D, Wheeler WG 3d, Seagraves A, Erdoes L, Lamis PA, Jones M, Clark MD, Pallos LL (1991) Nd:YAG iliac and femoropopliteal laser angioplasty: results with large probes as "sole therapy." J Cardiovasc Surg 32: 186–191.

Rosenthal E, Foussas S, Montarello JK, Boyd EG, Curry PV (1990) Laser thermal angioplasty probe ("hot tip") temperature: effects of flow. Lasers Surg Med 10: 124–132.

Rutter S, Ellis R (1986) Laser-assisted angioplasty. Nurs Times 82: 40–41.

Ryan TJ, Sanborn TA, Cumberland DC, Faxon DP, Haudenschild CC (1986) Laser thermal angioplasty: from the experimental model to early human experience. Trans Am Clin Climatol Assoc 98: 36–42.

Salvian AJ, Morris DC, Connell DG (1990) Laser-assisted transluminal angioplasty of the superficial femoral and popliteal arteries. Can J Surg 33: 213–215.

Sanborn TA (1988) Laser angioplasty: peripheral and coronary applications. Cardiovasc Clin 19: 181–195.

Sanborn TA (1989) Technical success, clinical success, and patency in laser angioplasty (letter; comment). Comment on: Radiology 1988 Aug; 168(2): 359–364. Radiology 170: 576–578.

Sanborn TA (1991) Primary success, long-term patency, reporting standards, and indications for peripheral angioplasty devices [editorial; comment]. Circulation 83: 350–352.

Sanborn TA, Cumberland DC, Greenfield AJ, Motarjeme A, Schwarten DE, Leachman DR, Ferris EJ, Myler RK, McCowan TC, Tatpati D, et al (1989) Peripheral laser-assisted balloon angioplasty. Initial multicenter experience in 219 peripheral arteries. Arch Surg 124: 1099–1103.

Sanborn TA, Cumberland DC, Greenfield AJ, Welsh CL, Guben JK (1988) Percutaneous laser thermal angioplasty: initial results and 1-year follow-up in 129 femoropopliteal lesions (see comments). Comment in: Radiology 1989 Sep;172(3 Pt 2): 941–942. Radiology 168: 121–125.

Sanborn TA, et al (1985) Acute and chronic results of angioplasty with a laser heated metallic tip fiber (Abstract). Lasers Med Surg 5: 169.

Sanborn TA, Greenfield AJ (1989) Response. Peripheral laser angioplasty: need for organized clinical trials. Radiology 172: 943.

Sanborn TA, Greenfield AJ, Guben JK, Menzoian JO, LoGerfo FW (1987) Human percutaneous and intraoperative laser thermal angioplasty: initial clinical results as an adjunct to balloon angioplasty. J Vasc Surg 5: 83–90.

Sanborn TA, Mitty HA, Train JS, Dan SJ (1989) Infrapopliteal and below-knee popliteal lesions: treatment with sole laser thermal angioplasty. Work in progress. Radiology 172: 89–93.

Sanfelippo PM (1989) The role of lasers in the management of peripheral vascular disease. Angiology 40: 982–986.

Sartori M, Henry PD, Sauerbrey R, Tittel FK, Weilbaecher D, Roberts R (1987) Tissue interactions and measurement of ablation rates with ultraviolet and visible lasers in canine and human arteries. Lasers Surg Med 7: 300–306.

Savolainen H, Keto P, Verkkala K, Schroder T, Mattila S (1992) Peripheral excimer laser-assisted angioplasty. Preliminary clinical experience. Ann Chir Gynaecol 81(1): 19–22.

Schaldach M (1990) Cardiovascular laser application. REVIEW ARTICLE: 30 REFS. Artif Organs 14: 28–40.

Scheu M, Kagel H, Zwaan M, Lebeau A, Engelhardt R (1991) A new concept for a realtime feedback system in angioplasty with a flashlamp pumped dye laser. Lasers Surg Med 11: 133–140.

SCVIR (Society of Cardiovascular and Interventional Radiology) (1989) position statement on thermal laser angioplasty. Radiology 172: 944.

Seeger JM (1991) Laser angioplasty. A vascular surgeon's view. Circulation 83: I97–98.

Seeger JM, Abela GS (1986) Angioscopy as an adjunct to arterial reconstructive surgery: a preliminary report. J Vasc Surg 4: 315–320.

Seeger JM, Abela GS, Silverman SH, Jablonski SK (1989) Initial results of laser recanalization in lower extremity arterial reconstruction. J Vasc Surg 9: 10–17.

Seeger JM, Kaelin LD, Barbeau G, Abela GS (1990) Laser recanalization in high risk patients. Lasers Surg Med 10: 105–111.

SenSarma PK, Tatpati DA, Erskin JT (1992) Human laser assisted angioplasty: clinical results of 42 case trial in peripheral vessels. J Indian Med Assoc 90(9): 247–248.

Silverman SH, Khoury AI, Seeger JM, Tomaru T, Hawkins IF Jr, Abela GS (1989) Effect of CO2 and blood media on laser probe temperature. Lasers Surg Med 9: 17–21.

Smithson PH, Jeans WD, Murphy P (1989) Installation requirements for an argon laser angioplasty system. Br J Radiol 62: 71–73.

Spears JR, James LM, Leonard BM, Sinclair IN, Jenkins RD, Motamedi M, Sinofsky EL (1988) Plaque-media rewelding with reversible tissue optical property changes during receptive cw Nd: YAG laser exposure (see comments). Comment in: Lasers Surg Med 1989;9(5): 506–508. Lasers Surg Med 8: 477–485.

Spears JR, Shropshire D, Paulin S (1983) Fluorescence of experimental atheromatous plaques with hematoporphyrin derivative. J Clin Invest 71: 395.

Spies JB, LeQuire MH, Brantley SD, Williams JE, Beckett WC, Mills JL (1990) Comparison of balloon angioplasty and laser thermal angioplasty in the treatment of femoropopliteal atherosclerotic disease: initial results of a prospective randomized trial. Work in progress (see comments). J Vasc Intervent Radiol 1(1): 39–42.

Steg PG, Menasche P (1989) Utilization of laser arterial angioplasty. Ann Vasc Surg 3: 86–94.

Strandness DE Jr, Barnes RW, Katzen B, Ring EJ (1989) Indiscriminate use of laser angioplasty (editorial). Radiology 172: 945–946.

Strandness DE Jr, Barnes RW, Katzen BT, Ring EJ (1989) Indiscriminate use of laser-assisted angioplasty (letter) (see comments). N Engl J Med 321: 1417.

Strikwerda S, Bott-Silverman C, Ratliff NB, Goormastic M, Cothren RM, Costello B, Kittrell C, Feld MS, Kramer JR (1988) Effects of varying argon ion laser intensity and exposure time on the ablation of atherosclerotic plaque. Lasers Surg Med 8: 66–71.

Stroh JA, Sanborn TA, Haudenschild CC (1990) Experimental argon laser thermal angioplasty as an adjunct to balloon angioplasty in peripheral arteriosclerotic disease. Cathet Cardiovasc Diagn 20: 63–70.

Tani M, Mizuno K, Midorikawa H, Igari T, Egawa M, Niimura S, Fukuchi S, et al. (1993) Thermal laser-assisted angioplasty of renal artery stenosis for renovascular hypertension. Cardiovasc Intervent Radiol 16(1): 52–54.

Tatpati DA, Sensarma PK, Erskin JT (1988) Angioscopy as an adjunct to laser-assisted angioplasty in seven peripheral vascular cases. Kans Med 89: 305–307.

Teitelbaum GP (1992) Holmium:YAG laser recanalization (letter). Lasers Surg Med 12(1): 112–113.

Tobis J, Smolin M, Mallery J, MacLeay L, Johnston WD, Connolly JE, Lewis G, Zuch B, Henry W, Berns M (1989) Laser-assisted thermal angioplasty in human peripheral artery occlusions: mechanism of recanalization. JACC 13: 1547–1554.

Tobis JM, Conroy R, Deutsch LS, Gordon I, Honye J, Andrews J, Profeta G, Chatzkel S, Berns M (1991) Laser-assisted versus mechanical recanalization of femoral arterial occlusions. Am J Cardiol 68: 1079–1086.

Tomaru T, Geschwind HJ, Boussignac G, Lange F, Tahk SJ (1992) Characteristics of shock waves induced by pulsed lasers and their effects on arterial tissue: comparison of excimer, pulse dye, and holmium YAG lasers. Am Heart J 123(4 Pt 1): 896–904.

Tomaru T, Geschwind HJ, Boussignac G, Lange F, Tahk SJ (1992) Comparison of ablation efficacy of excimer, pulsed-dye, and holmium-YAG lasers relevant to shock waves. Am Heart J 123(4 Pt 1): 886–895.

Torres JH, Motamedi M, Welch AJ (1990) Disparate absorption of argon laser radiation by fibrous versus fatty plaque: implications for laser angioplasty. Lasers Surg Med 10: 149–157.

Turnbull IW, Bannister CM (1992) Can laser angioplasty replace carotid endarterectomy in the management of nonstenotic atheromatous disease of the carotid bifurcation? Surg Neurol 38(1): 73–76.

Turnbull IW, Bannister CM, Armstrong G, Edwards P (1991) An experimental model to assess the value of laser angioplasty in the management of atheromatous disease of the carotid bifurcation. Br J Neurosurg 5: 25–30.

Verbunt RJ, Fitzmaurice MA, Kramer JR, Ratliff NB, Kittrell C, Taroni P, Cothren RM, Baraga J, Feld M (1992) Characterization of ultraviolet laser-induced autofluorescence of ceroid deposits and other structures in atherosclerotic plaques as a potential diagnostic for laser angiosurgery. Am Heart J 123(1): 208–216.

Verdaasdonk RM, Holstege FC, Jansen ED, Borst C (1991) Temperature along the surface of modified fiber tips for Nd:YAG laser angioplasty. Lasers Surg Med 11: 213–222.

Vorwerk D, Zolotas G, Hessel S, Adam G, Wondrazek F, Gunther RW (1991) In vitro ablation of normal and diseased vascular tissue by a fiber-transmitted holmium laser. Invest Radiol 26: 660–664.

Ward H (1987) Molding of laser energy by shaped optic fiber tips. Lasers Surg Med 7: 405–413.

Weber H, Enders S, Hessel S (1991) Thermal effects and histologic changes from Nd:YAG laser irradiation on normal and diseased aortic tissue using a novel angioplasty catheter with a mobile optical fiber: an in vitro assessment. Angiology 42: 597–606.

Webber M, Jenkins N (1988) Laser treatment of peripheral vascular disease. Implications for nursing care. Prog Cardiovasc Nurs 3: 81–88.

Wexler L (1989) Percutaneous transluminal angioplasty of peripheral vascular occlusions: a clinical perspective (editorial). JACC 13: 1555–1557.

White CJ, Ramee SR (1992) Options for percutaneous coronary and peripheral revascularization. Med Clin North Am 76(5): 1099–1124.

White GH, White RA, Colman PD, Kopchok GE (1989) Experimental and clinical applications of angioscopic guidance for laser angioplasty. Am J Surg 158: 495–500; discussion 500–501.

White RA, White GH (1989) Laser thermal probe recanalization of occluded arteries. REVIEW ARTICLE. 31 REFS. J Vasc Surg 9: 598–608.

White RA, White GH, Mehringer MC, Chaing FL, Wilson SE (1990) A clinical trial of laser thermal angioplasty in patients with advanced peripheral vascular disease. Ann Surg 212: 257–265.

White RA, White GH, Vlasak J, Fujitani R, Kopchok GE (1988) Histopathology of human laser thermal angioplasty recanalization. Lasers Surg Med 8: 469–476.

White RA, Wilson SE (1992) Laser-assisted balloon angioplasty. Adv Surg 25: 209–222.

Widlus DM, Osterman FA Jr (1989) Evaluation and percutaneous management of atherosclerotic peripheral vascular disease. JAMA 261: 3148–3154.

Wieman TJ (1986) Lasers and the surgeon. Am J Surg 151: 493–500.

Wollenek G, Laufer G (1989) Laser angioplasty in the treatment of peripheral vascular disease. Herz 14: 29–38.

Wollenek G, Laufer G, Grabenwoger F (1988) Percutaneous transluminal excimer laser angioplasty in total peripehral artery occlusion in man. Lasers Surg Med 8: 464–468.

Wright JG, Belkin M, Greenfield AJ, Guben JK, Sanborn TA, Menzoian JO (1989) Laser angioplasty for limb salvage: observations on early results (discussion 37–38). J Vasc Surg 10: 29–37.

Yamanashi WS, Patil AA, Hill DL, Lepage JR, Yassa NA, Valentine JL, Lester PD (1988) Precision surgery with an electromagnetically induced current convergence probe application in aneurysm treatment, angioplasty, and brain tumor resection in in vivo and in vitro models. Med Instrum 22: 205–216.

Yang X, Manninen H, Naukkarinen A, Ji H, Kankkunen JP, Suhonen M, Soimakallio S (1991) CO2 gas perfusion: improved efficiency and safety with sapphire-probe laser ablation of human artery. J Vasc Intervent Radiol 2(1): 159–165.

Yang XM, Manninen H, Soimakallio S (1991) Laser ablation ability of different fiber tips on human arteries. The role of photothermal effect. Chin Med J 104: 721–727.

Yang Y, Hashizume M, Arbutina D, Milewski LF, DuPree J, Matsumoto T (1987) Argon laser angioplasty with a laser probe. J Vasc Surg 6: 60–65.

Yared SF, Langsing AM, Norman JC, Masri ZH (1991) Laser-assisted balloon angioplasty in peripheral vascular surgery: a preliminary report. J Ky Med Assoc 89: 118–120.

Yu S, Wang DW, Hu XJ, Zhao ZS, Wang PL, Liu PT, Cui YB (1989) Choice of lasers for laser angioplasty. J Tongji Med Univ 9: 181–186.

Zeevi B, Gal D, Abramovici A, Berant M, Blieden LC, Katzir A (1987) Carbon dioxide fiberoptic laser for treatment of coarctation of the aorta. Am Heart J 113: 1518–1519.

Zwaan M, Weiss HD, Gothlin JH, Kummer D, Scheu M, Kagel H, Gmelin E, Rinast E (1992) Initial clinical experience with a new pulsed dye laser device in angioplasty of limb ischemia and shunt fistula obstructions. Eur J Radiol 14(1): 72–76.

VI. Lasers

B. Coronary

Abela G, Franzini D, Crea F, Pepine CJ, Conti CR (1984) No evidence of accelerated atherosclerosis following laser radiation (Abstract). Circulation 70 (Suppl II): 323.

Abela GS (1988) Laser recanalization: a basic and clinical perspective. REVIEW ARTICLE: 21 REFS. Thorac Cardiovasc Surg (Suppl 2): 137–141.

Abela GS, Conti CR (1983) Laser revascularization: what are its prospects? J Cardiovasc Med 8: 977–984.

Abela GS, et al (1986) Laser angioplasty with angioscopic guidance in man. JACC 8: 184.

Abela GS, et al (1985) "Hot-Tip": another method of laser vascular recanalization. Lasers Surg Med 5: 327.

Abela GS, et al (1985) In vitro effects of Argon laser radiation on blood: quantitative and morphologic analysis. JACC 5: 231.

Abela GS, et al (1985) Laser recanalizaiton of occluded atherosclerotic arteries: an in vivo and in vitro study. Circulation 71: 403.

Abela GS, et al (1985) Regeneration of endothelium and prostacyclin biosynthesis following laser radiation of atherosclerotic monkey arteries (Abstract). JACC 5: 544.

Abela GS, et al (1985) The healing process in normal canine arteries and in atherosclerotic monkey arteries after transluminal laser irradiation. Am J Cardiol 56: 983.

Abela GS, et al (1984) A new model for investigation of transluminal recanalization: human atherosclerotic coronary artery xenografts. Am J Cardiol 54: 200.

Abela GS, et al (1983) Immediate and long-term effects of laser radiation on the arterial wall: light and EM observations. Surg Forum 34: 454.

Abela, GS, et al (1983) Transvascular Argon laser-induced atrioventricular conduction ablation in dogs (Abstract). Circulation 68 (Suppl 3): 58.

Abela GS, Normann S, Cohen D, Feldman RL, Geiser EA, Conti CR (1982) Effects of carbon dioxide, Nd:YAG, and argon laser radiation on coronary atheromatous plaques. Am J Cardiol 50: 1199–1205.

Abela GS, Seeger JM, Barbieri E, Franzini D, Fenech A, Pepine CJ, Conti Cr (1986) Laser angioplasty with angioscopic guidance in humans. JACC 8: 184–192.

Agee K, Wells W (1987) Petroleum products and lasers do not mix (letter). AORN J 45: 1274.

Anand RK, Sinclair IN, Jenkins RD, Hiehle JF Jr, James L, Spears JR (1988) Laser balloon angioplasty: effect of constant temperature versus constant power on tissue weld strength. Lasers Surg Med 8: 40–44.

Anderson HV, King SB 3d (1988) Coronary artery laser therapy. AJR 150: 995–998.

Aretz HT, Martinelli MA, LeDet EG (1989) Intraluminal ultrasound guidance of transverse laser coronary atherectomy. Int J Card Imaging 4: 153–157.

Ashley S, Brooks SG, Gehani AA, Kester RC, Rees MR (1990) Experimental analysis of sapphire contact probes for Nd-YAG laser angioplasty. Angiology 41: 453–462.

Baumbach A, Haase KK, Voelker W, Mauser M, Karsch KR (1991) Effects of intracoronary nitroglycerin on lumen diameter during early follow-up angiography after coronary excimer laser atherectomy. Eur Heart J 12: 726–731.

Berger PB, Bresnahan J (1993) Use of excimer laser in the treatment of chronic total occlusion of a coronary artery that cannot be crossed with a balloon catheter. Cathet Cardiovasc Diagn 28(1): 44–46.

Bhatta KM, Rosen DI, Dretler SP (1989) Acoustic and plasma-guided laser angioplasty. Lasers Surg Med 9: 117–123.

Bittl JA, Sanborn TA (1992) Excimer laser-facilitated coronary angioplasty. Relative risk analysis of acute and follow-up results in 200 patients. Circulation 86(1): 71–80.

Bittl JA, Sanborn TA, Tcheng JE, Siegel RM, Ellis SG (1992) Clinical success, complications and restenosis rates with excimer laser coronary angioplasty. The Percutaneous Excimer Laser Coronary Angioplasty Registry [see comments]. Am J Cardiol 70(20): 1533–1539.

Bjork VO, Sternlieb JJ (1987) Prospects for laser application in cardiac operations. Cardiovasc Clin 17: 415–420.

Blakeslee S (1985) Laser is designed to clean arteries. New York Times: January 29.

Blanche C, Segalowitz J, Czer LS, Wong S, Matloff JM (1991) Excimer laser angioplasty during aortocoronary bypass grafting. Ann Thorac Surg 51: 670–672.

Bogen DK, Derbyshire GJ, Marchlinski FE, Josephson ME (1987) Is catheter ablation on target? Am J Cardiol 60: 1387–1392.

Bowker TJ, Cross FW, Fox KM, Poole-Wilson PA, Bown SG, Rickards AF (1988) Laser assisted coronary angioplasty. Eur Heart J 9 (Suppl C): 25–29.

Buchwald A, Werner G, Unterberg C, Voth A, Wiegand V (1990) Malignant restenosis after primary successful excimer laser coronary angioplasty. Clin Cardiol 13: 397–400.

Chan MC, Lee G, Brames WK, Tsoi D, Lee KK, Vazquez A, Seckinger D, Reis RL, Mason DT (1987) Differential photoabsorption using argon laser radiation on atherosclerotic plaque in non-hemolyzed and hemolyzed blood. Int J Clin Pharmacol Ther Toxicol 25: 527–529.

Chan MC, Lee G, Seckinger DI, et al (1984) Pretreatment with vital dyes to enhance or attenuate argon laser energy absorption in blood vessels (Abstract). Circulation 70 (Suppl II): 298.

Chen DX, Zheng DS, Zhang SH, Wu YX, Bao SH, Xia LL (1991) Factors influencing ablation of atherosclerotic plaque with argon laser. Chin Med J—Peking 104: 330–335.

Choy DS (1986) Laser revascularization, 1985: state of the art. Lasers Surg Med 6: 408–411.

Choy DS, Marco J, Fournial G, Stertzer S (1986) Argon laser recanalization of three totally occluded human right coronary arteries. Clin Cardiol 9: 296–298.

Choy DSJ (1980) Fiberoptic laser tunneling device: the laser catheter. In: Beijin/Ghanghai Proceedings of an International Conference on Lasers. New York, Wiley Interscience, pp 685–690.

Choy DSJ, Stertzer SH, Myler RK, Marco J, Fournial G (1984) Human coronary laser recanalization. Clin Cardiol 7: 377–381.

Choy DSJ, Stertzer SH, Rotterdam HZ, Sharrock N, Kaminow IP (1982) Transluminal laser catheter angioplasty. Am J Cardiol 50: 1206–1208.

Ciccone J, Saksena S, Pantopoulos D (1986) Comparative efficacy of continous and pulsed argon laser ablation of human diseased ventricle. PACE 9: 697–704.

Conacher ID, Paes ML, Morritt GN (1987) Carbon dioxide laser bronchoscopy. A review of problems and complications. Anaesthesia 42: 511–518.

Cook SL, Eigler NL, Shefer A, Goldenberg T, Forrester JS, Litvack F (1991) Percutaneous excimer laser coronary angioplasty of lesions not ideal for balloon angioplasty (comments). Circulation 84: 632–643.

Cooley DA (1987) Revascularization of the ischemic myocardium: current results and expectations for the future. Cardiology 74: 275–285.

Cothrem RM, Hayes GB, Kittrell C, Costello BJ, Sacks BA, Sheavin A, Kramer J, Feld MS (1985) A novel laser catheter for removing atherosclerotic plaque (Abstract). Circulation 72 (Suppl III): 111–402.

Crea F, Davies G, McKenna W, Pashazade M, Taylor K, Maseri A (1986) Percutaneous laser recanalization of coronary arteries (letter). Lancet 2: 214–215.

Crea F, et al (1985) Laser recanalization of acutely thrombosed coronary arteries in live dogs: early results. JACC 6: 1052.

Crea F, et at (1986) Transluminal laser irradiation of coronary arteries in live dogs: angiographic and morphologic study of acute effects. Am J Cardiol 57: 171.

Cross FW, Bowker TJ (1987) Percutaneous laser angioplasty with sapphire tips (letter). Lancet 1: 330.

Cross FW, Bowker TJ (1987) The physical properties of tissue ablation with excimer lasers. Med Instrum 21: 226–230.

Cumberland DC (1987) Laser coronary angioplasty (editorial). Br J Hosp Med 37: 281.

Cutruzzola FW, Stetz ML, O'Brien KM, Gindi GR, Laifer LI, Garrand TJ, Deckelbaum LI (1989) Change in laser-induced arterial fluorescence during ablation of atherosclerotic plague. Lasers Surg Med 9: 109–116.

Davis GS, Bott-Silverman C, Goormastic M, Gerrity RG, Kittrell C, Feld M, Kramer JR (1988) Gas volume quantitation during argon ion laser ablation of atheromatous aorta in blood and 0.9% saline media with an optically shielded catheter. Lasers Surg Med 8: 72–76.

Deckelbaum LI (1988) Laser angioplasty. Cardiol Clin 6: 345–356.

Deckelbaum, LI, et al (1985) Reduction of laser-induced pathologic tissue injury using pulsed energy delivery. Am J Cardiol 56: 662.

Deckelbaum LI, Isner JM, Donaldson RF, Laliberte SM, Clarke RH, Salem DN (1986) Use of pulsed energy delivery to minimize tissue injury resulting from carbon dioxide laser irradiation of cardiovascular tissues. J Am Coll Cardiol 7: 898–908.

Deckelbaum LI, Stetz ML, O'Brien KM, Cutruzzola FW, Gmitro AF, Laifer LI, Gindi GR (1989) Fluorescence spectroscopy guidance of laser ablation of atherosclerotic plague. Lasers Surg Med 9: 205–214.

Diethrich EB (1991) Has excimer coronary laser angioplasty finally found a niche? [editorial; comment]. Circulation 84: 939–941.

Diethrich EB (1991) Temperature monitoring during peripheral thermo-optical laser recanalization in humans [letter; comment]. Clin Cardiol 14: 95, 184.

Diethrich EB, Hanafy HM, Santiago OJ, Bahadir I (1991) Angioscopy after coronary excimer laser angioplasty [letter]. J Am Coll Cardiol 18: 643–644.

Downar E, Butany J, Jares A, Stoicheff BP (1986) Endocardial photoablation by excimer laser. JACC 7: 546–550.

Eagan J, Vitello-Cicciu J (1987) Laser thermal and balloon angioplasty. J Cardiovasc Nurs 1: 74–78.

Einstein, A (1917) Zur Quantentheorie der Strahlung. Phys S Z 18: 121.

Eldar M (1989) Laser angioplasty: a review. REVIEW ARTICLE: 68 REFS. Isr J Med Sci 25: 222–228.

Eldar M, Battler A, Gal D, Rath S, Rotstein Z, Neufeld HN, Akselrod S, Katzir A, Gaton E, Wolman M (1986) The effects of varying lengths and powers of CO2 laser pulses transmitted through an optical fiber on atherosclerotic plaques. Clin Cardiol 9: 89–91.

Eldar M, Battler A, Neufeld HN, Gaton E, Arieli R, Akselrod S, Levite A, Katzir A (1984) Transluminal carbon dioxide-laser catheter angioplasty for dissolution of atherosclerotic plaques. JACC 3: 135–137.

Faxon DP (1980) The impact of interventional techniques on the practice of cardiology. Keio J Med 38: 60–64.

Fenech A, et al (1985) A comparative study of laser beam characteristics in blood and saline media. Am J Cardiol 55: 1389.

Ferris EJ, McCowan TC, Baker ML (1986) Laser angioplasty. Compr Ther 12: 3–5.

Forrester JS (1988) Laser angioplasty. Now and in the future. Circulation 78: 777–779.

Forrester JS, Litvack F, Grundfest W (1988) Vaporization of atheroma in man: the role of lasers in the era of balloon angioplasty. REVIEW ARTICLE: 25 REFS. Int J Cardiol 20: 1–7.

Forrester JS, Litvack F, Grundfest WS (1986) Laser angioplasty and cardiovascular disease. Am J Cardiol 57: 990–992.

Foschi A, Myers G, Crick WF, Friedberg HD, Snyder D, Nordstrom LA (1989) Laser angioplasty of totally occluded coronary arteries and vein grafts: preliminary report on a current trial. Am J Cardiol 63 (Suppl): 9F-13F.

Fourrier JL, Brunetaud JM, Prat A, Marache P, Lablanche JM, Bertrand ME (1987) Percutaneous laser angioplasty with sapphire tip (letter). Lancet 1: 105.

Fox J (1986) Laser coronary angioplasty. J Cardiovasc Nurs 1: 57–66.

Frazier OH, Diethrich EB, Johansson B, Conger JL, Burnett CM, Bylock A, Kadipasaoglu KA (1992) Preliminary results of intraoperative excimer laser angioplasty: phase 1: an adjunct to coronary artery bypass surgery. Lasers Surg Med 12(1): 7–12.

Gaffney EJ, Clarke RH, Lucas AR, Isner JM (1989) Correlation of fluorescence emission with the plaque content and intimal thickness of atherosclerotic coronary arteries. Lasers Surg Med 9: 215–228.

Garcia AT (1989) Laser-enhanced angioplasty. Tex Med 85: 43–44.

Garnic JD (1986) An orderly approach: comments on the intravascular use of lasers. Cardiovasc Intervent Radiol 9: 318–319.

Garrand TJ, Stetz ML, O'Brien KM, Gindi GR, Sumpio BE, Deckelbaum

LI (1991) Design and evaluation of a fiberoptic fluorescence guided laser recanalization system. Lasers Surg Med 11: 106–116.

Garrison BJ, Srinivasan R (1984) Microscopic model for the ablation photodecomposition of polymer by far ultraviolet light. Appl Phys Lett 44: 851.

Gerrity RG, Loop FD, Golding LAR, Erhart LA, Argeny ZB (1983) Arterial response to laser operation for removal of atherosclerotic plaques. J Thorac Cardiovasc Surg 85: 409–421.

Geschwind H, Boussignac G, Teisseire B, Benhaiem N, Bittoun R, Laurent D (1984) Conditions for effective Nd-YAG laser angioplasty. Br Heart J 52: 484–489.

Geschwind H, Boussignac G, Teisseire B, Vieilledent C, Gaston A, Becquemin JP, Mayiolini P (1984) Percutaneous transluminal laser angioplasty in man (letter). Lancet 1: 844.

Geschwind HJ, Aptecar E, Boussignac G, Dubois-Rande JL, Zelinsky R, Poirot G, Tomaru T (1991) Results and follow-up after percutaneous pulsed laser-assisted balloon angioplasty guided by spectroscopy (comments). Circulation 83: 787–796.

Geschwind HJ, Blair JD, Mongkolsmai D, Kern MJ, Stern J, Deligonul U, Kennedy HL (1987) Development and experimental application of contact probe catheter for laser angioplasty. JACC 9: 101–107.

Geschwind HJ, Dubois-Rande JL, Murphy-Chutorian D, Tomaru T, Zelinsky R, Loisance D (1990) Percutaneous coronary angioplasty with mid-infrared laser and a new multifibre cathetre [letter]. Lancet 336: 245–246.

Geschwind HJ, Dubois-Rande JL, Shafton E, Boussignac G, Wexman M (1989) Percutaneous pulsed laser-assisted balloon angioplasty guided by spectroscopy. Am Heart J 117: 1147–1152.

Geschwind HJ, Dubois-Rande JL, Zelinsky R, Morelle JF, Boussignac G (1991) Percutaneous coronary mid-infrared laser angioplasty. Am Heart J 122: 552–558.

Geschwind HJ, Kern MJ, Vandormael MG, Blair JD, Deligonul U, Kennedy HL (1987) Efficiency and safety of optically modified fiber tips for laser angioplasty. JACC 10: 655–661.

Geschwind HJ, Nakamura F, Kvasnicka J, Dubois-Rande JL (1993) Excimer and holmium yttrium aluminum garnet laser coronary angioplasty. Am Heart J 125(2 Pt 1): 510–522.

Geschwind HJ, Teisseire B, Boussignac G, Vieilledent C (1986) Laser angioplasty of arterial stenoses. Cardiovasc Intervent Radiol 9: 313–317.

Gessman L, Reno C, Maranhao V (1984) Transcatheter laser dissolution of human atherosclerotic plaques: a model for testing catheters and techniques. Cathet Cardiovasc Diagn 10: 47–54.

Goodkind J, Coombs V, Golobic RA (1993) Excimer laser angioplasty. Heart Lung 22(1): 26–35.

Greenfield AJ (1991) Hot-tip laser. Results and complications. Circulation 83: I94–96.

Grundfest W, Litvack F. Forrester J, Fishbein M, Morgenstern L (1984) Pulsed ultraviolet lasers provide precise control of atheroma ablation (Abstract). Circulation 70 (Suppl II): II-35.

Grundfest WS, Litvack F, Forrester JS, Goldenberg T, Swan JHC, Morgenstern L, Fishbein M, McDermid IS, Rider DM, Pacala TJ, Laudenslager JB (1985) Laser ablation of human atherosclerotic plaque without adjacent tissue injury. JACC 5: 929–933.

Haavind R (1985) Lighting the way with lasers. High Technology 5: 39–41.

Halfman-Franey M, Coburn C (1990) Techniques in cardiac care: lasers, stents, and atherectomy devices. Clin Issues Crit Care Nurs 1: 87–109.

Hartnell GG (1991) Conventional angioplasty versus percutaneous transluminal laser angioplasty (letter). Circulation 84: 2204–2205.

Heuser RR, Mehta SS (1991) Holmium laser angioplasty after failed coronary balloon dilation: use of a new solid-state, infrared laser system. Cathet Cardiovasc Diagn 23: 187–189.

Holmes DR, et al (1984) Restenosis after percutaneous transluminal coronary angioplasty (PTCA). Registry of the National Heart, Lung and Blood Institute. Am J Cardiol 53: 77C.

Huether S (1986) Lasers in cardiovascular diseases. J Cardiovasc Nurs 1: 77–79.

Isner JM, Clarke RH (1986) Laser angioplasty: unraveling the Gordian knot. JACC 7: 705–708.

Isner JM, Clarke RL (1984) IEEE J Quantum Electron QE20: 1406.

Isner JM, Estes NA, Payne DD, Rastegar H, Clarke RH, Cleveland RJ (1987) Laser-assisted endocardiectomy for refractory ventricular tachyarrhythmias: preliminary intraoperative experience. Clin Cardiol 10: 201–204.

Isner JM, et al (1984) Laser myoplasty for hypertrophic cardiomyopathy: initial in vitro experience in human postmortem hearts and in vivo experience in a canine model and human patient. Am J Cardiol 53: 1620.

Isner JM, et al (1985) Identification of photo-products liberated by in vitro laser Argon irradiation of atherosclerotic plaque, calcified cardiac valves, and myocardium. Am J Cardiol 55: 1192.

Israel DH, Marmur JD, Sanborn TA (1991) Excimer laser-facilitated balloon angioplasty of a nondilatable lesion. J Am Coll Cardiol 18: 1118–1119.

Itoh A, Miyazaki S, Nonogi H, Ozono K, Daikoku S, Saito K, Goto Y, et al. (1993) Angioscopic and intravascular ultrasound imagings before and after percutaneous holmium-YAG laser coronary angioplasty. Am Heart J 125(2 Pt 1): 556–558.

Karsch KR, Haase KK, Mauser M, Ickrath O, Voelker W, Duda S, Seipel L (1989) Percutaneous coronary excimer laser angioplasty: initial clinical results. Lancet 2: 647–650.

Karsch KR, Haase KK, Wehrmann M, Hassenstein S, Hanke H (1991) Smooth muscle cell proliferation and restenosis after stand along coronary excimer laser angioplasty [comment]. J Am Coll Cardiol 17: 991–994.

Keogh B, Crea F, Davies G, Taylor K, Pashazadeh M, Foale R, Kidner P (1987) Angioscopy and intra-operative coronary laser angioplasty (letter). Lancet 2: 969.

Keogh BE, Crea F, Bull T, Blackie RA, Taylor KM (1989) Intravascular delivery of laser energy with metal-capped optical fibers: the potential hazard of distal embolism. Am Jeart J 118: 47–53.

Keogh BE, Taylor KM (1987) The pitfalls of laser coronary angioplasty research (letter). Br J Hosp Med 38: 81.

Kjellstrom BT, Cothren RM, Kramer JR (1987) The use of lasers in vascular and cardiac surgery. Clinical review. Acta Chir Scand 153: 493–499.

Kochs M, Haerer W, Eggeling T, Hoeher M, Schmidt A, Hombach V (1992) Excimer laser coronary angioplasty: experience with a prototype multifibre catheter in patients with stable anging pectoris. Eur Heart J 13(3): 338–347.

Kramer JR, Bott-Silverman C, Ratliff NB, Strikwerda S, Loop FD, Shearin A, Cothren RM, Kittrel C, Feld MS (1987) Removal of atherosclerotic plaque using multiple short exposures of argon ion laser light. Am Heart J 113: 1038–1040.

Krause PB, Schaer GL, Parrillo JE, Klein LW (1992) Excimer laser ablation before autoperfusion balloon inflation: a novel therapeutic approach to high grade stenoses in vessels supplying substantial myocardium at risk. Cathet Cardiovasc Diagn 27(3): 202–208.

Kuntz RE, Piana R, Pomerantz RM, Carrozza J, Fishman R, Mansour M, Safian RD, et al. (1992) Changing incidence and management of abrupt closure following coronary intervention in the new device era. Cathet Cardiovasc Diagn 27(3): 183–190.

Lablanche JM, Fourrier JL, Gommeaux A, Becquart J, Bertrand ME (1989) Percutaneous aspiration of a coronary thrombus. Cathet Cardiovasc Diagn 17: 97–98.

Laufer G, Wollenek G, Hohla K, Horvat R, Henke KH, Buchelt M, Wutzl G, Wolner E (1988) Excimer laser-induced simultaneous ablation and spectral identification of normal and atherosclerotic arterial tissue layers. Circulation 78: 1031–1039.

Lee BI, Fletcher RD, Cohen AI, Cutler DJ, Del Negro AA, Singh SN (1984)

Transcatheter endocardial ablation: comparison of laser photo ablation and electrode shock ablation (Abstract). JACC 3: 536.

Lee G, Argenal AJ, Rink DL, Lee MH, Mason DT (1988) Percutaneous coronary laser angioplasty: successful clinical application of a new thermal cap catheter coaxially guided over a steerable central guide wire. Am Heart J 116: 1637–1638.

Lee G, Chan MC, Garcia JM, Pichard AD, Corso PJ, Hannah H 3rd, Reis RL, Mason DT (1988) Effects of coronary laser radiation. REVIEW ARTICLE: 42 REFS. Cardiovasc Clin 18: 123–133.

Lee G, Chan MC, Rink DL, Beerline D, Lee MH, Reis RL, Mason DT (1987) Coronary revascularization by a new coaxially-guided laser-heated metal cap system. Am Heart J 113: 1507–1508.

Lee G, et al (1983) Effects of laser irradiation delivered by flexible fiberoptic system on the left ventricular internal myocardium. Am Heart J 106: 587.

Lee G, et al (1983) The qualitative effects of laser irradiation on human arteriosclerotic disease. Am Heart J 105: 885.

Lee G, et al (1984) Acute and chronic complications of laser angioplasty, vascular wall damage and formation of aneurysms in the atherosclerotic rabbit. Am J Cardiol 53: 290.

Lee G, Garcia JM, Chan MC, Corso PJ, Bacos J, Lee MH, Pichard A, Reis RL, Mason DT (1986) Clinically successful long-term laser coronary recanalization. Am Heart J 112: 1323–1325.

Lee G, Ikeda RM, Kozina J, Mason DT (1981) Laser dissolution of coronary atherosclerotic obstruction. Am Heart J 102: 1074–1075.

Lee G, Mason DT (1991) Laser angioplasty: a plea for modesty in the search for a real beginning [editorial; comment]. Circulation 83: 1093–1095.

Lee G, Pond G, Sacks E, Butman S, Rink D, Mason DT (1990) Single-passage laser recanalization plus subsequent balloon angioplasty by (1) a novel detachable fiberoptic guide wire device or (2) a balloon catheter over-the-fiberoptic wire system. Am Heart J 120: 1477–1481.

Lee G, Reis RL, Chan MC, Boggan MD, Lee MH, Low RI, Argenal A, Hannah H 3rd, Mason DT (1986) Clinical laser recanalization of coronary obstruction. Angioscopic and angiographic documentation. Chest 90: 770–772.

Lee G, Sommerhaug RG, Argenal A, Chan MC, Rink D, Mason DT (1987) Clinical laser revascularization of coronary obstruction with the coaxial-guided laser-heated metal cap catheter. Am Heart J 114: 1524–1526.

Leon MB, Lu DY, Prevosti LG, Macy WW Jr, Smith PD, Granovsky M, Bonner RF, Balaban RS (1988) Human arterial surface fluorescence: atherosclerotic plaque identification and effects of laser atheroma ablation. J Am Coll Cardiol 12: 94–102.

Linnemeier TJ, Cumberland DC (1989) Percutaneous laser coronary angioplasty without balloon angioplasty (letter). Lancet 1: 154–155.

Litvack F, Eigler NL, Margolis JR, Grundfest WS, Rothbaum D, Linnemeier T, Hestrin LB, Tsoi D, Cook SL, Krauthamer D et al. (1990) Percutaneous excimer laser coronary angioplasty. Am J Cardiol 66: 1027–1032.

Litvack F, et al (1985) Effects of hematoporphyrin derivative and photodynamic therapy on atherosclerotic rabbits. Am J Cardiol 56: 667.

Litvack F, Grundfast WS, Fishbein M, Rose H, Forrester J (1984) A standardized method for study of laser tissue interaction (Abstract). Circulation 70: (Suppl II): II-35.

Litvack F, Grundfest WS, Goldenberg T, Laudenslager J, Pacala T, Segalowitz J, Forrester JS (1988) Pulsed laser angioplasty: wavelength power and energy dependencies relevant to clinical application. Lasers Surg Med 8: 60–65.

Livesay JJ (1988) Intraoperative laser coronary angioplasty. Thorac Cardiovasc Surg 36: (Suppl 2): 150–154.

Livesay JJ, Leachman DR, Hogan PJ, et al (1985) Preliminary report on laser coronary endarterectomy in patients (Abstract). Circulation 72 (Suppl III): 111–302.

Lorenzi G, Domanin M, Constantini A (1991) PTA and laser-assisted PTA combined with simultaneous surgical revascularization. J Cardiovasc Surg 32: 456–462.

Margolis JR, Mehta S (1992) Excimer laser coronary angioplasty. Am J Cardiol 69(15): 3F–11F.

Matsumoto T, Okamura T, Rajyaguru V (1989) Laser arterial disobstructive procedures in 148 lower extremities. J Vasc Surg 10: 169–177.

Mirhoseini M, Cayton M (1981) Revascularization of the heart by laser. J Microsurg 2: 253.

Mirhoseini M, Cayton MM, Shelgikar S, Fisher JC (1986) Laser myocardial revascularization. Lasers Surg Med 6: 459–461.

Mohan SR, Hawker RJ, Wolinski AP, Grimley RP (1990) Detection of arterial thrombosis after laser angioplasty by platelet scintigraphy. Eur J Nucl Med 16: 865–868.

Morcos NC, Berns M, Henry WL (1988) Effect of laser-heated tip angioplasty on human atherosclerotic coronary arteries. Lasers Surg Med 8: 22–29.

Murphy-Chutorian D, et al (1985) Selective absorption of ultraviolet laser energy by atherosclerotic plaque treated with tetracycline. Am J Cardiol 55: 1,293.

Murphy-Chutorian D, Selzer P, Wexler L, et al (1986) Cardiovascular laser research at Stanford University. Semin Intervent Radiol 3: 61–63.

Narula O, et al (1985) Laser catheter-induced atrioventricular nodal delays and atrioventricular block in dogs: acute and chronic observations. J Am Coll Cardiol 5: 259.

Narula OS, Bharati S, Chan MC, Embi AA, Lev M (1984) Laser microtranssection of the His bundle: a pervenous catheter technique (Abstract). J Am Coll Cardiol 3: 537.

Nelson MJ, Enriquez RS, Guerra GG, Miller JT, Bogart DB (1991) Current therapy of impending myocardial infarction and acute cholecystitis. Missouri Medicine 88: 638–639.

Neubaur T, Klepzig M, Heintzen MP, Richter EI, Zeitler E, Strauer BE (1989) Peripheral percutaneous transluminal laser angioplasty in humans: in vitro investigations and clinical results with a novel laser catheter system. Clin Cardiol 12: 313–320.

Nilsson J, Herzfeld I, Grip L, Aberg B, Ryden L (1993) Immunohistochemical analysis of a human coronary artery exposed to excimer laser angioplasty in vivo: evidence for release of fibroblast growth factor at the site of injury. Am Heart J 125(3): 908–912.

Okada M, Ikuta H, Shimizu K, Horii H, Nakamura K (1986) Alternatives method of myocardial revascularization by laser: experimental and clinical study. Kobe J Med Sci 32: 151–161.

Parker JD, Ganz P, Selwyn AP, Bittl JA (1991) Successful treatment of an excimer laser-associated coronary artery perforation with the Stack perfusion catheter. Cathet Cardiovasc Diagn 22: 118–123.

Peene P, Wilms G, Piessens J, Baert AL (1991) Percutaneous transluminal laser angioplasty with balloon centered direct argon laser light. Experience with 12 patients and a minimal follow-up of 6 months. Rofo 154: 176–179.

Petrone S (1990) Laser-assisted balloon angioplasty: bypassing the traditional methods. Todays OR Nurse 12: 22–27.

Petrosyan YS, Kipshidze NN, Putilin SA (1989) Clinical experience with the use of laser radiation energy in the treatment of atherosclerosis. Cor Vasa 31: 118–127.

Preisack MB, Athanasiadis A, Voelker W, Baumbach A, Karsch KR (1993) Acute closure during coronary excimer laser angioplasty and conventional balloon dilatation: a comparison of management outcome and prediction. Eur Heart J 14(2): 195–204.

Prince MR, Deutsch TF, Shapiro AH, Margolis RJ, Oseroff AR, Fallon JT, Parrish JA, Anderson RR (1986) Selective ablation of atheromas using a flashlamp-excited dye laser at 465 nm. Proc Natl Acad Sci USA 83: 7064–7068.

Prince MR, et al (1985) Selective light absorption in atheromas (Abstract). Clin Res 33: 218A.

Prince MR, LaMuraglia GM, MacNichol EF Jr (1988) Increased preferential absorption in human atherosclerotic plaque with oral beta carotene. Implications for laser endarterectomy. Circulation 78: 338–344.

Reeder GS, Bresnahan JF, Holmes DR Jr, Litvack F (1992) Excimer laser coronary angioplasty: results in restenosis versus de novo coronary lesions. Excimer Laser Coronary Angioplasty Investigators. Cathet Cardiovasc Diagn 25(3): 195–199.

Reekers JA, Sprangers RL, van de Kley AJ (1991) Angioplasty after laser perforation. Cardiovasc Intervent Radiol 14: 113–114.

Reis GJ, Pomerantz RM, Jenkins RD, Kuntz RE, Baim DS, Diver DJ, Schnitt SJ, Safian RD (1991) Laser balloon angioplasty: clinical, angiographic and histologic results. J Am Coll Cardiol 18: 193–202.

Richens D, Rees M, Watson DA (1987) Laser coronary angioplasty under direct vision (letter). Lancet 2: 683.

Rosenthal E, Montarello JK, Palmer T, Curry PV (1989) Thermal effects of stationary "hot tip" laser coronary probes: an in vitro assessment. Lasers Surg Med 9: 229–236.

Sakallaris BR (1987) Laser therapy for cardiovascular disease. REVIEW ARTICLE: 29 REFS. Heart Lung 16: 465–471.

Saksena S, Ciccone JM, Chandran P, Pantopoulos D, Lee B, Rothbart ST (1986) Laser ablation of normal and diseased human ventricle. Am Heart J 112: 52–60.

Saksena S, Gadhoke A (1986) Laser therapy for tachyarrhythmias: a new frontier. REVIEW ARTICLE: 30 REFS. PACE 9: 531–550.

Saksena S, Hussain SM, Gielchinsky I, Gadhoke A, Pantopoulos D (1987) Intraoperative mapping-guided argon laser ablation of malignant ventricular tachycardia. Am J Cardiol 59: 78–83.

Saksena S, Hussain SM, Gielchinsky I, Pantopoulos D (1987) Intraoperative mapping-guided argon laser ablation of supraventricular tachycardia in the Wolff-Parkinson-White syndrome. Am J Cardiol 60: 196–199.

Sanborn TA (1988) Experimental and clinical angioplasty with a laser probe fiberoptic catheter system. REVIEW ARTICLE: 19 REFS. Thorac Cardiovasc Surg 36: 133–136.

Sanborn TA (1988) Laser angioplasty: peripheral and coronary applications. Cardiovasc Clin 19: 181–195.

Sanborn TA (1988) Laser angioplasty. What has been learned from experimental studies and clinical trials? Circulation 78: 769–774.

Sanborn TA (1989) Recanalization of arterial occlusions: pathologic basis and contributing factors. JACC 13: 1558–1560.

Sanborn TA (1991) Early limitations of coronary excimer laser angioplasty [editorial; comment]. J Am Coll Cardiol 17: 995–996.

Sanborn TA, Bittl JA, Hershman RA, Siegel RM (1991) Percutaneous coronary excimer laser-assisted angioplasty: initial multicenter experience in 141 patients. J Am Coll Cardiol 17: 169B–173B.

Sanborn TA, Faxon DP, Huadenschild CC, Ryan TJ (1985) Experimental angioplasty: circumferential distribution of laser thermal injury with a laser probe. JACC 5: 934–938.

Sanborn TA, Faxon DP, Kellett MA, Ryan TJ (1986) Percutaneous coronary laser thermal angioplasty. JACC 8: 1437–1440.

Sanborn TA, Hershman RA, Torre SR, Sherman W, Cohen M, Amborse JA (1989) Percutaneous excimer laser coronary angioplasty (letter). Lancet 2: 616.

Sanborn TA, Torre SR, Sharma SK, Hershman RA, Cohen M, Sherman W, Ambrose JA (1991) Percutaneous coronary excimer laser-assisted balloon angioplasty: initial clinical and quantitative angiographic results in 50 patients. J Am Coll Cardiol 17: 94–99.

Scriven AJ, Lidbury PS, Nathan AW (1991) Effects of laser-generated tissue debris on aggregation of human platelets. Am Heart J 122: 802–808.

Selle JG, Svenson RH, Sealy WC, Gallagher JJ, Zimmern SH, Fedor JM, Marroum MC Robicsek F (1986) Successful clinical laser ablation of ventricular tachycardia: a promising new therapeutic method. Ann Thorac Surg 42: 380–384.

Serruys PW, Breeman A (1992) Coronary angioplasty—long-term follow-up results and detection of restenosis: guidelines for aviation cardiology. A European view. Eur Heart J 13(Suppl H): 76–88.

Shelton ME, Hoxworth B, Shelton JA, Virmani R, Friesinger GC (1986) A new model to study quantitative effects of laser angioplasty on human atherosclerotic plaque. J Am Cardiol 7: 909–915.

Spears JR (1986) Percutaneous laser treatment of atherosclerosis: an overview of emerging techniques. Cardiovasc Intervent Radiol 9: 303–312.

Spears JR, Marais HJ, Serur J (1983) In vivo coronary angioscopy. JACC 1: 1311–1314.

Spears JR, Reyes VP, Wynne J, Fromm BS, Sinofsky EL, Andrus S, Sinclair IN, Hopkins BE, Schwartz L, Aldridge HE, et al. Percutaneous coronary laser balloon angioplasty: initial results of a multicenter experience. J Am Coll Cardiol 16: 293–303.

Steenkiste AR, Baim DS, Sipperly ME, Desvigne-Nickens P, Robertson T, Detre K (1991) The NACI Registry: an instrument for the evaluation of new approaches to coronary intervention. The NACI Investigators. Cathet Cardiovasc Diagn 23: 270–281.

Svenson RH, Gallagher JJ, Selle JG, Zimmern SH, Fedor JM, Robicsek F (1987) Neodymium:Yag laser photocoagulation: a successful new map-guided technique for the intraoperative ablation of ventricular tachycardia. Circulation 76: 1319–1328.

Tayler DI, Cumberland DC (1985) Laser assisted balloon angioplasty (Abstract). Circulation 72 (Suppl 3): 371.

Tibi PR, Simmons D, Hicks GL (1987) Improving argon ion laser atheroablation using microlens fibers. Curr Surg 44: 216–218.

Tick PA, Thompson DA (1985) IR fibres: at the frontier. Photon Spectra 19: 65–68.

Tomaru T, Geschwind HJ, Boussignac G, Lange F, Tahk SJ (1991) The role of shock waves in pulsed-dye laser angioplasty. Am Heart J 122: 255–258.

Tomaru T, Geschwind HJ, Lange F, Boussignac G (1991) Enhancement of pulsed-dye laser ablation of arterial tissues with blood medium: effects of laser-induced shock waves. Am Heart J 122: 809–817.

Topaz O, Rozenbaum EA, Battista S, Peterson C, Wysham DG (1993) Laser facilitated angioplasty and thrombolysis in acute myocardial infarction complicated by prolonged or recurrent chest pain. Cathet Cardiovasc Diagn 28(1): 7–16.

Umans VA, Strauss BH, Rensing BJ, de Jaegere P, de Feyter PJ, Serruys PW (1991) Comparative angiographic quantitative analysis of the immediate efficacy of coronary atherectomy with balloon angioplasty, stenting, and rotational ablation. Am Heart J 122: 836–843.

Veith FJ, Bakal CW, Cynamon J, Gupta SK, Keeley J, Greenberg M, Mennigus MA, Wengerter KR, Dietzek AM (1991) Early experience with the smart laser in the treatment of atherosclerotic occlusions: Am Heart J 121: 1531–1538.

Weinstein GS (1986) Laser angioplasty and atherosclerosis (letter). J Am Coll Cardiol 8: 254.

Welch AJ, Bradley AB, Torres JH, Motamedi M, Ghidoni JJ, Pearch JA, Hussein H, O'Rourke RA (1987) Laser probe ablation of normal and atherosclerotic human aorta in vitro: a first thermographic and histologic analysis. Circulation 76: 1353–1363.

Werner G, Buchwald A, Unterberg C, Voth E, Kreuzer H, Wiegand V (1991) Excimer laser angioplasty in coronary artery disease. Eur Heart J 12: 24–29.

White CJ, Ramee SR (1992) Options for percutaneous coronary and peripheral revascularization. Med Clin North Am 76(5): 1099–1124.

White GH (1988) Angioscopy and lasers in cardiovascular surgery: current applications and future prospects. REVIEW ARTICLE. 52 REFS. Aust N Z J Surg 58: 217–274.

White P (1985) Chalcogenide fibres make their debut. Photon Spectra 19: 70–71.

Wollenek G, Laufer G (1988) Comparative study of different laser systems with special regard to angioplasty. Thorac Cardiovasc Surg 36(Suppl 2): 126–132.

VII. Stents

Adams PS, Jr. (1987) Iliac artery-ureteral fistula developing after dilatation and stent placement. Radiology 153: 647–648.

Anderson PG, Bajaj RK, Baxley WA, Roubin GS (1992) Vascular pathology of balloon-expandable flexible coil stents in humans. J Am Coll Cardiol 19(2): 372–381.

Antonucci F, Salomonowitz E, Stuckmann G, Stiefel M, Largiader J, Zollikofer CL (1992) Placement of venous stents: clinical experience with a self-expanding prosthesis. Radiology 183(2): 493–497.

Bach RG, Kern MJ, Bell C, Donohue TJ, Aguirre F (1993) Clinical application of coronary flow velocity for stent placement during coronary angioplasty. Am Heart J 125(3): 873–877.

Baim DS (1991) Intracoronary stenting—hope or hype? [editorial; comment]. Mayo Clin Proc 66: 332–335.

Baim DS, Levine MJ, Leon MB, Levine S, Ellis SG, Schatz RA (1993) Management of restenosis within the Palmaz-Schatz coronary stent (the U.S. multicenter experience. The U.S. Palmaz-Schatz Stent Investigators. Am J Cardiol 71(4): 364–366.

Barnes RW, Fleisher HL, 3d, Redman JF, Smith JW, Harshfield DL, Ferris EJ (1988) Mesoaortic compression of the left renal vein (the so-called nutcracker syndrome): repair by a new stenting procedure. J Vasc Surg 8: 415–421.

Becker GJ (1991) Intravascular stents. General principles and status of lower-extremity arterial applications. Circulation 83: I122–136.

Becker GJ, Cikrit DF, Lalka SG, Benenati JF, Ehrman KO, Waller BF, Palmaz JC (1989) Early experience with the Palmaz stent in human iliac angioplasty. Indiana Med 82: 286–292.

Becker GJ, Palmaz JC, Rees CR (1990) Angioplasty-induced dissections in human iliac arteries: management with Palmaz balloon-expandable intraluminal stents. Radiology 176: 31–38.

Becker GJ, Palmaz JC, Rees CR, Ehrman KO, Lalka SG, Dalsing MC, Cikrit DF, McLean GK, Burke DR, Richter GM, et al (1990) Angioplasty-induced dissections in human iliac arteries: management with Palmaz balloon-expandable intraluminal stents. Radiology 176: 31–38.

Belli AM, Cumberland DC, Procter AE, Welsh CL (1991) Follow-up of conventional angioplasty versus laser thermal angioplasty for total femoropopliteal artery occlusions: results of a randomized trial. J Vasc Intervent Radiol 2(4): 485–488.

Bergeron P, Rudondy P, Poyen V, Pinot JJ, Alessandri C, Martelet JP (1991)

Long-term peripheral stent evaluation using angioscopy. Int Angiol 10(3): 182–186.

Bilodeau M, Rioux L, Willems B, Pomier-Layrargues G (1992) Transjugular intrahepatic portacaval stent shunt as a rescue treatment for life-threatening variceal bleeding in a cirrhotic patient with severe liver failure. Am J Gastroenterol 87(3): 369–371.

Block PC (1991) Coronary-artery stents and other endoluminal devices [editorial; comment]. N Engl J Med 324: 52–53.

Bonn J, Gardiner GA, Jr, Shapiro MJ, Sullivan KL, Levin DC (1990) Palmaz vascular stent: initial clinical experience. Radiology 174: 741–745.

Bowerman RE, Pinkerton CA, Kirk B, Waller BF (1991) Disruption of a coronary stent during atherectomy for restenosis. Cathet Cardiovasc Diagn 24(4): 248–251.

Brothers TE, Greenfield LJ (1990) Long-term results of aortoiliac reconstruction. J Vasc Intervent Radiol 1(1): 49–55.

Brown RI, Galligan L, Penn IM (1991) Balloon expandable stents for acute closure post failed coronary angioplasty: case report and review of the literature. Can J Cardiol 7: 311–315.

Buchwald A, Unterberg C, Werner G, Voth E, Kreuzer H, Wiegand V (1991) Initial clinical results with the Wiktor stent: a new balloon-expandable coronary stent. Clin Cardiol 14: 374–379.

Bucx JJ, de Scheerder I, Beatt K, van den Brand M, Suryapranata H, de Feyter PF, Serruys PW (1991) The importance of adequate anticoagulation to prevent early thrombosis after stenting of stenosed venous bypass grafts. Am Heart J 121: 1389–1396.

Capek P, Rocco M, McGahan J, Frey C (1992) Direct aneurysm puncture and coil occlusion: a new approach to peripancreatic arterial pseudoaneurysms. J Vasc Intervent Radiol 3(4): 653–656.

Carrozza JP Jr, Kuntz RE, Levine MJ, Pomerantz RM, Fishman RF, Mansour M, Gibson CM, Senerchia CC, Diver DJ, Safian RD, et al (1992) Angiographic and clinical outcome of intracoronary stenting: immediate and long-term results from a large single-center experience. J Am Coll Cardiol 20(2): 328–337.

Cavaye DM, Tabbara MR, Kopchok GE, Termin P, White RA (1991) Intraluminal ultrasound assessment of vascular stent deployment. Ann Vasc Surg 5: 241–246.

Chalmers N, Redhead DN, Simpson KJ, Hayes PC (1992) Transjugular intrahepatic portosystemic stent shunt (TIPSS): early clinical experience. Clin Radiol 46(3): 166–169.

Chatelain P, Meier B, Friedle B (1991) Stenting of superior vena cava and inferior vena cava for symptomatic narrowing after repeated atrial surgery for D-transposition of the great vessels. Br Heart J 66(6): 466–468.

Cheong WF, Spears JR, Welch AJ (1991) Laser balloon angioplasty. Crit Rev Biomed Eng 19(2-3): 113–146.

Cikrit DF, Becker GJ, Dalsing MC, Ehrman KO, et al (1991) Early experience with the Palmaz expandable intraluminal stent in the iliac artery stenoses. Ann Vasc Surg 5: 150–155.

Cikrit DF, Becker GJ, Dalsing MC, Ehrman KO, Lalka SG, Sawchuk AP (1991) Early experience with the Palmaz expandable intraluminal stent in iliac artery stenosis. Ann Vasc Surg 5: 150–155.

Colombo A, Hall P, Thomas J, Almagor Y, Finci L (1992) Initial experience with the disarticulated (one-half) Palmaz-Schatz stent: a technical report. Cathet Cardiovasc Diagn 25(4): 304–308.

Dake MD (1990) Peripheral angiography, angioplasty, atherectomy, laser techniques, thrombolysis, and stents. Curr Opin Radiol 2: 239–249.

Darcy MD, Vesely TM, Picus D, Middleton WD, Hicks ME (1992) Percutaneous revision of an acutely thrombosed transjugular intrahepatic portosystemic shunt. J Vasc Intervent Radiol 3(1): 77–80; discussion 81–82.

Davies RP, Voyvodic F (1992) Percutaneous retrieval of a partially expanded iliac artery stent: case report. Cardiovasc Intervent Radiol 15(2): 120–122.

De Feyter PJ, DeScheerder I, van den Brand M, Laarman G, Suryapranata H, Serruys PW (1990) Emergency stenting for refractory acute coronary artery occlusion during coronary angioplasty. Am J Cardiol 66: 1147–1150.

De Jaegere PP, Hermans WR, Rensing BJ, Strauss BH, de Feyter PJ, Serruys PW (1993) Matching based on quantitative coronary angiography as a surrogate for randomized studies: comparison between stent implantation and balloon angioplasty of native coronary artery lesions. Am Heart J 125(2 Pt 1): 310–319.

De Jaegere PP, Serruys PW, Bertrand M, Wiegand V, Kober G, Marquis JF, Valeix B, Uebis R, Piessens J (1992) Wiktor stent implantation in patients with restenosis following balloon angioplasty of a native coronary artery. Am J Cardiol 69(6): 598–602.

Dick R, Hobbs KE (1991) Metal stents in Budd-Chiari syndrome [letter]. Lancet 338: 1075.

Dick RJ, Popma JJ, Muller DW, Burek KA, Topol EJ (1991) In-hospital costs associated with new percutaneous coronary devices. Am J Cardiol 68: 879–885.

Diethrich EB, Santiago O, Gustafson G, Heuser RR (1993) Preliminary observations on the use of the Palmaz stent in the distal portion of the abdominal aorta. Am Heart J 125(2 Pt 1): 490–501.

Do-dai-Do, Triller J, Walpoth BH, Stirnemann P, Mahler F (1992) A comparison study of self-expandable stents vs balloon angioplasty alone in femoropopliteal artery occlusions. Cardiovasc Intervent Radiol 15(5): 306–312.

Dorros G, Hall P, Prince C (1993) Successful limb salvage after recanalization of an occluded infrapopliteal artery utilizing a balloon expandable (Palmaz-Schatz) stent. Cathet Cardiovasc Diagn 28(1): 83–88.

Dorros G, Mathiak L (1993) Direct deployment of the iliofemoral balloon expandable (Palmaz) stent utilizing a small (7.5 French) arterial puncture. Cathet Cardiovasc Diagn 28(1): 80–82.

Doty DB, Doty JR, Jones KW (1990) Bypass of superior vena cava. Fifteen years' experience with spiral vein graft for obstruction of superior vena cava caused by benign disease. J Thorac Cardiovasc Surg 99: 889–895; discussion 895–896.

Douek PC, Leon MB, Geschwind H, Cook PS, Selzer P, Miller DL, Bonner RF (1991) Occlusive peripheral vascular disease: a multicenter trial of fluorescence-guided, pulsed dye laser-assisted balloon angioplasty. Radiology 180: 127–133.

Duda SH, Karsch KR, Haase KK, Huppert PE, Claussen CD (1990) Laser ring catheters in excimer laser angioplasty. Radiology 175: 269–270.

Edwards RD, Cassidy J, Taylor A (1992) Case report: superior vena cava obstruction complicated by central venous thrombosis—treatment with thrombolysis and Gianturco-Z stents. Clin Radiol 45(4): 278–280.

Ellis SG, Savage M, Fischman D, Baim DS, Leon M, Goldberg S, Hirshfeld JW, et al. (1992) Restenosis after placement of Palmaz-Schatz stents in native coronary arteries. Initial results of a multicenter experience. Circulation 86(6): 1836–1844.

Ellis SG, Topol EJ (1989) Intracoronary stents: will they fulfill their promise as an adjunct to angioplasty? [published erratum appears in J Am Coll Cardiol 1989 Jul;14(1): 264]. REVIEW ARTICLE: 58 REFS. J Am Coll Cardiol 13: 1425–1430.

Elson JD, Becker GJ, Wholey MH, Ehrman KO (1991) Vena caval and central venous stenoses: management with Palmaz balloon-expandable intraluminal stents. J Vasc Intervent Radiol 2(2): 215–232.

Erbel R, Haude M, Dietz U, Rupprecht HJ, Zotz R, Meyer J (1990) New mechanical devices for treatment of coronary artery disease. Z Kardiol 79 (Suppl 3): 121–129.

Escorcia E, Hollman J (1992) Current status of stents (editorial). Am J Cardiol 69(6): 687–689.

Fajadet JC, Jenny DB, Robert GP, Cassagneau BG, Marco J (1992) Clinical use of disarticulated Palmaz-Schatz stents [letter; comment]. Cathet Cardiovasc Diagn 27(3): 246–247.

Fallone BG, Wallace S, Gianturco C (1988) Elastic characteristics of the self-expanding metallic stents. Invest Radiol 23: 370–376.

Finch IJ (1992) Use of the Palmaz stent in ostial celiac artery stenosis. J Vasc Intervent Radiol 3(4): 633–635; discussion 636–637.

Fischell TA, Stadius ML, New technologies for the treatment of obstructive arterial disease. Cathet Cardiovasc Diagn 22: 205–233.

Foley JB, Penn IM, Brown RI, Murray-Parsons N, White J, Galligan L, MacDonald C (1993) Safety, success, and restenosis after elective coronary implantation of the Palmaz-Schatz stent in 100 patients at a single center. Am Heart J 125(3): 686–694.

Freedman AM, Sanyal AJ, Tisnado J, Shiffman ML, Luketic VA, Fisher RA, Posner MP (1993) Results with percutaneous transjugular intrahepatic portosystemic stent-shunts for control of variceal hemorrhage in patients awaiting liver transplantation. Transplant Proc 25(1 Pt 2): 1087–1089.

Furui S, Sawada S, Irie T, Makita K, Yamauchi T, Kusano S, Ibukuro K, Nakamura H, Takenaka E (1990) Hepatic inferior vena cava obstruction: treatment of two types with Gianturco expandable metallic stents [see comments]. Radiology 176: 665–670.

Gardiner G, Jr, Schwarten D, Schatz RA, Root HD, Rogers W (1989) Angioplasty and stenting of completely occluded iliac arteries. Radiology 172: 953–959.

Garratt KN, Holmes DR Jr, Roubin GS (1991) Early outcome after placement of a metallic intracoronary stent: initial Mayo Clinic experience [comments]. Mayo Clin Proc 66: 268–275.

Gillams A, Dick R, Platts A, Irving D, Hobbs K (1991) Dilatation of the inferior vena cava using an expandable metal stent in Budd-Chiari syndrome. J Hepatol 13: 149–151.

Goldsmith MF (1988) Artery-expanding stents widen hopes for patients with atherosclerosis (news). JAMA 259: 327–329.

Goy JJ, Sigwart U, Vogt P, Stauffer JC, Kappenberger L (1992) Long-term clinical and angiographic follow-up of patients treated with the self-expanding coronary stent for acute occlusion during balloon angioplasty of the right coronary artery. J Am Coll Cardiol 19(7): 1593–1596.

Goy JJ, Sigwart U, Vogt P, Stauffer JC, Kauffman U, Urban P, Kappenberger L (1991) Long-term follow-up of the first 56 patients treated with intracoronary self-expanding stents (the Lausanne experience). Am J Cardiol 67: 569–572.

Greenberg MA, Menegus MA, Issenberg H, Spindola-Franco H (1990) Advances in interventional cardiology: coronary balloon angioplasty and alternative techniques. Curr Opin Radiol 2: 602–615.

Gunther RW, Vorwerk D, Antonucci F, Beyssen B, Essinger A, Gaux JC, Joffre F, Raynaud A, Rousseau H, Zollikofer CL (1991) Iliac artery stenosis or obstruction after unsuccessful balloon angioplasty: treatment with a self-expandable stent. AJR 156: 389–393.

Gunther RW, Vorwerk D, Bohndorf K, Klose KC, Kistler D, Mann H, Sieberth HG, el-Din A (1989) Venous stenoses in dialysis shunts: treatment with self-expanding metallic stents. Radiology 170: 401–405.

Gunther RW, Vorwerk D, Bohndorf K, Peters I, el Din A, Messmer B (1989) Iliac and femoral artery stenoses and occlusions: treatment with intravascular stents. Radiology 172: 725–730.

Gunther RW, Vorwerk D, Klose KC, Bohndorf K, Kistler D, Mann H, Sieberth HG (1989) Self-expanding stents for the treatment of a long venous stenosis in a dialysis shunt: case report. Cardiovasc Intervent Radiol 12: 29–31.

Halfman-Franey M, Coburn C (1990) Techniques in cardiac care: lasers, stents, and atherectomy devices. REVIEW ARTICLE: 128 REFS. AACN Clin Issues Crit Care Nurs 1: 87–109.

Halfman-Franey M, Levine S (1989) Intracoronary stents. REVIEW ARTICLE: 59 REFS. Crit Care Nurs Clin North Am 1: 327–337.

Halfman-Franey M, Tukan T, Bergstrom D, Hoffman M (1991) Using stents in the coronary circulation: nursing perspectives. Focus on Critical Care 18: 132–133, 135–136, 138–140 passim.

Harville LE, Rivera FJ, Palmaz JC, Levine BA (1992) Variceal hemorrhage associated with portal vein thrombosis: treatment with a unique portal venous stent. Surgery 111(5): 585–590.

Haude M, Erbel R, Straub U, Dietz U, Meyer J (1991) Short and long term results after intracoronary stenting in human coronary arteries: monocentre experience with the balloon-expandable Palmaz-Schatz stent. Br Heart J 66: 337–345.

Haude M, Erbel R, Straub U, Dietz U, Schatz R, Meyer J (1990) Coronary stent implantation in acute vessel closure 48 hours after an unsatisfactory coronary angioplasty. Cathet Cardiovasc Diagn 21: 263–265.

Haude M, Erbel R, Straub U, Dietz U, Schatz R, Meyer J (1991) Results of intracoronary stents for management of coronary dissection after balloon angioplasty. Am J Cardiol 67: 691–696.

Hausegger KA, Lammer J, Hagen B, Fluckiger F, Lafer M, Klein GE, Pilger E (1992) Iliac artery stenting—clinical experience with the Palmaz stent, Wallstent, and Strecker stent. Acta Radiol 33(4): 292–296.

Herrmann HC, Buchbinder M, Clemen MW, Fischman D, Goldberg S, Leon MB, Schatz RA, et al. (1992) Emergent use of balloon-expandable coronary artery stenting for failed percutaneous transluminal coronary angioplasty. Circulation 86(3): 812–819.

Heuser RR, Mehta S, Strumpf RK (1992) ACS RX flow support catheter as a temporary stent for dissection or occlusion during balloon angioplasty: initial experience. Cathet Cardiovasc Diagn 27(1): 66–74.

Heuser RR, Mehta SS, Strumpf RK, Ponder R (1992) Intracoronary stent implantation via the brachial approach: a technique to reduce vascular bleeding complications. Cathet Cardiovasc Diagn 25(4): 300–303.

Holmes DR Jr, Bresnahan JF (1991) Interventional cardiology. Cardiol Clin 9: 115–134.

Holmes DR Jr, Vlietstra RE, Reiter SJ, Bresnahan DR (1990) Advances in interventional cardiology. REVIEW ARTICLE: 79 REFS. Mayo Clin Proc 65: 565–583.

Hontz RA, Tripp MD, Kline LP (1991) Stents keep occluded vessels open. Rn 54: 50–54.

Hosking MC, Benson LN, Nakanishi T, Burrows PE, Williams WG, Freedom RM (1992) Intravascular stent prosthesis for right ventricular outflow obstruction. J Am Coll Cardiol 20(2): 373–380.

Hsu RK, Lo KK, Lai CW, Leung JW (1992) Late stent blockage by blood clot successfully treated by urokinase. Gastrointest Endosc 38(5): 604–605.

Irving JD, Dondelinger RF, Reidy JF, Schild H, Dick R, Adam A, Maynar M, et al (1992) Gianturco self-expanding stents: clinical experience in the vena cava and large veins. Cardiovasc Intervent Radiol 15(5): 328–333.

Ishiguchi T, Fukatsu H, Itoh S, Shimamoto K, Sakuma S (1992) Budd-Chiari syndrome with long segmental inferior vena cava obstruction: treatment with thrombolysis, angioplasty, and intravascular stents. J Vasc Intervent Radiol 3(2): 421–425.

Isner JM, Rosenfield K, Losordo DW, Kelly S, Palefski P, Langevin RE, Razvi S, Pastore JO, Kosowsky BD (1990) Percutaneous intravascular US as adjunct to catheter-based interventions: preliminary experience in patients with peripheral vascular disease. Radiology 175: 61–70.

Jaeger HJ, Kerin MJ, Kruegener GH, MacFie J (1991) Rupture of false aneurysm secondary to passage of ureteric stent. Br J Urol 68: 101–102.

Jenny DB, Robert GP, Fajadet JC, Cassagneau BG, Marco J (1992) Intracoronary stent implantation: new approach using a monorail system and new large-lumen 7F catheters from the brachial route. Cathet Cardiovasc Diagn 25(4): 297–299.

Joffre F, Rousseau H, Bernadet P, Nomblot C, Montoy JC, Chemali R, Knight C (1992) Midterm results of renal artery stenting. Cardiovasc Intervent Radiol 15(5): 313–318.

Kar A, Angwafo FF, Jhunjhunwala JS (1984) Ureteroarterial and ureterosigmoid fistula associated with polyethylene indwelling ureteral stents. J Urol 132: 755–757.

Karsch KR, Haase KK, Mauser M, Voelker W (1989) Initial angiographic results in ablation of atherosclerotic plaque by percutaneous coronary excimer laser angioplasty without subsequent balloon dilatation. Am J Cardiol 64: 1253–1257.

Katzen B (1991) Refinements widen utility of interventional devices. Diagn Imaging 100–107.

Katzen BT, Becker GJ (1992) Intravascular stents. Status of development and clinical application. Surg Clin North Am 72(4): 941–957.

Kichikawa K, Uchida H, Yoshioka T, Maeda M, Nishimine K, Kubota Y, Sakaguchi S, Ohishi H, Iwasaki S (1990) Iliac artery stenosis and occlusion: preliminary results of treatment with Gianturco expandable metallic stents. Radiology 177: 799–802.

Kidd RV, 3d, Confer DJ, Ball TP, Jr (1980) Ureteral and renal vein perforation with placement into the renal vein as a complication of the pigtail ureteral stent. J Urol 124: 424–426.

King SB, 3d (1990) Prediction of acute closure in percutaneous transluminal coronary angioplasty. Circulation 81(3 Suppl): IV5–IV8.

Kuffer G, Spengel F, Steckmeier B (1991) Percutaneous reconstruction of the aortic bifurcation with Palmaz stents: case report. Cardiovasc Intervent Radiol 14: 170–172.

Kuhn FP, Kutkuhn B, Torsello G, Modder U (1991) Renal artery stenosis: preliminary results of treatment with the Strecker stent. Radiology 180: 367–372.

Kuntz RE, Gibson CM, Nobuyoshi M, Baim DS (1993) Generalized model of restenosis after conventional balloon angioplasty, stenting and directional atherectomy. J Am Coll Cardiol 21(1): 15–25.

Kuntz RE, Hinohara T, Robertson GC, Safian RD, Simpson JB, Baim DS (1992) Influence of vessel selection on the observed restenosis rate after endoluminal stenting or directional atherectomy. Am J Cardiol 70(13): 1101–1108.

Kuntz RE, Piana R, Pomerantz RM, Carrozza J, Fishman R, Mansour M, Safian RD, et al. (1992) Changing incidence and management of abupt closure following coronary intervention in the new device era. Cathet Cardiovasc Diagn 27(3): 183–190.

Kuntz RE, Safian RD, Carrozza JP, Fishman RF, Mansour M, Baim DS (1992) The importance of acute luminal diameter in determining restenosis after coronary atherectomy or stenting. Circulation 86(6): 1827–1835.

Kuntz RE, Safian RD, Levine MJ, Reis GJ, Diver DJ, Baim DS (1992) Novel approach to the analysis of restenosis after the use of three new coronary devices. J Am Coll Cardiol 19(7): 1493–1499.

Lalude AO, Conroy RM (1983) Vascular complication of percutaneously placed pigtail ureteral stent. J Urol 130: 553–554.

Lammer J (1990) Biliary endoprostheses. Plastic versus metal stents. Radiol Clin North Am 28: 1211–1222.

Lau KW, Gunnes P, Williams M, Rickards A, Sigwart U (1992) Angiographic restenosis after successful Wallstent stent implantation: an analysis of risk predictors. Am Heart J 124(6): 1473–1477.

Lau KW, Sigwart U (1992) The current status of intracoronary stent: an overview. Singapore Med J 33(2): 143–149.

Lembo NJ, Roubin GS (1989) Intravascular stents. REVIEW ARTICLE: 18 REFS. Cardiol Clin 7: 877–894.

Levin DC (1988) The Palmaz stent: a possible technique for prevention of postangioplasty restenosis (editorial). Radiology 168: 873–874.

Levine MJ, Leonard BM, Burke JA, Nash ID, Safian RD, Diver DJ, Baim DS (1990) Clinical and angiographic results of balloon-expandable intracoronary stents in right coronary artery stenoses. J Am Coll Cardiol 16: 332–339.

Liermann D, Strecker EP, Peters J (1992) The Strecker stent: indications and results in iliac and femoropopliteal arteries. Cardiovasc Intervent Radiol 15(5): 298–305.

Litvack F (1989) Intravascular stenting for prevention of restenosis: in search of the magic bullet. J Am Coll Cardiol 13: 1092–1093.

Lopez RR Jr, Benner KG, Hall L, Rosch J, Pinson CW (1991) Expandable venous stents for treatment of the Budd-Chiari syndrome. Gastroenterology 100: 1435–1441.

Macaya C, Alfonso F, Iniguez A, Goicolea J, Hernandez R, Zarco P (1992) Stenting for elastic recoil during coronary angioplasty of the left main coronary artery. Am J Cardiol 70(1): 105–107.

Maiello L, Colombo A, Almagor Y, Bouzon R, Thomas J, Zerboni S, Finci L (1992) Coronary stenting with a balloon-expandable stent after the recanalization of chronic total occlusions. Cathet Cardiovasc Diagn 25(4): 293–296.

Mali WP (1990) Follow-up of endovascular stented renal artery [letter]. AJR Am J Roentgenol 154: 902.

Mali WP, Geyskes GG, Thalman R (1989) Dissecting renal artery aneurysm: treatment with an endovascular stent. AJR Am J Roentgenol 153: 623–624.

Mehl JK, Schieman G, Dittrich H, Buchbinder M (1990) Emergent saphenous vein graft stenting for acute occlusion during percutaneous transluminal coronary angioplasty. Cathet Cardiovasc Diagn 21: 266–270.

Montgomery TA (1992) TIPSS: use of metallic stents offers non-surgical alternative. Radiol Technol 64(1): 38–45.

Mulcahy D, Sigwart U, Somerville J (1991) Successful stenting of a life threatening pulmonary arterial stenosis. Br Heart J 66(6): 463–465.

Muller DW, Ellis SG, Debowey DL, Topol EJ (1990) Quantitative angiographic comparison of the immediate success of coronary angioplasty, coronary atherectomy and endoluminal stenting. Am J Cardiol 66: 938–942.

Nath FC, Muller DW, Ellis SG, Rosenschein U, Chapekis A, Quain L, Zimmerman C, et al. (1993) Thrombosis of a flexible coil coronary stent: frequency, predictors and clinical outcome. J Am Coll Cardiol 21(3): 622–627.

Nawa S, Yamada M, Irie H, Teramoto S (1988) Magnetic resonance evaluation of patency of stented polytetrafluoroethylene graft connecting right atrium to pulmonary artery. Chest 94: 1105–1107.

Noeldge G, Richter GM, Roessle M, Haag K, Katzen BT, Becker GJ, Palmaz JC (1992) Morphologic and clinical results of the transjugular intrahepatic portosystemic stent-shunt (TIPSS). Cardiovasc Intervent Radiol 15(5): 342–348.

O'Laughlin MP, Perry SB, Lock JE, Mullins CE (1991) Use of endovascular stents in congenital heart disease. Circulation 83: 1923–1939.

Olcott EW, Ring EJ, Roberts JP, Ascher NL, Lake JR, Gordon RL (1990) Percutaneous transhepatic portal vein angioplasty and stent placement after liver transplantation: early experience. J Vasc Intervent Radiol 1(1): 17–22.

Olsen ER, Michielsen C, Thomas A (1971) Intra and extraluminal vascular stents for perfusion during anastomosis. Vasc Surg 5: 109–114.

Oudkerk M, Heystraten FM, Stoter G (1993) Stenting in malignant vena caval obstruction. Cancer 71(1): 142–146.

Palmaz JC (1992) Intravascular stenting: from basic research to clinical application. Cardiovasc Intervent Radiol 15(5): 279–284.

Palmaz JC (1988) Balloon-expandable intravascular stent. REVIEW ARTICLE: 64 REFS. AJR Am J Roentgenol 150: 1263–1269.

Palmaz JC, Encarnacion CE et al. (1991) Aortic bifurcation stenosis: treatment with intravascular stents. Radiology IVIR, 2: 319–323.

Palmaz JC, Garcia OJ, Schatz RA, Rees CR, Roeren T, Richter GM, Noeldge G, Gardiner GA, Jr, Becker GJ, Walker C, et al (1990) Placement of balloon-expandable intraluminal stents in iliac arteries: first 171 procedures. Radiology 174: 969–975.

Palmaz JC, Laborde JC, Rivera FJ, Encarnacion CE, Lutz JD, Moss JG (1992) Stenting of the iliac arteries with the Palmaz stent: experience from a multicenter trial. Cardiovasc Intervent Radiol 15(5): 291–297.

Palmaz JC, Richter GM, Noeldge G, Schatz RA, Robinson PD, Gardiner GA Jr, Becker GJ, McLean GK, Denny DF Jr, Lammer J, et al (1988) Intraluminal stents in atherosclerotic iliac artery stenosis: preliminary report of a multicenter study. Radiology 168: 727–731.

Pan M, Medina A, Romero M, Suarez de Lezo J, Hernandez E, Pavlovic D, Melian F, et al. (1992) Peripheral stent recovery after failed intracoronary delivery. Cathet Cardiovasc Diagn 27(3): 230–233.

Perry SB, Rome J, Keane JF, Baim DS, Lock JE (1992) Transcatheter closure of coronary artery fistulas. J Am Coll Cardiol 20(1): 205–209.

Pomerantz RM, Kuntz RE, Carrozza JP, Fishman RF, Mansour M, Schnitt SJ, Safian RD, Baim DS (1992) Acute and long-term outcome of narrowed saphenous venous grafts treated by endoluminal stenting and directional atherectomy. Am J Cardiol 70(2): 161–167.

Popma JJ, Ellis SG (1990) Intracoronary stents: clinical and angiographic results. Herz 15: 307–318.

Porter J, Ahsan A, Mulcahy D, Sigwart U (1992) Coronary stents. Br J Hosp Med 47(6): 411, 414, 417–419.

Potkin B, Mintz G, Matar F, Keren G, Akbari M, Douek P, Lindsay J, Satler L (1991) A mechanistic comparison of transcatheter therapies assessed by intravascular ultrasound. Circulation 84 (Suppl II): I-541.

Pucillo AL, Schechter AG, Moggio RA, Kay RH, Tenner MS, Herman MV (1990) Postoperative evaluation of ascending aortic prosthetic conduits by magnetic resonance imaging. Chest 97: 106–110.

Puel J, Juilliere Y, Bertrand ME, Rickards AF, Sigwart U, Serruys PW (1988) Early and late assessment of stenosis geometry after coronary arterial stenting. Am J Cardiol 61: 546–553.

Putnam JS, Uchida BT, Antonovic R, Rosch J (1988) Superior vena cava syndrome associated with massive thrombosis: treatment with expandable wire stents. Radiology 167: 727–728.

Quinn SF, Schuman ES, Hall L, Gross GF, Uchida BT, Standage BA, Rosch J, Ivancev K (1992) Venous stenoses in patients who undergo hemodialysis: treatment with self-expandable endovascular stents. Radiology 183(2): 499–504.

Rab St, King SB 3d, Roubin GS, Carlin S, Hearn JA, Douglas JS Jr (1991) Coronary aneurysms after stent placement: a suggestion of altered vessel wall healing in the presence of anti-inflammatory agents. JACC 18: 1524–1528.

Raillat C, Rousseau H, Joffre F, Roux D (1990) Treatment of iliac artery stenoses with the Wallstent endoprosthesis. AJR Am J Roentgenol 154: 613–616.

Rees CR, Palmaz JC, Becker GJ, Ehrman KO, Richter GM, Noeldge G, Katzen BT, Dake MD, Schwarten DE (1991) Palmaz stent in atherosclerotic stenoses involving the ostia of the renal arteries: preliminary report of a multicenter study. Radiology 181: 507–514.

Rees CR, Palmaz JC, Garcia O, et al (1989) Angioplasty and stenting of completely occluded iliac arteries. Radiology 172: 953–959.

Rees CR, Palmaz JC, Garcia O, Roeren T, Richter GM, Gardiner G, Jr, Schwarten D, Schatz RA, Root HD, Rogers W (1989) Angioplasty and stenting of completely occluded iliac arteries. Radiology 172: 953–959.

Resar JR, Brinker J (1992) Early coronary artery stent restenosis: utility of percutaneous coronary angioscopy. Cathet Cardiovasc Diagn 27(4): 276–279.

Richter GM, Roeren T, Roessle M, Palmaz JC (1992) Transjugular intrahepatic portosystemic stent shunt. Baillieres Clin Gastroenterol 6(2): 403–419.

Rosch J, Putnam JS, Uchida BT (1988) Modified Gianturco expandable wire stents in experimental and clinical use. Ann Radiol (Paris) 31: 100–103.

Rosch J, Uchida BT, Hall LD, Antonovic R, Petersen BD, Ivancev K, Barton RE, et al. (1992) Gianturco-Rosch expandable Z-stents in the treatment of superior vena cava syndrome. Cardiovasc Intervent Radiol 15(5): 319–327.

Rosenthal E, Qureshi SA (1992) Stent implantation in congenital heart disease (editorial; comment). Br Heart J 67(3): 211–212.

Roubin GS, Cannon AD, Agrawal SK, Macander PJ, Dean LS, Baxley WA, Breland J (1992) Intracoronary stenting for acute and threatened closure complicating percutaneous transluminal coronary angioplasty. Circulation 85(3): 916–927.

Roubin GS, King SB, 3d, Douglas JS, Jr, Lembo NJ, Robinson KA (1990) Intracoronary stenting during percutaneous transluminal coronary angioplasty. Circulation 81(3 Suppl): IV92–IV100.

Rousseau H, Joffre J, Puel J, Imbert C, Puech JL, Duboucher C, Wallsten H (1987) Percutaneous vascular stent: experimental studies and preliminary clinical results in peripheral arterial diseases. Int Angiol 6: 153–161.

Rousseau H, Joffre F, Raillat C, Duboucher C, Glock Y, Escourrou G (1989) Iliac artery endoprosthesis: radiologic and histologic findings after 2 years. AJR Am J Roentgenol 153: 1075–1076.

San Nicolo M, Achammer T, Flora G (1990) Duodenal fistula after reconstruction of the inferior vena cava with an externally stented PTFE graft. J Cardiovasc Surg (Torino) 31: 382–384.

Sapoval MR, Long AL, Raynaud AC, Beyssen BM, Fiessinger JN, Gaux JC (1992) Femoropopliteal stent placement: long-term results. Radiology 184(3): 833–839.

Schafers HJ, Hamm M, Wagner TO (1992) Gianturco self-expanding metallic stents (letter). Eur J Cardiothorac Surg 6(5): 278.

Schatz RA (1989) A view of vascular stents. REVIEW ARTICLE: 49 REFS. Circulation 79: 445–457.

Schatz RA, Baim DS, Leon M, Ellis SG, Goldberg S, Hirshfeld JW, Cleman MW, Cabin HS, Walker C, Stagg J, et al. Clinical experience with the Palmaz-Schatz coronary stent. Initial results of a multicenter study. Circulation 83: 148–161.

Schatz RA, Goldberg S, Leon M, Baim D, Hirshfeld J, Cleman M, Ellis S,

Topol E (1991) Clinical experience with the Palmaz-Schatz coronary stent. J Am Coll Cardiol 17: 155B–159B.

Schatz RA, Palmaz JC (1987) Intravascular stents for angioplasty. Cardio. 4: 270.

Schryver TE, Popma JJ, Kent KM, Leon MB, Eldredge S, Mintz GS (1992) Use of intracoronary ultrasound to identify the "true" coronary lumen in chronic coronary dissection treated with intracoronary stenting. Am J Cardiol 69(12): 1107–1108.

Serruys P, De Jaegere P, Bertrand M, Kober G, Marquis JF, Piessens J, Uebis R, Valeix B, Wiegand V (1991) Morphologic change in coronary artery stenosis with the Medtronic Wiktor stent: initial results from the core laboratory for quantitative angiography. Cathet Cardiovasc Diagn 24(4): 237–245.

Serruys PW, Beatt KJ, van der Giessen WJ (1989) Stenting of coronary arteries. Are we the sorcerer's apprentice? REVIEW ARTICLE: 54 REFS. Eur Heart J 10: 774–782.

Serruys PW, Juilliere Y, Bertrand ME, Puel J, Rickards AF, Sigwart U (1988) Additional improvement of stenosis geometry in human coronary arteries by stenting after balloon dilatation. Am J Cardiol 61: 71G–76G.

Serruys PW, Strauss BH, Beatt KJ, Bertrand ME, Puel J, Rickards AF, Meier B, Goy JJ, Vogt P, Kappenberger L, et al. Angiographic follow-up after placement of a self-expanding coronary-artery stent [see comments]. N Engl J Med 324: 13–17.

Serruys PW, Strauss BH, van Beusekom HM, van der Giessen WJ (1991) Stenting of coronary arteries: has a modern Pandora's box been opened? JACC 17 (6 Suppl B): 143B–154B.

Sigwart U, Kaufmann U, Goy JJ, Grbic M, Golf S, Essinger A, Fischer A, Sadeghi H, Mirkovitch V, Kappenberger L (1988) Prevention of coronary restenosis by stenting. Eur Heart J 9:(Suppl C) 31–37.

Sigwart U, Puel J, Mirkovitch V, Joffre F, Kappenberger L (1987) Intravascular stents to prevent occlusion and restenosis after transluminal angioplasty. N Engl J Med 316: 701–706.

Sigwart U, Urban P, Gold S, Kaufmann U, Imbert C, Fischer A, Kappenberger L (1988) Emergency stenting for acute occlusion after coronary balloon angioplasty. Circulation 78: 1121–1127.

Smith RB (1984) Ureteral common iliac artery fistula: a complication of internal double-J ureteral stent. J Urol 132: 113.

Solomon N, Wholey MH, Jarmolowski CR (1991) Intravascular stents in the management of superior vena cava syndrome. Cathet Cardiovasc Diagn 23: 245–252.

Stauffer JC, Sigwart U, Goy JJ, Kappenberger L (1991) Milking dissection:

an unusual complication of emergency coronary artery stenting for acute occlusion. Am Heart J 121: 1539–1542.

Steenkiste AR, Baim DS, Sipperly ME, Desvigne-Nickens P, Robertson T, Detre K (1991) The NACI Registry: an instrument for the evaluation of new approaches to coronary intervention. The NACI Investigators. Cathet Cardiovasc Diagn 23: 270–281.

St. Goar FG, Giacomini JC, Fischell TA (1991) Coronary occlusion following diagnostic angiography: salvage by intracoronary stenting. Cathet Cardiovasc Diagn 23: 294–296.

Strauss BH, Juilliere Y, Rensing BJ, Reiber JH, Serruys PW (1991) Edge detection versus densitometry for assessing coronary stenting quantitatively. Am J Cardiol 67: 484–490.

Strauss BH, Leborgne O, De Scheerder IK, Serruys PW (1990) Implantation of an endoluminal prosthesis at the distal anastomosis of a bypass graft for abrupt closure following balloon angioplasty. Cathet Cardiovasc Diagn 21: 271–274.

Strauss BH, Serruys PW, Bertrand ME, Puel J, Meier B, Goy JJ, Kappenberger L, Rickards AF, Sigwart U (1992) Quantitative angiographic follow-up of the coronary Wallstent in native vessels and bypass grafts (European experience—March 1986 to March 1990). Am J Cardiol 69(5): 475–481.

Strauss BH, Serruys PW, de Scheerder IK, Tijssen JG, Bertrand ME, Puel J, Meier B, Kaufmann U, Stauffer JC, Rickards AF et al (1991) Relative risk analysis of angiographic predictors of restenosis within the coronary Wallstent. Circulation 84: 1636–1643.

Strauss BH, Umans VA, van Suylen RJ, de Feyter PJ, Marco J, Robertson GC, Renkin J, et al. (1992) Directional atherectomy for treatment of restenosis within coronary stents: clinical, angiographic and histologic results. J Am Coll Cardiol 20(7): 1465–1473.

Strecker EP, Liermann D, Barth KH, Wolf HR, Freudenberg N, Berg G, Westphal M, Tsikuras P, Savin M, Schneider B (1990) Expandable tubular stents for treatment of arterial occlusive diseases: experimental and clinical results. Work in progress. Radiology 175: 97–102.

Strumpf RK, Mehta SS, Ponder R, Heuser RR (1992) Palmaz-Schatz stent implantation in stenosed saphenous vein grafts: clinical and angiographic follow-up. Am Heart J 123(5): 1329–1336.

Swars H, Hafner G, Erbel R, Ehrenthal W, Rupprecht HJ, Prellwitz W, Meyer J (1991) Prothrombin fragments and thrombotic occlusion of coronary stents [letter]. Lancet 337: 59–60.

Swenson WM, Javid H (1980) Use of an intraluminal catheter as a stent in femoropopliteal arterial procedures. Surg Gynecol Obstet 151: 107.

Toolin E, Pollack HM, McLean GK, Banner MP, Wein AJ (1984) Ureteroarterial fistula: a case report. J Urol 132: 553–554.

Topol EJ (1991) Promises and pitfalls of new devices for coronary artery disease [editorial]. Circulation 83: 689–694.

Umans VA, Strauss BH, Rensing BJ, de Jaegere P, de Feyter PJ, Serruys PW (1991) Comparative angiographic quantitative analysis of the immediate efficacy of coronary atherectomy with balloon angioplasty, stenting, and rotational ablation. Am Heart J 122: 836–843.

Urban P, Meier B, Haine E, Verine V, Mehan V (1993) Coronary stenting through 6 French guiding catheters. Cathet Cardiovasc Diagn 28(3): 263–266.

Urban P, Sigwart U, Golf S, Kaufmann U, Sadeghi H, Kappenberger L (1989) Intravascular stenting for stenosis of aortocoronary venous bypass grafts. J Am Coll Cardiol 13: 1085–1091.

Van Oppen J, Van Ommen V, Bar FW, De Swart JB, Van der Veen FH, Wellens HJ (1992) Complications after intracoronary stent implantation: three cases. Cardiology 80(2): 126–131.

Vassanelli C, Turri M, Morando G, Menegatti G, Zardini P (1989) Open-ended guidewire: new technique for balloon angioplasty of chronically occluded coronary arteries. Cathet Cardiovasc Diagn 17: 224–227.

Vignan H (1992) Nonsurgical portosystemic shunting: a radiologic breakthrough. Am J Gastroenterol 87(9): 1220–1221.

Vlietstra RE (1989) Management of acute occlusion after percutaneous transluminal coronary angioplasty. Eur Heart J 10(Suppl H): 101–103.

Volodos NL, Karpovich IP, Troyan VI, Kalashnikova YuV, Shekhanin VE, Ternyuk NE, Neoneta AS, Ustinov NI, Yakovenko LF (1991) Clinical experience of the use of self-fixing synthetic prostheses for remote endoprosthetics of the thoracic and the abdominal aorta and iliac arteries through the femoral artery and as intraoperative endoprosthesis for aorta reconstruction. Vasa Suppl 33: 93–95.

Vorwerk D, Guenther RW (1990) Mechanical revascularization of occluded iliac arteries with use of self-expandable endoprostheses. Radiology 175: 411–415.

Vorwerk D, Guenther RW (1990) Removal of intimal hyperplasia in vascular endoprostheses by atherectomy and balloon dilatation. AJR Am J Roentgenol 154: 617–619.

Vorwerk D, Guenther RW (1990) Self-expandable endoprostheses. Radiology 175: 411–415.

Vorwerk D, Gunther RW (1992) Stent placement in iliac arterial lesions: three years of clinical experience with the Wallstent. Cardiovasc Intervent Radiol 15(5): 285–290.

Vorwerk D, Guenther RW, Bohndorf K, Keulers P (1991) Stent placement for failed angioplasty of aortic stenoses: report of two cases. Cardiovasc Intervent Radiol 14: 316–319.

Walker CM, Stagg SJ, 3d (1990) Coronary stents: a review of recent developments. REVIEW ARTICLE: 21 REFS. J La State Med Soc 142: 25–32.

Walker HS, Rholl KS, Register TE, Van Breda A (1990) Percutaneous placement of a hepatic vein stent in the treatment of Budd-Chiari syndrome. J Vasc Intervent Radiol 1(1): 23–27.

Weernink EE, Huisman AB, ten Napel CH (1991) Treatment of Budd-Chiari syndrome by insertion of wall-stent in hepatic vein [letter]. Lancet 338: 644.

Wilms G, Peene P, Baert AL (1991) Modified delivery catheter for Wallstent treatment of renal artery stenosis [letter]. AJR 156: 640.

Wright KC (1990) Percutaneous transcatheter stent placement [editorial; comment]. Radiology 176: 620–621.

Zahn EM, Lima VC, Benson LN, Freedom RM (1992) Use of endovascular stents to increase pulmonary blood flow in pulmonary atresia with ventricular septal defect. Am J Cardiol 70(3): 411–412.

Zemel G, Becker GJ, Bancroft JW, Benenati JF, Katzen BT (1992) Technical advances in transjugular intrahepatic portosystemic shunts. Radiographics 12(4): 615–622; discussion 623–624.

Zollikofer CL, Antonucci F, Pfyffer M, Redha F, Salomonowitz E, Stuckmann G, Largiader I, Marty A (1991) Arterial stent placement with use of the Wallstent: midterm results of clinical experience. Radiology 179: 449–456.

Zollikofer CL, Antonucci F, Stuckmann G, Mattias P, Bruhlmann WF, Salomonowitz EK (1992) Use of the Wallstent in the venous system including hemodialysis-related stenoses. Cardiovasc Intervent Radiol 15(5): 334–341.

Zollikofer CL, Antonucci F, Stuckmann G, Mattias P, Salomonowitz EK (1992) Historical overview on the development and characteristics of stents and future outlooks. Cardiovasc Intervent Radiol 15(5): 272–278.

Zollikofer CL, Largiader I, Bruhlmann WF, Uhlschmid GK, Marty AH (1988) Endovascular stenting of veins and grafts: preliminary clinical experience. Radiology 167: 707–712.

VIII. Selected References on Contrast Agents

Iodixanol—a new nonionic dimer—in aortofemoral angiography.
Albrechtsson U; Larusdottir H; Norgren L; Lundby B. Acta Radiol 1992; 33(6): 611–613.

In 26 patients iodixanol, a new nonionic dimer, isotonic to blood in all concentrations, was used as contrast medium in aortofemoral angiography. Half of the patients received contrast medium in a concentration of 270 mg I/ml and the other half 320 mg I/ml. The aim of the trial was to evaluate the safety and tolerability of iodixanol and the radiographic efficacy of the two concentrations. The degree of discomfort, adverse events, changes in serum chemistry parameters, and diagnostic information were assessed. There were no changes or trends of clinical importance in serum chemistry parameters. The side effects were mild and consisted mostly of some sensation of warmth of short duration. No other adverse events were seen. The overall radiographic efficacy did not show any significant difference between the two concentrations. This indicates that iodixanol is safe and well tolerated when used in adult femoral angiography.

MR angiography of peripheral, carotid, and coronary arteries.
Alfidi RJ; Masaryk TJ; Haacke EM; Lenz GW; Ross JS; Modic MT; Nelson AD; LiPuma JP; Cohen AM. AJR 1987; 149(6): 1097–1109.

[Digital arteriography using an intra-arterial route in vertebrobasilar insufficiency. Comparison of iopromide 300 and ioxaglate 320 mgI/ml] Arteriographie numerisee par voie intra-arterielle dans l'insuffisance vertebro-basilaire. Comparison de l'iopromide 300 et de l'ioxaglate 320 mgI/ml.
Arnaud O; Salamon G. Ann Radiol (Paris) 1989; 32(4 Pt 2): 339–341.

During intra-arterial digital subtraction angiography of the vertebral and basilar arteries, 24 patients were included in a prospective double-blind randomized trial comparing a new non-ionic contrast medium, iopromide 300 and an ionic low osmolar medium, ioxaglate 320 mgI/ml. There was a statistically significant reduction in the number of adverse effects observed with Iopromide 300, particularly in terms of unwanted movements, source of image quality degradation.

Decrease of plasma prekallikrein and kallikrein inhibitors during intravenous phlebography.
Aronen HJ; Torstila I; Vahtera E; Suoranta HT. Eur J Radiol 1988; 8(1): 30–33.

Complex contact activation systems may have major involvement in side effects of i.v. contrast media. To investigate this, quantitative measurements of several factors (plasma prekallikrein, kallikrein inhibitory activity, haematocrit, alpha-2 macroglobulin, antithrombin III, alpha-1 antitrypsin and beta-thromboglobulin) were made before and after i.v. contrast phlebography in two groups of patients (each containing 21 patients) with no thrombosis, using a high- (meglumine iodamide) and a low-osmolality (ioxaglate) contrast medium. A statistically significant decrease in plasma prekallikrein was observed after the high-osmolality contrast medium, which is a sign of the activation of the kallikrein-kinin system and an indicator of the activation of the intrinsic coagulation. These events may play an important role in the adverse effects of contrast media.

[Evaluation of cardiac tolerance of intravenous digital angiography] Evaluation de la tolerance cardiaque des angiographies numerisees par voie veineuse.
Baudouy P; Lasry JL; Lagneau P. J Mal Vasc 1987; 12(2): 208–212.

Cardiac tolerance to intravenous digital subtraction angiography (ANVV) was evaluated by a prospective study in a continuous series of patients of both sexes investigated for various arterial diseases and classified initially into "cardiac" and "non-cardiac" cases. Ischemic and rhythmic electrocardiographic modifications were monitored, the contrast medium (PC) used being randomly selected between Ioxaglate and Iopamidol. Of the first 46 patients studied, 40% had had more than one auricular and/or ventricular extrasystole (ES), 18% had painless depression of the ST segment (greater than or equal to 0.5 mm) and 46.7% both effects. In the 17 "cardiac" patients, depression of ST and the ES were more frequent (p less than 0.02 and p less than 0.05 respectively) than in the 29 "non-cardiac" cases. There was absence of difference between Ioxaglate and Iopamidol with respect to frequency of disorders of repolarization, but Ioxaglate appeared to provoke more ES than Iopamidol (respectively 13 of 23 and 5 of 22 cases, p = 0.02). Major cardiac complications were not reported, and it is concluded, after discussion of cardiovascular effects of PC injection, that intravenous digital subtraction angiography is generally well tolerated but requires some precautions in patients with cardiac affections.

[Evaluation of the myocardial ischemic and arrhythmogenic risk of digitalized angiography by venous route. Apropos of a comparative trial of ioxaglate and iopamidol] Evaluation du risque ischemique myocardique et arythmogene des angiographies numerisees par voie veineuse. A propos d'un essai comparatif de Ioxaglate et de Iopamidol.
Baudouy PY; Lasry JL; Lagneau P; Abassade P; Valleteau de Moulliac M. J Radiol 1988; 69(3): 211–216.

Cardiac tolerance to digital subtraction angiography by venous route (DSAV) was evaluated during a prospective study of a continuous series of 100 patients of both sexes investigated for various arterial diseases, and classified previously as "cardiac" and "non-cardiac". A permanent 12 lead ECE recording by sequences of 3 allowed study of ischemic and rhythmic changes provoked by randomly allocated injections of contrast media, Ioxaglate or Iopamidol. Major cardiac complications were not observed in the 98 patients studied (2 excluded), but in 32.6% auricular extrasystoles (AES) and/or ventricular extrasystoles (VES) were noted and in 19.4% a painless widening of the ST segment of 0.5 mm or more. The and ST widening were more frequent in the VES 40 patients classed as "cardiac" than in the 58 "non cardiac" (35% against 8.6%, p less than 0.01 and 37.5% against 6.9%, p less than 0.001 respectively). The two products did not differ with respect to their effect on frequency of repolarization anomalies, whereas Ioxaglate provoked more VES than Iopamidol (30% against 8%, p less than 0.02). It is concluded that cardiac tolerance to DSAV is good, but that the frequency of VES and painless repolarization ischemic disorders observed, even with only weakly hypertonic contrast media of non ionic type, suggests that their indications be limited and that certain precautions are necessary in cardiac patients.

Ioversol clinical safety summary.
Benamor M; Aten EM; McElvany KD; Lankin DG; James MA; Buy Gandal T; Harashe LT; Weinandt WJ. Invest Radiol 1989; 24(Suppl 1): S67–72.

The authors evaluated double-blind comparative and open-label clinical trials in 1,186 patients who received ioversol to evaluate the safety and efficacy of ioversol, new nonionic low-osmolality contrast medium, at iodine concentrations of 32%, 24%, and 16%. The results indicate that ioversol was well tolerated in all patients and showed fewer adverse effects than conventional ionic agents. The diagnostic efficacy of ioversol was comparable to both conventional and other nonionic agents with respect to diagnostic quality. However, the improved patient tolerance may contribute to higher quality radiographs. The effects on renal function were monitored at 24, 48, 72, and 96 hours and did not reveal any clinically or statistically significant changes.

Clinical experience with ioversol for angiography.
Bettmann MA. Invest Radiol 1989; 24(Suppl 1): S61–66.

Ioversol, the new nonionic, low-osmolality contrast agent, has been well characterized chemically and in terms of basic toxicity testing. Ioversol has a formula similar to that of other nonionic agents, and has been used in a variety of clinical studies. These have been reviewed in detail in other papers. This article reviews the worldwide experience to date with the intra-arterial use of this contrast agent. Ioversol has been given to more than 500 patients for studies including intra-arterial digital subtraction angiography, and cerebral, visceral, peripheral, and cardiac angiography. In 23 carefully monitored studies, ioversol was shown to be safe and diagnostically efficacious, as compared with several high- and low-osmolality agents. To date, there have been no deaths or other severe reactions with this new nonionic formulation. Ioversol is likely to provide a useful addition to the current formulary of low-osmolality agents.

Contrast venography of the leg: diagnostic efficacy, tolerance, and complication rates with ionic and nonionic contrast media.
Bettmann MA; Robbins A; Braun SD; Wetzner S; Dunnick NR; Finkelstein J. Radiology 1987; 165(1): 113–116.

A prospective, three-center study of two contrast agents for leg venography was performed to evaluate both the relative frequency of adverse effects and whether low-osmolality agents provided significant advantages for this procedure. Fifty-four patients were studied with the standard preparation (iothalamate meglumine) and 57 with a nonionic agent (iopamidol). Both were used at an iodine concentration of 200 mg/mL, and there were no differences in volume of contrast material, duration of infusion, percentage of positive studies, or overall diagnostic adequacy. Patient discomfort was less with iopamidol than with iothalamate (18% vs. 44%), although discomfort was generally mild in both groups. By objective follow-up studies, the frequency of postvenographic thrombosis was not significantly different in the two groups (8% vs. 9%). Contrast venography, then, had a low frequency of complications when either a dilute conventional or a low-osmolality agent was employed. Although the frequency of postvenographic thrombosis was low with both agents, patient discomfort was less with the low-osmolality formulation.

Arterial phlebography of the leg.
Bjork L. Acta Radiol 1991; 32(2): 141–142.

On conventional ascending phlebography of the leg the deep femoral and pelvic veins are poorly visualized or not visualized at all. These veins are presumed to be the site of thrombosis and a source of pulmonary embolism in many instances. Diagnostic images of deep femoral and pelvic veins were obtained in 4 patients using injection of 30 ml of iopromide 300 mg I/ml into the iliac artery and DSA imaging of the venous phase of the angiogram.

Glomerular filtration rate estimated after multiple injections of contrast medium during angiography.
Boijsen M; Granerus G; Jacobsson L; Bjorneld L; Aurell M; Tylen U. Acta Radiol 1988; 29(6): 669–674.

In twenty-six patients referred for angiography, clearance of contrast medium was determined with x-ray fluorescence analysis after multiple injections of contrast medium. A formula for correction of the injected amount, which takes into consideration the different times of contrast medium injections, approximating the total injected amount into one injection, was used. A single injection clearance of 51Cr-EDTA was determined at the same time. The results showed a good correlation between the clearance of contrast medium after multiple injections and the 51Cr-EDTA clearance after a single injection (r = 0.945). The correlation between contrast medium clearance calculated without correction for the different injection times, and 51Cr-EDTA clearance was the same (r = 0.946), due to short angiography time and rather low clearance values in our patients. It is concluded that total plasma clearance of contrast medium can easily be estimated after multiple injections. In this way patients with a risk of developing post-angiographic renal failure can be found.

Safety and tolerability of iodixanol. A dimeric, nonionic contrast medium: an emphasis on European clinical phases I and II.
Bolstad B; Borch KW; Grynne BH; Lundby B; Nossen JO; Kloster YF; Kristoffersen DT; Andrew E. Invest Radiol 1991; 26(Suppl 1): S201–204; discussion S208.

Identification and minimization of risk factors in angiography.
Bonomo L; De Pascale A; Salute L; Cattaneo G; Spinazzi A. Rays 1988; 13(3): 81–86.

[Iopromide in angiography. Review of the literature] Le iopromide en angiographie. Revue de la litterature.
Brossel R. Am Radiol (Paris) 1989; 32(4 Pt 2): 361–368.

A comparative study of the nephrotoxicity of iohexol, iopamidol and ioxaglate in peripheral angiography (see comments).
Campbell DR; Flemming BK; Mason WF; Jackson SA; Hirsch DJ; Mac Donald KJ. Can Assoc Radiol J 1990; 41(3): 133–137.

Iohexol (Omnipaque 350) and iopamidol (Isovue 370) are nonionic monomers; ioxaglate (Hexabrix 320) is an ionic dimer. We compared the nephrotoxicity of these three media by a prospective double-blind evaluation in 500 patients who underwent peripheral angiography during a 6-month period. Serum creatinine levels were determined before injection of the contrast medium and 72 hours after in 478 patients. In 308 (64%) patients there was an average increase in the serum creatinine level of 18.1 mumol/L after injection of an average volume of 123 ml of contrast medium. A subset of 80 patients who had an elevated baseline creatinine level (more than 110 mumol/L) had an average increase in the serum creatinine level of 40.45 mumol/L. Of patients who had arterial injections, 182 (72%) had an increase in serum creatinine level (20.7 mumol/L), but of those who had peripheral venous injections, only 43 (45%) had an elevated creatinine level (9.2 mumol/L), and of those who had central venous injections, 83 (63.8%) had an elevated level (17.0 mumol/L). In most patients elevation of the serum creatinine level was not of clinical importance. High-risk patients with an elevated serum creatinine level were found to be most vulnerable to contrast nephrotoxicity. Although mean differences were not statistically significant, there were consistent trends which suggested that ioxaglate was the least nephrotoxic of the three agents studied.

Magnetic resonance angiography in peripheral artery disease.
Carpenter P. Hosp Pract [Off] 1992; 27(10): 79–82, 85–86, 92.

Magnetic resonance angiography of peripheral runoff vessels.
Carpenter JP; Owen RS; Baum RA; Cope C; Barker CF; Berkowitz HD; Golden MA; Perloff LJ. J Vasc Surg 1992; 16(6): 807–813; discussion 813–815.

Recent improvements in magnetic resonance imaging techniques have made magnetic resonance angiography (MRA) a very useful adjunct to invasive angiography. Fifty-five limbs in 51 patients with occlusive peripheral vascular disease were studied with both MRA and contrast arteriography. The magnetic resonance and contrast arteriograms were read by radiologists and surgeons and separate interventional plans were based on each study. The MRA findings differed significantly from those of conventional arteriography in 26 limbs (48%). In every case MRA visualized all of the same vessels and hemodynamic stenoses seen on the contrast arteriogram. In

48% of the cases, however, MRA revealed additional findings. Thus the discrepancies in the two studies were always the result of the failure of the arteriogram to reveal all of the patent vessels seen on MRA. The additional information provided by MRA resulted in alteration of the interventional plan in 11 cases (22%). In nine cases (18%) target vessels suitable for use in a limb-salvage procedure were identified by MRA, although they had been missed by conventional arteriography. In all of these cases, intraoperative arteriograms confirmed the suitability of these vessels for use in technically successful bypass procedures. In two cases (4%) additional information provided by MRA identified a target runoff vessel for bypass grafting that proved to be a better alternative than the one that would have been chosen on the basis of contrast arteriography. (ABSTRACT TRUNCATED AT 250 WORDS)

Role of low-osmolality contrast media in thromboembolic complications: scanning electron microscopy study.
Casalini E. Radiology 1992; 183(3): 741–744.

Numerous in vitro studies have found that clot formation may occur when blood is mixed directly with nonionic low-osmolality contrast media during angiographic procedures because of activation of hemostasis in the catheter; ionic contrast media, on the other hand, inhibit clot formation. Thirty patients were injected with low-osmolality contrast media—15 with ioxaglate, an ionic dimer, and 15 with iopamidol, a nonionic monomer. The inner wall of the angiographic catheter was studied with electron microscopy after selective catheterization of supraaortic vessels. Clot formation of various extent was observed in nine (60%) of the patients administered iopamidol. No coagulation process was found in the catheters of the patients administered ioxaglate. Results indicate that nonionic, low-osmolality contrast media may play a role in the formation of thromboembolisms.

Intravenous contrast media: use and associated mortality.
Cashman JD; McCredie J; Henry DA. Med J Aust 1991; 155(9): 618–623. Comment in: Med J Aust 1992; 156(3): 218–219; Comment in: Med J Aust 1992; 156(3): 218; discussion 219.

OBJECTIVE: To determine the extent of use and mortality associated with peripheral intravenous injections of radiocontrast media. DESIGN: A retrospective study of injection data was made for the three and a half year period from January 1987 to June 1990 using the Health Insurance Commission database and the records of public hospital x-ray departments. Information about deaths associated with the injections was obtained from a survey of all radiologists and from other relevant sources. SETTING AND PARTICIPANTS: The study related to the entire population of New South Wales and the Australian Capital Territory, approximately 6 million people. INTERVENTIONS: Intravenous injections of radiographic contrast medium for computed tomographic scans, intravenous pyelograms and venograms. MAIN OUTCOME: A comprehensive record of intravenous contrast usage and associated mortality in a large community. RESULTS: Between January 1987 and June 1990, 613 581 intravenous injections of radiocontrast media were administered in New South Wales and the Australian Capital

Territory. The overall annual incidence of use was estimated to be 2.9% and was markedly age dependent being more than 7% in subjects over 65 years. Eight deaths were documented, representing an overall mortality of 13 per million injections (95% confidence interval (CI), 5.6-25.7). Mortality appeared to be age related being 35 per million (95% CI, 12.7-75.6) in those over 65 years compared with 4.5 per million (95% CI, 0.6-16.4) in those under 65 years. Two of the deaths involved low osmolar contrast media. CONCLUSIONS: Death after injection of intravenous contrast medium is a rare event. There was no evidence that mortality was lower with the newer, low osmolar media than with the older, high osmolar media.

Acute thrombocytopenia after i.v. administration of a radiographic contrast medium.
Chang JC; Lee D; Gross HM. AJR 1989; 152(5): 947–949.

Dosing of contrast material to prevent contrast nephropathy in patients with renal disease.
Cigarroa RG; Lange RA; Williams RH; Hillis LD. Am J Med 1989; 86(6 Pt 1): 649–652.

PURPOSE: Contrast-induced renal dysfunction has been reported to occur in 15% to 42% of patients with underlying azotemia, but there is disagreement as to whether its incidence is reduced by limiting the amount of contrast material. To adjust the amount of contrast material to the severity of azotemia, we have utilized the following formula to calculate a contrast material "limit" in patients with renal disease: Contrast material limit = (formula; see text) PATIENTS AND METHODS: Over a 10-year period, 115 patients (53 men, 62 women, aged 61 +/− 11 (mean +/− SD) years) with renal dysfunction (baseline serum creatinine level greater than or equal to 1.8 mg/dL) underwent cardiac catheterization and angiography, after which the level of serum creatinine was measured daily for five days. The amount of contrast material that was given adhered to the limit in 86 patients (Group I) and exceeded it in 29 (Group II). RESULTS: Contrast-induced renal dysfunction (an increase in serum creatinine greater than or equal to 1.0 mg/dL) occurred in two (2%) patients in Group I and in six (21%) patients in Group II (p less than 0.001). Of the 48 patients with concomitant diabetes mellitus, the contrast limit was surpassed in 16, six (38%) of whom had contrast nephropathy. Only two of the 32 (6%) diabetic patients in whom the contrast limit was not exceeded had contrast nephropathy (p less than 0.001). CONCLUSIONS: Thus, contrast-induced renal dysfunction occurs infrequently if the amount of contrast material is limited in accordance with the degree of azotemia. Diabetic patients have a high incidence of contrast nephropathy, particularly when they receive an excessive amount of contrast. In patients with diabetes and renal impairment, it may be preferable to perform angiography as a staged procedure or to utilize alternative (non-contrast) techniques to obtain the desired information rather than to exceed the prescribed contrast limit.

Case report: deep venous thrombosis following iopamidol venography.
Cope LH. Clin Radiol 1992; 45(1): 44–45.

A case of deep venous thrombosis following iopamidol venography is presented. This complication has not previously been reported.

Contrast media-related thromboembolic risks: effects of blood mixed with contrast media in contact with angiographic catheters.
Corot C; Belleville J; Amiel M; Eloy R. Semin Hematol 1991; 28(4 Suppl 7): 54–59; discussion 66–68.

Scanning electron microscopic analysis of catheters during routine angiographic procedures. Role of the contrast agent. The European Clotting Group.
Corot C; Cornillac A; Belleville J; Eloy R. Invest Radiol 1991; 26(Suppl 1): S96–100; discussion S107–109.

Renal failure following radiologic procedures.
Cronin RE. Am J Med Sci 1989; 298(5): 342–356.

Radiologic procedures that employ intravascular contrast material with or without angiography may lead to renal failure. In procedures that use intravenous contrast alone, the mechanism of renal injury is not precisely known, but direct toxicity to renal tubular cells is likely to be a major factor. Ionic and nonionic contrast agents are both capable of causing this adverse reaction. Renal failure occurring during angiography may also be secondary to the effects of radiocontrast, but the additional possibility that micro cholesterol emboli have been dislodged from atheroma located on the intima of large vessels must be considered. The acute or subacute development of renal failure in the presence of skin changes (livido reticularis), hypertension, multiple organ failure or dysfunction, and a fatal outcome favors the later diagnosis.

Contrast agents, red cells, coagulation, and the angiographer.
Dawson P. Invest Radiol 1990; 25(Suppl 1): S117–118.

Iodinated intravascular contrast agents past and present. Toxicity considerations.
Dawson P. Invest Radiol 1990; 25(Suppl 1): S11.

Embolic problems in angiography.
Dawson P. Semin Hematol 1991; 28(4 Suppl 7): 31–37; 38–41.

All contrast agents, including the non-ionic variety, are anticoagulant and have antiplatelet effects. There is absolutely no evidence from any source, in vitro or in vivo, that non-ionic contrast agents have any "prothrombotic" or "procoagulant" or "thrombogenic" potential, as has been suggested in some quarters. They simply have a lesser anticoagulant effect than do the ionic agents old or new, which is entirely predictable and in line with their generally greater inertness and biocompatibility. Although there may still be scope for greater understanding of structure-toxicity relationships in contrast agent design, currently it is believed that it would be impossible to restore a stronger anticoagulant effect to a non-ionic contrast agent without simultaneously restoring other aspects of toxicity. The angiographer who calls for more anticoagulant contrast agents is calling for more toxic contrast agents. It has been our clinical experience, and that of many others throughout Europe, that there has been no increase in clinically apparent thromboembolic phenomena since the introduction of non-ionic agents. Furthermore, it has been our experimental experience that, although contrast agents of all kinds play a role (inhibitory) in thromboembolism, the role of other materials used by the angiographer are of greater importance. Thus, the materials of and, indeed, the method of preparation of, the catheters and guidewires used has a great bearing on the phenomenon. Heparinization of the patient should surely be beneficial in some cases, but there is, surprisingly, no firm consensus or data on this and the individual requirements of patients vary, necessitating some method of monitoring and control. (ABSTRACT TRUNCATED AT 250 WORDS)

Magnetic resonance versus conventional angiography in peripheral arterial occlusive disease (letter).
Druy EM. N Engl J Med 1992; 327(18): 1319; discussion 1320.

Thrombogenic potential of nonionic contrast media? (see comments).
Fareed J; Walenga JM; Saravia GE; Moncada RM. Radiology 1990; 174(2): 321–325.

Comment in: Radiology 1990; 177(1): 280–285.

Iodixanol in excretory urography: initial clinical experience with a nonionic, dimeric (ratio 6:1) contrast medium. Work in progress.
Gavant ML; Siegle RL. Radiology 1992; 183(2): 515–518.

The authors report the first clinical experience in the United States with the highly water soluble, nonionic dimer (6:1 ratio) contrast medium iodixanol (5,5'-((2-hydroxyl-1,3-propanediyl)bis(acetylimino))bis(N,N'-bis(2,3dihydroxypropyl)-2,4,6-triodo 1,3-benzenedicarbooxa mide)). Iodixanol has an osmolality less than half that of monomeric, nonionic equivalent contrast media. Sodium, calcium, and magnesium ions were added to iodixanol to make the injected solution isosmotic to blood (290 mosm/kg H2O), with levels of free calcium and magnesium equivalent to levels found in the blood. Forty patients undergoing elective excretory urography were studied after bolus injection of doses of iodixanol with either 27 or 32 g of iodine. No adverse event or idiosyncratic reaction occurred. Seven patients felt coolness at the site of injection. Diagnostically adequate urographic examinations were routinely obtained with both doses. Further clinical investigation with iodixanol is warranted to determine if its beneficial chemical properties minimize both the chemotoxic and osmotoxic side effects and the disruption of physiologic functions that are seen with use of other ionic and nonionic contrast media.

Acute renal dysfunction in high-risk patients after angiography: comparison of ionic and nonionic contrast media.
Gomes AS; Lois JF; Baker JD; McGlade CT; Bunnell DH; Hartzman S. Radiology 1989; 170(1 Pt 1): 65–68.

A group of 145 high-risk patients who underwent angiography after administration of the nonionic contrast agent iohexol were monitored for the development of acute renal dysfunction. The results in this group were compared with those in 202 high-risk historical control subjects who had undergone angiography after administration of ionic contrast material. All patients in both groups received similar pre- and postangiographic treatment. A greater number of patients in the ionic group had preexisting renal disease, were of advanced age, and had received large volumes of contrast material. Acute renal dysfunction occurred in 20 of the 202 (10%) patients in the ionic group, compared with eight of the 145 (5.5%) patients in the nonionic group; this difference is not statistically significant. Five patients in the ionic group, but none of the patients in the nonionic group, ultimately required dialysis; this difference is not statistically significant. The findings suggest that a randomized trial in high-risk patients should be undertaken before a clinical advantage of the nonionic contrast agent iohexol with regard to renal function can be assumed.

Anticoagulant effects of nonionic versus ionic contrast media in angiography syringes.
Grabowski EF; Kaplan KL; Halpern EF. Invest Radiol 1991; 26(5): 417–421.

To determine whether nonionic contrast media present a clotting hazard when plastic or glass injection syringes are contaminated with aspirated blood, we evaluated two nonionic (iohexol and iopamidol) and two ionic (ioxaglate and diatrizoate) contrast agents. We used a blood:contrast media ratio of 2 mL:5 mL and ten normal donors, each studied at 10, 20, 30, and 60 minutes, a parallel study of clotting and fibrinopeptide A (FPA) generation in plastic tubes, and life table analysis to estimate more accurately donor-based early clotting probabilities. While ionic contrast media are stronger anticoagulants, both nonionic and ionic media retard clotting in plastic tubes, and clotting in plastic and glass angiography syringes in comparison to saline controls. A clotting probability of 1% for nonionic agents in plastic syringes was not reached until a time (mean +/− SD) of 21.5 +/− 3.2 minutes. This contrasts with a time of 8.7 +/− 2.5 minutes for saline control. With plastic syringes, no clotting at all was observed at 10 and 20 minutes with either class of agents. Neither class of agents hastened the generation of FPA. We found no evidence, therefore, that nonionic agents either cause clots or are procoagulant.

Ioversol. Double-blind study of a new low osmolar contrast agent for peripheral and visceral arteriography.
Grassi CJ; Bettmann MA; Finkelstein J; Reagan K. Invest Radiol 1989; 24(2): 133–137.

The new low-osmolar contrast agent ioversol was compared with the conventional ionic contrast agent diatrizoate in 60 patients undergoing routine abdominal (21 patients) and peripheral (39 patients) arteriography. The effects on hemodynamics, various laboratory parameters, and patient comfort were evaluated. In peripheral arteriography, there was less discomfort with ioversol as well as decreased magnitude and incidence of hypotension (P less than .001) after injection. In visceral arteriography, there was no significant difference between the two agents. Overall, the incidence of ECG changes was small in both groups (ioversol 2%, diatrizoate 8%). The two media were equivalent in incidence of adverse reactions (eg, nausea, vomiting, urticaria), the effect on laboratory parameters, and in the diagnostic adequacy of the radiographs. We conclude that ioversol is safe and efficacious for peripheral and visceral arteriography. In peripheral arteriography it causes less patient discomfort and, perhaps more importantly, fewer hemodynamic alterations than diatrizoate. These differences in hemodynamic effects may be important in patients with hemodynamic instability or limited cardiovascular reserve.

[Acute adverse effects and complications of central venous digital subtraction angiography (DSA). Results of 2,600 studies] Akute Nebenwirkungen und Komplikationen der zentralvenosen DSA. Ergebnisse bei 2600 Untersuchungen.
Gross Fengels W; Beyer D; Fischbach R; Lanfermann H. Med Klin 1991; 86(11): 561–565.

Side-effects and complications from 2,600 intravenous digital-subtraction-angiographies (IV-DSA) are reported. All studies were performed in a standardized technique using a non-ionic contrast agent (Iopromid 370 mg J/ml). Side-effects or complications were noted in 2.5% of all IV-DSA. Most often nausea (0.92%), urticaria (0.5%), angina pectoris (0.5%) and symptomatic alterations of blood-pressure (0.27%) were recorded. 8.4% of all reactions occurred with a delay of at least one hour. All side-effects and complications resolved, partly under symptomatic therapy. In one (0.04%) out of 2,600 studies a severe allergoid reaction occurred, affording intensive-care therapy. With proper patient selection and a suitable technique, IV-DSA may be regarded—within the angiographic methods—as a procedure of relatively low risk.

[Complications of intravenous digital subtraction angiography—results in 500 patients] Komplikationen der IV-DSA—Ergebnisse bei 500 Patienten.
Gross Fengels W; Neufang KF; Beyer D; Steinbrich W. Rontgenblatter 1987; 40(9): 281–285.

500 patients were studied respectively for complications of intravenous digital subtraction angiography (IV-DSA) performed with non-ionic contrast media, using a central venous injection technique. In 21 patients (4.2%) during or shortly after the procedure 23 systemic, 1 neurologic, and 7 local complications occurred. In addition 1 patient developed acute renal failure 26 hours after the IV-DSA, whereas 4 patients later showed on thromboses of the catheterised vein. No permanent neurologic or systemic complications and severe allergic reactions were seen.

[Undersirable side effects of contrast media during i.v. DSA—a comparison of 2 nonionic contrast media] Unerwunschte Kontrastmittelnebenwirkungen bei der i.v. DSA—Vergleich von zwei nicht-ionischen Kontrastmitteln.
Gross Fengels W; Neufang KF; Siebert C; Lanfermann H; Steinbrich W. Rontgenblatter 1990; 43(4): 144–149.

For the first time a controlled double-blind study was performed to compare side effects and complications of i.v. DSA with central venous application of iopamidol and iopromide. 200 consecutive patients 15–85 years of age were studied. The randomisation brought up two homogeneously structured groups of 100 patients each. Using a given protocol, 66% of the patients were classified as high-risk patients. Side-effects and complications were registered by an extensive, standardised protocol. In 71 (35.5%) of 200 patients contrast-media related side effects and complications were noted. 37 reactions in 24 patients (9 iopamidol, 15 iopromide group) were classified as clinically relevant. In four patients (4%) of each group a drug therapy was initiated. Contrast-media related reactions occurred with delay in 5.5% of initially symptom-free patients. In no case intensive care of hospital admission became necessary. There were no significant differences between the two non-ionic contrast media in the incidence of side effects and complications. Both substances were well tolerated in i.v. DSA. In the total population patients with diseases known as auto-immune diseases and prior drug reactions demonstrated clinically relevant reactions significantly more often.

Selective cerebral intraarterial DSA. Complication rate and control of risk factors.
Grzyska U; Freitag J; Zeumer H. Neuroradiology 1990; 32(4): 296–299.

In 1095 patients 2770 brain supplying arteries have been studied by i.a.-DSA. Definitive neurological deficits occurred in 0.09%, transient deficits were observed in 0.45%. The reduced complication rate in comparison to former studies seems to be a continued effect of technical progress (DSA) and the use of new isoosmotic contrast media. In order to reduce the "training hospital effect" as to complication rate careful supervision of trainees is necessary. The average fluoroscopy time per vessel is proposed as an objective measure of the investigational skill of a neuroradiologist.

Renal dysfunction after angiography; a risk factor analysis in patients with peripheral vascular disease.
Gussenhoven MJ; Ravensbergen J; Van Bockel JH; Feuth JD; Aarts JC. J Cardiovasc Surg (Torino) 1991; 32(1): 81–86.

Angiography is required for a detailed anatomical investigation before reconstructive surgery or percutaneous transluminal angioplasty can be performed. Although angiography is a safe procedure, it is associated with renal dysfunction, usually transient, in about 10% of the cases. This study concentrates on the evaluation of renal dysfunction induced by "conventional" (i.e. film-screen) Seldinger angiography and a consecutive series of 396 angiographic procedures have been evaluated. Induced Renal Dysfunction was defined as an increase of more than 10% in the serum creatinine after angiography. To identify "risk factors" for Induced Renal Dysfunction we have studied whether clinical and angiographical variables were associated with the occurrence of Induced Renal Dysfunction. These variables included: age, hypertension, the use of antihypertensive drugs, diabetes mellitus, technique of angiography, site of contrast injection and type and quantity of contrast medium. Induced Renal Dysfunction was found in 21 cases (5.7%) and appeared to be associated with age above 70, hypertension, administration of more than 150 ml contrast medium and the presence of renal disease prior to angiography. More than 95% of the 21 patients with dysfunction had two or more of these "risk factors". The presence of diabetes was not clearly associated with Induced Renal Dysfunction and haemodialyses was not required in any of the patients. The incidence of Induced Renal Dysfunction after angiography was 5.7% which is low but not negligible. However, renal dysfunction was always transient and never severe. Furthermore, the identification of "risk factors" allows the prompt identification of patients at risk before angiography, which may help to reduce the incidence of Induced Renal Dysfunction.

Initial experience with a nonionic, dimeric contrast medium (iotrolan) in direct and indirect arteriography: a randomized, intraindividual double-blind study in 60 patients.
Hagen G; Wenzel Hora BI. Fortschr Geb Rontgenstr Nuklearmed Erganzungsband 1989; 128: 54–60.

The new isotonic contrast medium iotrolan has been compared with iopromide in aortofemoral arteriography, selective femoral arteriography, and intravenous digital substraction angiography (DSA). In each case a crossover study design has been chosen with special emphasis on patient comfort. Despite problems in the interpretation of results due to a "hangover" effect in selective peripheral arteriography, it may be concluded: (1) Iotrolan causes significantly less discomfort, such as the feeling of heat and most likely also pain, than iopromide. However, one patient reported slight pain after the injection of iotrolan even when no previous injection of iopromide had been performed; (2) in intravenous DSA contrast appeared 1 to 2 seconds later in the region of interest after the injection of iotrolan compared with iopromide, probably due to the slightly higher viscosity of the former agent; (3) otherwise, no differences between the two agents have been observed. No cardiovascular or other kind of side effects occurred with the exception of one slight allergy-like reaction in 60 patients.

Contrast-induced nephrotoxicity: the effects of vasodilator therapy.
Hall KA; Wong RW; Hunter GC; Camazine BM; Rappaport WA; Smyth SH; Bull DA; McIntyre KE; Bernhard VM; Misiorowski RL. J Surg Res 1992; 53(4): 317–320.

The increasingly frequent use of contrast-enhanced imaging for diagnosis or intervention in patients with peripheral vascular disease has generated concern about the incidence and avoidance of contrast-induced nephrotoxicity (CIN). In this prospective study, we sought to identify those patients at greater risk of developing CIN and to evaluate the efficacy of vasodilator therapy with dopamine in limiting this complication. Baseline serum creatinine (Cr) concentrations were obtained on admission and daily for up to 72 hr after angiography in 222 patients undergoing 232 angiographic procedures. The preangiographic treatment was varied at 2-month intervals for 1 year. All patients received an intravenous infusion of 5% dextrose and 0.45% normal saline at a rate of 75 to 125 ml/hr. During the first interval patients received 12.5 g of 25% mannitol immediately prior to their contrast load, in addition to intravenous fluids. During the next 2-month period the patients were given renal dose dopamine intravenously (3 micrograms/kg/

min) commencing the evening before angiography and continued to the next morning. During the latter half of the study the treatment regimens were modified so that the use of mannitol was restricted to patients with diabetes mellitus and dopamine to patients with serum creatinine concentrations of > or = 2 mg/dl. Postangiographic elevation in Cr occurred in 2, 10.4, and 62% of studies in patients with baseline creatinine levels of < or = 1.2 mg/dl, 1.3 to 1.9 mg/dl, and > or = 2.0 mg/dl, respectively. None of the patients receiving dopamine experienced an elevation in creatinine. There was no statistical correlation between age, diabetes, or medication with calcium channel blockers and CIN. (ABSTRACT TRUNCATED AT 250 WORDS)

Renal functional response to dopamine during and after arteriography in patients with chronic renal insufficiency.
Hans B; Hans SS; Mittal VK; Khan TA; Patel N; Dahn MS. Radiology 1990; 176(3): 651–654.

The potential renal vasodilatory effect of dopamine in improving renal function after arteriography was studied. Sixty patients with preexisting renal insufficiency were prospectively randomized into two groups. Patients in the treated group (n = 30) received an infusion of dopamine for 12 hours starting at the beginning of arteriography. Patients who received placebo infusion with arteriography (n = 30) served as controls. The study was conducted in two different time intervals. In the first interval, serum creatinine levels and 12-hour creatinine clearance values were obtained before and immediately after arteriography in 12 patients in the dopamine group and 13 patients in the control group. In the second interval, the same variables were measured before arteriography and for 3 consecutive days after arteriography in 18 patients in the dopamine group and 17 patients in the control group. Serum creatinine levels became significantly elevated in the control group on the 1st day and remained so on the 3rd day after arteriography, whereas the dopamine group did not show significant elevation of these levels. Creatinine clearance decreased in the control group on the 1st day, but this deterioration was not sustained on the 3rd day. In the dopamine group, there was no deterioration in creatinine clearance on either day, and mean effective renal plasma flow during and after arteriography was greater.

Contrast medium reactions—does Buscopan reduce them? (letter).
Hartnell GG; Hemingway AP. Br J Radiol 1988; 61(727): 652.

The potential role of magnetic resonance imaging in ischemic vascular disease (editorial; comment).
Higgins CB. N Engl J Med 1992; 326(24): 1624–1626.

Anaphylactoid reactions to iodinated contrast media.
Hildreth EA. Hosp Pract [Off] 1987; 22(5A): 77–85, 89–90, 95.

[Changes in the kallikrein-kinin and complement system in angiography using non-ionic contrast media] Veranderungen des Kallikrein-Kinin- und des Komplement-Systems bei Angiographien mit nicht-ionischen Kontrastmitteln.
Hoffmeister HM; Fuhrer G; Pirschel J; Heller W. Klin Wochenschr 1988; 66(17): 760–763.

To examine alterations of the kallikrein-kinin system and of the complement due to the bolus injection of newer non-ionic contrast agents, venous blood samples were taken before and 3 min after angiography. There were no adverse contrast reactions clinically evident. Prekallikrein, kallikrein inhibition, beta-factor XIIa inhibition, C1-esterase inhibitor, C1q, C3, ATIII, HMW-kininogen fibrinogen and factor XII were determined. Bolus injection of the contrast medium caused an activation of the kallikrein-kinin system (p less than 0.05) with reduction of prekallikrein, kallikrein-inhibition, beta-factor XIIa inhibition and C1-esterase inhibitor. The levels of C1q and C3 were also decreased (p less than 0.05) indicating an activation of the complement. Our results demonstrate, that angiography causes a significant activation of the kallikrein-kinin as well as of the complement system in spite of the use of newer non-ionic contrast agents.

[Long-term results using a nonionic contrast medium—a report of clinical experiences] Langzeitergebnisse mit einem nichtionischen Kontrastmittel—Ein klinischer Erfahrungsbericht.
Hruby W; Stellamor K. Rontgenblatter 1987; 40(3): 73–77.

Between January 1982 and May 1986 more than 50,000 patients were examined radiologically with water-soluble (ionic and nonionic) contrast media at the Department of Radiology Rudolfsstifung, Vienna. In 1983 only 2.2% of the contrast agents used were nonionic, in 1985 the share had increased to 53.3%. During this period the rate of drug-related side effects (DRSE) decreased from 6.9% (1983) to 3.3% (1985). From 1983 to 1985 DRSE were observed with 1952 patients after administration of ionic agents, whereas after application of nonionic media adverse reactions occurred in only 6 cases, so that DRSE rates of 6.98% respectively 0.07% resulted for ionic respectively nonionic contrast media. These results are discussed with regard to the physicochemical properties and physiological actions of ionic and nonionic contrast agents.

Non-ionic contrast media: a comparison of iodine delivery rates during manual injection angiography.
Hughes PM; Bisset R. Br J Radiol 1991; 64(761): 417–419.

Iodine delivery rates (IDR) of five commonly used non-ionic contrast media were determined at room temperature (24 degrees C) and body temperature (37 degrees C). Contrast media of strength 300 mgI/ml were also evaluated at 50% dilution (150 mgI/ml) with N-saline. Iodine delivery differed significantly (p less than 0.005) between samples at room temperature: Omnipaque 350 (1163) mg/s) less than Niopam 370 (1311 mg/s) less than Omnipaque 300 (1422 mg/s) less than Niopam 300 (1635 mg/s) and Ultravist 300 (1636 mg/s). Niopam 300 and Ultravist 300 delivered 41% more iodine per second than Omnipaque 350 at room temperature. Similar differences were identified at body temperature, while delivery of individual media was on average 23.5% greater than at room temperature. No significant difference between iodine delivery rates of diluted media at room temperature or body temperature was identified. The results demonstrate that iodine delivery and hence vascular opacification are better achieved during hand-injection arteriography by using relatively low viscosity media such as Niopam 300 or Ultravist 300. In digital subtraction arteriography all 300 strength contrast media diluted to 150 strength are equally effective.

Evaluation of renal function with delayed CT after injection of nonionic monomeric and dimeric contrast media in healthy volunteers.
Jakobsen JA; Lundby B; Kristoffersen DT; Borch KW; Hald JK; Berg KJ. Radiology 1992; 182(2): 419–424.

A new nonionic dimeric contrast medium (CM), iodixanol, was intravenously administered to 40 healthy male volunteers in doses of 0.3–1.2 g of iodine per kilogram of body weight, nonionic monomeric iopamidol and iopentol were administered to 20 others, and the renal effects were studied up to 120 hours after administration. Computed tomography of the kidneys was performed up to 80 hours after injection. Creatinine clearance as an index of the glomerular filtration rate was unchanged with all CM. Urine volume and osmolar clearance increased most with the monomeric CM. The proximal tubular brush border enzyme alkaline phosphatase increased with all CM. The lysosomal enzyme N-acetyl-beta-glucosaminidase increased more with the monomeric CM than with iodixanol. A persistent increased attenuation in the region of the cortex was observed with all CM. Attenuation returned to baseline within 80 hours, with the slowest decline with iodixanol. This delayed cortical enhancement did not correlate with the effects of the CM on the tubular enzyme excretion.

Eosinophilic pneumonia associated with reaction to radiographic contrast medium.
Jennings CA; Deveikis J; Azumi N; Yeager H Jr. South Med J 1991; 84(1): 92–95.

We have described what we believe to be the first published case of a reaction to radiographic contrast medium followed by a diffuse eosinophilic pneumonia. This association seems to confirm what is known about the immunologic mechanisms of such reactions, and though further verification of causation is needed, we found it to be the most plausible explanation.

Elimination of variable vasomotor tone in studies with repeated quantitative coronary angiography.
Jost S; Rafflenbeul W; Reil GH; Trappe HJ; Gulba D; Hecker H; Gerhardt U; Knop I. Int J Card Imaging 1990; 5(2-3): 125–134.

In quantitative coronary angiographic studies, unintentional changes of coronary vasomotor tone may have a significant influence on the coronary artery diameters, thereby increasing the variability in the measurements. To obtain objective data on these measurement variabilities, two protocols were designed to assess the influences of ionic and nonionic radiographic contrast media on the mean diameters of angiographically normal coronary arteries. The vessel sizes were determined with the CAAS using automated edge detection techniques. In 21 patients (study no. I), coronary angiograms were taken in identical angiographic projections before (control), and immediately following several (at average 7) subsequent diagnostic dye injections administered over a period of about 7 min. The ionic contrast agent diatrizoate 76% induced a coronary dilation of 19 +/− 7% (mean +/− s.d., p less than 0.001; n = 10); the nonionic agent iopromide 370 increased the coronary artery diameters by only 6 +/− 4% (p less than 0.01; n = 11). In another 11 patients (study no. II) coronary angiograms were obtained using the nonionic contrast medium iopamidol 300 at 5, 8, 10 and 11 min after the control acquisition; this protocol was repeated in the same patients with diatrizoate 76%. With iopamidol, coronary diameter changes were not significant at any time; with diatrizoate, however, coronary dilation was measured at 10 min (2 +/− 2%; p less than 0.01) and at 11 min (10 +/− 3%; p less than 0.001). In a third study it was tested, whether standardization of coronary vasomotor tone (e.g. in coronary angiographic follow-up studies) is possible by the induction of a reproducible maximum coronary dilation with nitrocompounds. In 12 patients, the mean diameters of angiographically normal coronary segments were analyzed before and at various times after i.v. administration (over 4 min) of 0.025 mg SIN-1/kg bodyweight. Coronary dilation was maximal at 10 or 15 min after the onset of the SIN-1-infusion (29 +/− 5%; p less than 0.001). 0.8 mg nitroglycerin given s.l. at 15 min did not further dilate the coronary arteries (28 +/− 7%). One hour after SIN-1, coronary dilation still amounted to an average of 24 +/− 8% (p less than 0.001) and became 'maximal' again, when 0.8 mg nitroglycerin was again administered sublingually (28 +/− 8%; p less than 0.001). In conclusion, short-term variability of coronary vasomotor tone induced by ionic radiographic contrast media can be eliminated by the use of nonionic contrast agents and observation of injection intervals of at least 2 min. In quantitative coronary angiographic follow-up studies, as well as during acute interventions (e.g., PTCA), identical baseline vasomotor tone can be achieved by induction of the maximal coronary dilation using nitrocompounds.

Adverse reactions to low osmolar iodine contrast media.

Katayama H; Kuwatsuru R; Sumie H; Sumi Y. Nippon Igaku Hoshasen Gakkai Zasshi 1991; VOL: 51(6): 632–642.

From January 1989 to December 1989, we performed a prospective survey of adverse reactions to contrast media at three institutes of Juntendo University. We collected a total of 4365 case cards during the period. Low osmolar iodine contrast media were given in all but one case. Procedures using contrast media included computed tomography, intravenous urography, arteriography, venography and myelography. The overall incidence of adverse reactions was 6.6%, and there were no severe or fatal reactions. The incidence of adverse reactions was about the same in both sexes. However, in males, the incidence was higher in the fifth decade, and in females, it was higher in the third and seventh decades. There was no relation between the dose of contrast medium and adverse reactions. Intravenous bolus injections caused adverse reactions more often, followed by intra-arterial injections and then usual intravenous injections. The incidence of adverse reactions in patients with a history of allergy or previous reactions was higher. Pretesting was performed in 48.9% of the cases.

Adverse reactions to ionic and nonionic contrast media. A report from the Japanese Committee on the Safety of Contrast Media (see comments).
Katayama H; Yamaguchi K; Kozuka T; Takashima T; Seez P; Matsuura K. Radiology 1990; 175(3): 621–628.

A large-scale (337,647 cases), nationwide comparative clinical study in Japan on adverse drug reactions (ADRs) to high-osmolar ionic contrast media and low-osmolar nonionic contrast media was performed prospectively. Ionic contrast media were administered in 169,284 cases (50.1%) and nonionic contrast media in 168,363 cases (49.9%). The overall prevalence of ADRs was 12.66% in the ionic contrast media group and 3.13% in the nonionic contrast media group. Severe ADRs occurred in 0.22% of the ionic and 0.04% of the nonionic contrast media examinations. One death occurred in each group, but a causal relationship to the contrast medium could not be established. It is concluded that nonionic contrast media significantly reduce the frequency of severe and potentially life-threatening ADRs to contrast media at all levels of risk and that use of these media represents the most effective means of increasing the safety of contrast media examinations.

Magnetic resonance versus conventional angiography in peripheral arterial occlusive disease (letter).
Kaufman SL. N Engl J Med 1992; 327(18): 1319–1320.

Contrast media adversely affect oxyhemoglobin dissociation.
Kim SJ; Salem MR; Joseph NJ; Madayag MA; Cavallino RP; Crystal GJ. Anesth Analg 1990; 71(1): 73–76.

Effects of ionic (Hypaque-76) and nonionic (Isovue-370 and Omnipaque-350) contrast media on oxyhemoglobin dissociation of normal human red blood cells were evaluated. In series 1, 4-mL venous blood samples were obtained from 15 normal human volunteers. One blood sample served as control, and 1 mL of either of the three contrast media was added in vitro to the other 4-mL blood samples. P50 values were estimated from the linear portion of the oxyhemoglobin dissociation curve obtained by tonometry. Determinations of P50 were performed at either pH 7.4 or 7.2. At pH 7.4, P50 in the absence of contrast media was 26.3 +/− 0.4 mm Hg (mean +/− SEM). The contrast media caused comparable decreases in P50 from this value (Hypaque-76, 20.0 +/− 0.5 mm Hg; Omnipaque-350, 21.6 +/− 0.4 mm Hg; Isovue-370, 20.7 +/− 0.4 mm Hg). Reducing pH to 7.2 in the absence of contrast media increased P50 to 33.3 +/− 1.0 mm Hg, evidence of the Bohr effect. The presence of contrast media either completely abolished (Hypaque-76 and Omnipaque-350) or markedly attenuated (Isovue-370) this effect. In series 2 (five patients), blood samples were withdrawn from the external iliac artery during injection of Isovue-370 (60–78 mL) into the proximal abdominal aorta to evaluate peripheral vascular disease. Measurement of P50 of these samples yielded findings consistent with those of series 1. The present findings demonstrate that both ionic and nonionic contrast media increase the affinity of hemoglobin for oxygen and, therefore, that they may inhibit oxygen delivery to body tissues.

Diagnostic imaging in peripheral vascular disease.
Kozak BE. Ann Vasc Surg 1992; 6(4): 393–401.

Adverse reactions to low osmolar iodine contrast media (second report).
Kuwatsuru R; Katayama H; Tomita T; Naoi Y; Hirano A; Miyauchi T; Takeuchi N; Ozaki Y; Nakanishi A; Sumie H; et al. Nippon Igaku Hoshasen Gakkai Zasshi 1992; 52(9): 1233–1246.

From January to December 1990, we performed a prospective survey of adverse reactions to contrast media at two different institutes of Juntendo University. We collected a total of 4555 case sheets during the period. The radiological procedures we investigated were computed tomography, intravenous urography, arteriography, venography and myelography. Low osmolar iodine contrast medium was used almost exclusively (except for five cases). The overall incidence of adverse reactions was 7.0%, and there were no severe or fatal reactions. The incidence of adverse reactions was higher in females (8.5%) than in males (6.1%). The incidence of adverse reactions increased according to the dose of contrast medium, especially when more than 101 ml was injected. Intra-arterial injection caused adverse reactions most often, followed by regular intravenous injections, followed by bolus intravenous injections. Adverse reactions occurred most often during injection. The next occurred in 5 minutes after injection, and then, 5–10 minutes after the injection of contrast medium. The incidence of adverse reactions was higher in patients with a history of allergy or previous reactions. Allergic adverse reactions were observed at a higher frequency. Pretesting was performed in 56.7% of the cases.

Renal and hepatic tolerance of nonionic and ionic contrast media in intravenous digital subtraction angiography.
Langer M; Junge W; Keysser R; Hasford J; Janicke UA. Fortschr Geb Rontgenstr Nuklearmed Erganzungsband 1989; 128: 95–100.

The liver and kidney tolerance of iopromide 370 in comparison to that of sodium meglumine diatrizoate 370 or iopamidol 370 in doses of 2 ml/kg body weight was examined in two controlled double-blind studies with intravenous digital subtraction angiography on the basis of enzyme assays in serum and urine. In patients with normal kidney function no changes were observed in the levels of the liver enzymes GPT, GOT, and gamma glutamyl transpeptidase (GGT) serum up to 72 hours after injection of iopromide or sodium meglumine diatrizoate. Among the kidney-specific enzymes, the excretion of GGT in urine increased after injection of iopromide and iopamidol. The maximum increase of GGT excretion was, however, statistically significantly lower in the group treated with iopromide than in the iopami-dol group. Within 72 hours, the activities had been returned to the initial values in both groups.

Analysis of renal and hepatic impairment by ionic and nonionic contrast media.
Langer M; Langer R; Felix R; Speck U; Behrends B; Mutzel W. Invest Radiol 1990; 25(Suppl 1): S125–126.

Radiocontrast-associated renal dysfunction: a comparison of lower-osmolality and conventional high-osmolality contrast media (published erratum appears in AJR 1991; 157(4): 895) (see comments).
Lautin EM; Freeman NJ; Schoenfeld AH; Bakal CW; Haramati N; Friedman AC; Lautin JL; Braha S; Kadish EG; Haramanti N; et al. AJR 1991; 157(1): 59–65.

Nephropathy is an established untoward event associated with intravascular administration of conventional high-osmolality contrast media (HOM). It has not been shown previously that lower-osmolality contrast media (LOM) are less nephrotoxic in a clinical setting. We evaluate the ability to replace HOM with LOM (in lower-extremity angiography) to reduce the incidence of nephropathy. We use multiple definitions for contrast-induced nephropathy (six different magnitudes of rise of serum levels of creatinine or blood urea nitrogen in various periods). The incidences of nephrotoxic effects with LOM vs HOM in patients with presumed risk factors, including preexisting renal insufficiency and diabetes, are evaluated also. When all patients are considered, the incidence of contrast-induced nephropathy for LOM vs HOM (defined as an increase in serum creatinine level greater than 0.3 mg/dl and greater than 20% on day 1, 2 or 3 and on day 5, 6, or 7) is 7% vs 26% (p = .001). When only patients with preangiography azotemia are considered, the incidence of contrast-induced nephropathy for LOM vs HOM is 10% vs 41% (p = .017); for diabetic patients, regardless of preangiography creatinine level, the incidence is 10% vs 31% (p = .012). Although contrast-induced nephropathy may develop even in a patient with no risk factors who receives LOM, LOM is associated with a decreased incidence of this condition, to various degrees, depending on the presence of risk factors.

Radiocontrast-associated renal dysfunction: incidence and risk factors.
Lautin EM; Freeman NJ; Schoenfeld AH; Bakal CW; Haramati N; Friedman AC; Lautin JL; Braha S; Kadish EG; Sprayregen S; et al. AJR 1991; 157(1): 49–58.

Contrast-induced nephropathy is a potentially serious untoward reaction to radiologic contrast media. The incidence of this nephropathy and the predisposing conditions are not well established, possibly because of methodologic differences between studies. We evaluated the incidence of contrast-induced nephropathy after femoral arteriography in 394 patients by using multiple definitions (different increases in serum creatinine or blood urea nitrogen levels at various times). When an increase in the level of serum creatinine of greater than 0.3 mg/dl and greater than 20% on day 1, 2, or 3 and on day 5, 6, or 7 was used to define the disorder, the incidence in our group of patients was 10% for nonazotemic patients vs 30% for azotemic patients (p less than .001); 2% for nondiabetic, nonazotemic patients vs 16% for diabetic, nonazotemic patients (p = .003); and 38% for patients who were both diabetic and azotemic vs 16% for diabetic, nonazotemic patients (p = .022). Baseline renal insufficiency and diabetes mellitus (especially when insulin dependent) were significant predisposing factors. The effects of dehydration and increased volume of contrast medium on the incidence of contrast-induced nephropathy were not clear; the age and sex of the patient were not important risk factors. The incidence of contrast-induced nephropathy depends on the definition used. Although contrast-induced nephropathy may develop in any patient, diabetes, renal insufficiency, and, possibly, dehydration and dose of contrast medium are risk factors.

Preliminary European intravenous clinical experience with a new, low osmolar, nonionic contrast medium: ioversol (Optiray).

Le Mignon MM: Azau C; Arthaud A; Bonnemain B. Eur J Radiol 1991; 13(2): 126–133.

The intravenous clinical trial program of ioversol (Optiray), a low osmolar, nonionic, monomeric contrast agent characterized by high hydrophilicity, is evaluated on the basis of results from the first clinical trials conducted in Europe as part of the development of the 300 and 350 mgI/ml formulations: 7 double-blind, comparative trials and 5 single trials were performed in a total of 743 patients, of whom 472 received ioversol and 271 a monomeric nonionic reference product. The diagnostic efficacy of ioversol was equivalent or superior to that of the reference products and tolerance was comparable to that of nonionic agents in terms of pain and heat sensations. No significant difference in adverse reactions was found and all the contrast agents studied were well tolerated by the patients.

Lower extremity venography with iohexol: results and complications.

Lensing AW; Prandoni P; Buller HR; Casara D; Cogo A; Ten Cate JW. Radiology 1990; 177(2): 503–505.

The frequency of side effects of a nonionic contrast agent (iohexol) was studied in 463 consecutive patients who underwent venography for clinically suspected deep-vein thrombosis (DVT) and compared with the frequency of adverse reactions of another series in which patients received either the same contrast material or a high-osmolar ionic compound. Minor side effects, including local pain and discomfort, nausea and vomiting, dizziness, skin reactions, superficial phlebitis, and edema, occurred in 83 patients (17.9%; 95% confidence interval (CI), 15%–22%). The only serious adverse reaction (bronchospasm) was seen in two patients (0.4%; 95% CI, 0.1%–1.4%). Postvenographic thrombosis confirmed by means of repeat venography occurred in one of 41 consecutive patients with a previous normal venogram (incidence, 2%; 95% CI, 0%–13%). The frequency of side effects appears to be significantly less than when conventional high-osmolar contrast agents are used. Use of iohexol for venography is associated with minor side effects in approximately one-fifth of patients, and serious adverse reactions necessitating therapy are rare.

Intravascular contrast media. Ionic versus nonionic: current status.
McClennan BL; Stolberg HO. Radiol Clin North Am 1991; 29(3): 437–454.

The development of LOCM is one of the most important medical discoveries made at the end of this century. In developing nonionic compounds, Almen showed that it was possible to decrease the osmolality by a factor of 2 and also thereby reduce the chemotoxicity by as much as a factor of 20. Serious adverse side effects after the intravascular administration of contrast material are caused by a combination of osmotoxic and chemotoxic properties of an individual contrast media molecule as well as the ionic composition of the agent when in solution. Worldwide clinical experience with the use of LOCM, ionic and nonionic, consistently has shown the new material to be safer and more comfortable in clinical practice. Some form of limited use of LOCM is now part of virtually every radiologist's daily practice, and the focus is turning to the low-risk-no-risk group. There are gray areas between risk categories, with some evidence even suggesting that the 20- to 40-year-old age group may be at risk to the same or even a greater degree than other commonly accepted risk groups such as the elderly. The future promises even better and safer but, in all likelihood, expensive, contrast agents for intravascular use. The ultimate decision on choice of contrast or the fate of LOCM rests with public policy makers, organized medicine, and the individual physician and patient. Based on penetration of the marketplace (nearly 50%) in terms of LOCM sales in 1990, there is a growing awareness within our specialty as well as the public sector of the improvements offered by LOCM. It is unlikely that a major conversion back to the universal use of HOCM will ever occur. As long as cost remains the major focus of the debate over the choice, however, physicians need to be informed advocates, familiar with the science, yet sensitive to the economic implications of the decisions they make to best serve the interests of their patients.

[Osmolality of contrast media—a risk factor in radiological endovascular procedures in children] Osmolialnoct' rentgenokontrastynkh veshchestv—faktor agressii pri rentgenoendovackuliarnykh vmeshchatel'stvakh u detei.
Mikhel son BA: Guliev ND; Lazarev VV; Poliaev IuA; Vodolazov IuA. Khirurgiia (Mosk) 1991: Aug (8): 85–89.

The study was conducted in 90 children aged from 5 months to 14 years during radiologically-guided endovascular (RIV) interventions with bolus injection of radiocontrast agents (RCA) in a dose of 2–3 ml/kg for 2–3 sec. High-osmolality RCA were used in 80 children, and nonionic low-osmolality RCA omnipaque-300 in 10 children. Injection of RCA bolus was attended by marked acute disorders of blood colloidoosmotic equilibrium (COE) which depended on the initial status of the latter and were greater when high osmolality RCA were used. On the basis of the study results, the authors developed and tested a method of modulator infusion therapy with consideration for the initial blood COE (hyper-, normo-, hypoosmolality). The suggested therapy makes it possible to reduce the degree of blood COE disorders considerably and prevent the development of complications associated with disturbed osmoregulation.

Frequency and determinants of adverse reactions induced by high-osmolality contrast media.

Moore RD; Steinberg EP; Powe NR; White RI Jr: Brinker JA; Fishman EK; Zinreich SJ; Smith CR. Radiology 1989; 170(3 Pt 1): 727–732.

To determine the frequency of and risk factors for adverse reactions to high-osmolality contrast media, the authors prospectively studied hospitalized patients undergoing cardiac catheterization. The authors also studied patients undergoing peripheral angiography and contrast material-enhanced computed tomography (CT) of the head or body who met at least one of the following criteria thought to increase the risk of adverse reactions: age of more than 60 years, diabetes, renal or liver disease, concurrent nephrotoxic drug use, or a history of allergic reactions (n = 795). Criteria were defined and used to group adverse reactions into three classes of clinical severity. Overall, class I (mild), class II (moderate), and class III (severe) reactions occurred in 362 (45%), 44 (5.5%), and three (0.4%) patients, respectively. Class II reactions were relatively common (25%) in patients undergoing cardiac catheterization yet were uncommon (2%) in patients undergoing the other three procedures. Nephrotoxicity occurred in 18 of 651 patients who had follow-up creatinine levels obtained at 48–72 hours. With multivariate regression analysis, the only risk factor (P less than .05) for combined class II and III reactions was diabetes. Diabetes, furosemide use, and a history of atopy (odds ratio = 2.8) were associated with nephrotoxicity (P less than .05). Underlying renal insufficiency was not a risk factor for nephrotoxicity.

Peripheral arterial occlusive disease: prospective comparison of MR angiography and color duplex US with conventional angiography.

Mulligan SA; Matsuda T; Lanzer P; Gross GM; Routh WD; Keller FS; Koslin DB; Berland LL; Fields MD; Doyle M, et al. Radiology 1991; 178(3): 695–700.

Conventional angiography, two-dimensional inflow magnetic resonance (MR) angiography, and color duplex ultrasound (US) were performed on 12 patients in a blinded, prospective study. The ability to grade arterial lesions and plan revascularization interventions were compared. Arterial lesions were categorized as nonsignificant (0%–49% diameter reduction) or significant (50%–100% diameter reduction). Determination of nonsignificant and significant lesions with MR angiography was in agreement with that at conventional angiography in 100 of 140 lesions (71%). Agreement between results of conventional angiography and color duplex US occurred with 114 of 123 infrainguinal lesions (93%). Twenty-one vascular interventions were planned by using conventional angiography; there was agreement with color duplex US in 11 cases and MR angiography in five. Color duplex US performed well in the assessment of infrainguinal disease but was limited in the evaluation of the iliac segments because of nonvisualization. The iliac region was visualized in more patients with MR angiography than with color duplex US, but image quality with MR angiography was inconsistent. Strategies to improve MR angiography of the peripheral vasculature merit further study.

Pain in peripheral arteriography: an assessment of conventional versus ionic and non-ionic low-osmolality contrast agents.
Murphy G; Campbell DR; Fraser DB. Can Assoc Radiol 1988; 39(2): 103–106.

Transfemoral digital subtraction aortography. Are diluted high osmolar contrast media acceptable?
Naisby GP; Owen JP; Alexander TW; Cope L; Laker MF; Hamilton PJ. Acta Radiol 1991; 32(2): 137–140.

The ionic monomer, sodium diatrizoate at 150 mg I/ml (726 mosmol/kg) and the non-ionic monomer, iopamidol, diluted to the same iodine concentration but at 324.3 mosmol/kg, were randomly allocated to patients undergoing transfemoral intra-arterial digital subtraction angiography for lower limb peripheral vascular disease. The agents produced images of comparable quality and diagnostic efficacy. There were no significant differences between the media regarding sensations of pain and warmth. Minor neurological symptoms (headache and dizziness) occurred 7 times more frequently with the ionic monomer. There was a slight but temporary rise in plasma potassium one hour after injection of the ionic monomer but no evidence of appreciable intravascular haemolysis. The non-ionic monomer caused a slight fall in haemoglobin and haematocrit one hour after injection which is attributed to osmotic haemodilution. It is concluded that a diluted high osmolar contrast agent is an acceptable alternative to a low osmolar agent in transfemoral digital subtraction lower limb aortography.

Computer-assisted femoral arteriography in serial assessment of atherosclerosis. A methodologic study.
Nilsson S. Acta Radiol Suppl (Stockh) 1992; 378(Pt 3): 31–50.

Simple isocratic high-performance liquid chromatographic method for measurement of iodixanol in human plasma.
Nomura H; Teshima E; Hakusui H. J Chromatogr 1991; 572(1–2): 333–338.

Experience with iodixanol, a new nonionic dimeric contrast medium. Preliminary results from the human phase I study.
Nossen JO; Aakhus T; Berg KJ; Jorgensen NP; Andrew E. Invest Radiol 1990; 25(Suppl 1): S113–114.

[Iodixanol. A new isotonic x-ray contrast medium] Iodixanol. Et nytt isotont rontgenkontrastmiddel.
Nossen JO; Andrew E; Aakhaus T; Berg KJ; Jorgensen NP. Tidsskr Nor Laegeforen 1991; 111(9): 1108–1111.

In this phase I study, safety, tolerance and pharmacokinetics of iodixanol 300 mg I/ml, were evaluated in 40 healthy male volunteers using four dose levels. No clinically important influences on renal function parameters, hemodynamics, ECG or clinical-chemical parameters in blood and urine were observed. 17 adverse events including discomfort were reported, but only three of them (sensation of warmth) were classified as related to iodixanol. CT-investigations revealed a dose-related, reversible increase in kidney cortex density. However, iodixanol caused no changes in glomerular function, and the increase in excretion of tubular enzymes was less than caused by other nonionic x-ray contrast media. Further investigations will focus on the safety and efficacy of iodixanol in patients.

Comparison of iopromide versus iohexol in aortobifemoral arteriography. A Swedish multi-center study of 446 patients.
Ohlsen H; Albrechtsson U; Billstrom A; Calissendorff B; Gustavsson S; Jenson R; Johnsson K; Nyberg P; Strindberg L. Acta Radiol 1991; 32(2): 130–133.

A double-blind randomized, clinical trial was conducted in 9 hospitals comparing the use of non-ionic contrast media (CM) iopromide 300 (Ultravist) and iohexol 300 (Omnipaque) during peripheral arteriography in a total of 446 patients. After premedication with morphine-scopolamine each patient was given two consecutive injections of 50 ml CM at a rate of 12 ml/s above the aortic bifurcation. Both CM were well tolerated. There were no differences between the two substances as far as general tolerance, pulse rate, blood pressure, sensation of heat or pain after CM injection were concerned.

Magnetic resonance imaging of angiographically occult runoff vessels in peripheral arterial occlusive disease (see comments).
Owen RS; Carpenter JP; Baum RA; Perloff LJ; Cope C. N Engl J Med 1992; 326(24): 1577–1581.

BACKGROUND. Bypass grafting to arteries of the lower leg has become standard surgical management of advanced peripheral vascular disease. Its success depends on identifying suitable distal vessels. Preoperative preparation includes imaging of the arteries of the lower leg, usually by conventional contrast arteriography. An alternative procedure, magnetic resonance (MR) angiography, has been successfully employed in patients with various cardiovascular diseases, but its possible value in patients with peripheral vascular disease has received little attention. METHODS. We used both conventional and MR angiography in preoperative studies of the lower-leg vessels of 23 patients (25 legs) with peripheral arteriosclerosis and arterial insufficiency, and developed independent therapeutic plans based on the information provided by each technique. When the plans differed, the interventional procedure judged more likely to save the limb was performed. The findings of conventional and MR angiography were verified by intraoperative arteriography, postinterventional arteriography, or direct operative exploration. RESULTS. MR angiography detected all vessels identified by conventional angiography, whereas conventional arteriography failed to detect 22 percent of the runoff vessels identified by MR angiography. The detection by MR angiography of vessels not identified by conventional angiography altered the surgical management of the disorders of four patients (17 percent) and guided successful bypass procedures. CONCLUSIONS. MR angiography is a noninvasive technique with greater sensitivity than conventional contrast arteriography for detecting distal runoff vessels in patients with peripheral arterial occlusive disease.

Induction of mitotic micronuclei by X-ray contrast media in human peripheral lymphocytes.
Parvez Z; Kormano M; Satokari K; Moncada R; Eklund R. Mutat Res 1987; 188(3): 233–239.

Pain during angiography: a randomized double-blind trial comparing ioxaglate and diatrizoate.
Pathria M; Somers S; Gill G. Can Assoc Radiol J 1987; 38(1): 32–34.

We performed a randomized, double-blind prospective study comparing pain experienced during peripheral and aortic angiography with two different contrast agents. Sixty patients, receiving a total of 107 injections, were randomized to receive either ioxaglate (Hexabrix) or sodium-meglumine diatrizoate (Renografin-76). Subjects scored the pain they experienced on a 10-point visual analog scale, and the physician also scored their discomfort on a five point scale. Hemodynamic parameters were monitored during the procedure in all patients, and subsequent hematology, serum chemistry, and urinalysis were performed in 19 of the 60 patients. There was a significant reduction in the degree of pain experienced by the Ioxaglate group compared to the reference group (p less than 0.001). The patients in the Hexabrix group had a mean pain score of 1.3 compared to the patients in the Renografin-76 group who had a mean pain score of 6.1. The two groups did not differ in their hemodynamic responses to the contrast agents, and no significant differences were noted in the subsequent laboratory measures.

Invasive diagnostic imaging of the lower extremities.
Plecha DM; Plecha FM; King TA. Clin Podiatr Med Surg 1992; 9(1): 57–68.

Invasive arterial imaging techniques are crucial to the preoperative evaluation of patients requiring arterial surgery. Venography is important in patients who are candidates for venous reconstruction, and it is also useful in the difficult diagnosis of deep venous thrombosis. The authors discuss the development of angiographic techniques, indications for use, patient preparation, and potential complications. Several examples of these tests are illustrated.

Changes in platelet activity and tissue plasminogen activator during arteriography in patients with chronic limb ischaemia.
Polanowska R; Wilczynska M; Slawinski W; Goch JH; Augustyniak W; Cierniewski CS. Thromb Res 1992; 65(4–5): 663–665.

Contrast medium-induced adverse reactions: economic outcome.
Powe NR; Steinberg EP; Erickson JE; Moore RD; Smith CR; White RI Jr; Brinker JA; Fishman EK; Zinreich SJ; Kinnison ML; et al. Radiology 1988; 169(1): 163–168.

Because the cost of managing an expected greater number of adverse reactions when high-osmolality contrast media (HOM) are used could offset the higher material cost of low-osmolality contrast media (LOM), a prospective study was done of 795 inpatients undergoing any of four procedures involving intravascular injection of HOM: cardiac catheterization, peripheral angiography, head computed tomography (CT), or body CT. The resources used in managing HOM-induced adverse reactions were measured, and the costs of these resources were estimated. Four hundred five patients (51%) had adverse reactions. Reactions were grouped into three classes according to their severity. Class 1 (mild) reactions occurred in 358 patients (45%), class 2 (moderate) reactions occurred in 44 patients (6%), and class 3 (severe) reactions occurred in three patients (0.4%). Ninety-nine patients (12%) consumed resources as a result of an adverse reaction. The average cost of these resources per patient undergoing examination was $1.07 to the radiology department, $5.83 to the hospital, and $12.93 to a charge-paying insurer. Mean (+/− standard deviation) cost to the hospital for managing class 1, class 2 and class 3 reactions were $2.52 +/− $5.33, $24 +/− $54, and $910 +/− $749, respectively. By comparison, the difference in material cost of HOM versus LOM ranged from $93 for body CT to $179 for cardiac catheterization. Even if LOM were to induce no adverse reactions, the increased material cost associated with universal substitution of LOM for HOM would be greater than the expected cost of managing adverse reactions when HOM are used.

The effect of iodixanol, new isotonic contrast agent, on femoral blood flow in man.
Pugh ND; Sissons GR; Ruttley M. Clin Radiol 1992; 45(4): 243–245.

Both ionic and non-ionic contrast media (CM) injected intra-arterially produce peripheral vasodilation and a sensation of heat or even pain. This effect has been considered to be predominantly related to the osmolality of the CM used. Iodixanol is a non-ionic dimeric CM which can be made isotonic with blood at iodine concentrations up to 400 mg/ml. To assess the degree of peripheral vasodilation following aortic injection of iodixanol, the change in femoral artery blood flow has been assessed non-invasively. Dupex ultrasound flow-velocity records were taken from the contralateral femoral artery in 10 patients undergoing transfemoral aortography. Volume flow, mean velocity, pulsatility index and peak systolic velocity were continuously recorded before and up to 2 min after injection of 60 ml of iodixanol at an iodine concentration of 320 mg/ml (iodixanol 320). Transient changes consistent with vasodilatation were observed in all patients. The greatest changes were observed during the time period 18–24 s after injection. Volume flow, mean velocity and pulsatility index all changed significantly from baseline (mean changes of 80.6%, 73% and −42.7% respectively). Peak systolic velocity did not change significantly. Intra-arterial injections of isotonic iodixanol 320 produces a significant increase in femoral blood flow in man. Factors other than hypertonicity must therefore be implicated in the vasodilatory effect of contrast media.

Blood clot formation in angiographic catheters. In vitro tests with various contrast media.
Raininko R; Riihela M. Acta Radiol 1990; 31(2): 217–220.

Human blood was injected into angiographic catheters filled with contrast media or flushing media. The catheters were allowed to stand at 37 degrees

C for 10, 20 or 30 min. Physiologic saline was then injected through the catheters, the catheter contents were shaken and filtered, and any clots were identified. Diatrizoate, ioxaglate, iohexol, iopamidol and iopromide were tested. Physiologic and heparinized saline were used as controls. At 10 min, clots were found in 65 percent of the catheters filled with physiologic saline, in 25 percent with non-ionic media, in 19 percent with heparinized saline, and in 4 percent with ionic contrast media. At 30 min, all catheters with physiologic saline, 85 percent with non-ionic contrast media, 46 percent with heparinized saline and 23 percent with ionic contrast media contained a clot. Although all the contrast media were anticoagulants, a more careful angiographic technique is needed for non-ionic media. All the non-ionic agents showed equal results. Physiologic saline without heparin is not suitable for flushing during angiography.

MR imaging of symptomatic peripheral vascular malformations.
Rak KM; Yakes WF; Ray RL; Dreisbach JN; Parker SH; Luethke JM; Stavros AT; Slater DD; Burke BJ. AJR 1992; 159(1): 107–112.

We performed a retrospective study of symptomatic peripheral vascular malformations to determine if MR imaging can be used to distinguish slow-flow venous malformations from high-flow arteriovenous malformations and arteriovenous fistulas. Twenty-seven MR examinations in 25 patients with malformations outside the CNS were reviewed. Sixteen venous malformations, nine arteriovenous malformations, and two arteriovenous fistulas were included. In all cases, the MR findings were correlated with the results of angiography. The distinction between slow-flow venous malformations and high-flow arteriovenous malformations and arteriovenous fistulas was made primarily on T2-weighted MR images, which showed high signal intensity in venous malformations and flow voids in high-flow lesions. In addition to the previously described MR features of venous malformations (serpentine pattern with septations, associated muscle atrophy, and typical T1 and T2 signal intensities), several new MR features were apparent. Venous malformations had a propensity for multifocal involvement (37%), orientation along the long axis of extremities or affected muscles (78%), and adherence to neurovascular distributions (64%). Prominent subcutaneous fat was commonly seen adjacent to the malformation. MR images of arteriovenous malformations and arteriovenous fistulas also commonly showed muscle atrophy and subcutaneous fatty prominence. Our results show that slow-flow venous malformations can be distinguished from high-flow arteriovenous malformations and fistulas on the basis of spin-echo MR signal characteristics. The associated imaging characteristics help in the differential diagnosis in problematic cases.

Altered urinary beta 2-microglobulin excretion as an index of nephrotoxicity.
Rashad FA; Vacca CV; Speroff T; Hall PW. Kidney Int Suppl 1991; 34: S18–20.

The experimental and clinical evidence indicate that beta 2-microglobulin (beta 2m) is actively reabsorbed from the glomerular filtrate by receptors on the brush border located in the proximal third of the proximal tubule.

Increased beta 2m excretion in the absence of increased filtered load of beta 2m is indicative of nephrotoxicity. The data presented show that urine beta 2m increases and creatinine concentrations decrease within four hours of administration of diatrizoate megalumine (DMG). In 9 of the 20 patients, the urinary excretion of beta 2m (U beta 2m) increased to clearly abnormal values. In 12 of the 20 patients, the beta 2m excretion expressed as mg per g creatinine (Cr), increased from normal (less than 0.30) to an abnormal beta 2m excretion rate. The increased beta 2m excretion per g Cr occurring immediately after DMG administration lead us to conclude that this effect occurs when the nephrotoxic agent is present in the kidney. Based on these data we believe that the onset of abnormal urinary beta 2m excretion coincides with the presence of the causative agent. This criterion therefore, should prove to be useful in determining the time to conduct studies designed to search for the causative agent(s) in Balkan endemic nephropathy.

Radiographic contrast media and release of neutrophil specific proteins in vitro and after intravenous injection.
Rasmussen F; Antonsen S; Georgsen J; Christensen JK. Acta Radiol 1992; 33(5): 495–499.

Blood clot formation in angiographic syringes containing nonionic contrast media.
Robertson HJ. Radiology 1987; 162(3): 621–622.

Spontaneous thrombus formation may occur if blood is allowed to mix with a nonionic contrast medium in the injection syringe or angiographic catheter. This is probably due to the absence of significant inhibition of the normal blood coagulation mechanism by currently used nonionic contrast media. Careful angiographic techniques will prevent blood from mixing with the contrast medium before injection. The use of a three-way stopcock and connecting tube between catheter and syringe is suggested. Contrast material should be flushed from the catheter immediately after injection. Systemic anticoagulation is not justified as a means of preventing thrombus formation. The potential prophylactic use of heparin added to the contrast medium during angiography or premedication with aspirin, and the attendant risks of these techniques, are discussed.

Nonionic contrast media in radiology. Procedural considerations.
Robertson HJ. Invest Radiol 1988; 23(Suppl 2): S374–377.

Thrombogenic potential of nonionic contrast media (letter; comment).
Robertson HJ. Mayo Clin Proc 1990; 65(4): 603–604.

Comment on: Mayo Clin Proc 1989; 64(8): 976–985.

Nephrotoxicity of high and low osmolar contrast media: case control studies following digital subtraction angiography in potential risk patients.
Scherberich JE; Fischer A; Rautschka E; Kollath J; Riemann H. Fortschr Geb Rontgenstr Nuklearmed Erganzungsband 1989: 128: 91–94.

The urinary excretion of kidney-specific marker proteins before and 120 hours after intravenous injection of either high- or low-osmolar contrast media (CM; diatrizoate, iopamidol 370) was monitored in patients after digital vascular imaging. Inclusion criteria for the randomized clinical study in a total of 40 patients (15 women, 25 men; mean age, 64.5 years) were at least 50 years of age or diabetes mellitus with normal creatinine concentration in serum. Compared with the control period, the elimination of tubular indicator enzymes alanine aminopeptidase, gamma-glutamyltranspeptidase, alkaline phosphatase, as well as of glomerular localized angiotensinase A was significantly higher in all patients after injection of the CM. The most significant differences were observed after 48 hours. In contrast, lysosomal N-acetyl-beta-D-glucosaminidase activity in urine specimens reacted less clearly and appears to be a less sensitive parameter in assessing CM nephrotoxicity. Elimination of brush border as well as of glomerular marker proteins was significantly lower after intravenous injection of low-osmolar CM iopamidol 370 (832 mOsm/kg) than after meglumine diatrizoate 76 (2100 mOsm/kg). In all 40 patients a significant decrease in creatinine clearance was observed; however, patients receiving diatrizoate had a significant decrease in creatinine clearance (period 0 versus 24 to 48 hours after CM), whereas patients after administration of iopamidol had not. No difference was found between creatinine clearance after 48 hours of CM injection within both groups of CM. Due to noninvasive parameters of kidney damage nonionic, low-osmolar CM are less nephrotoxic in potential risk patients, and should be preferred to conventional CM.

Tubular histuria: clinical evaluation of the different nephrotoxic potential of X-ray contrast media.
Scherberich JE; Rautschka E; Fischer A; Kollath J; Riemann HE. Contrib Nephrol 1990; 83: 229–236.

[Pharmacokinetics and tolerance of roentgen contrast media] Pharmakodynamik und Vertraglichkeit von Rontgenkontrastmitteln.
Schmiedel E. Rontgenblatter 1987; 40(1): 1–8.

Complications of imaging procedures in six elderly patients.
Scott D; Christenson L. Postgrad Med 1989; 85(4): 145–148.

Ioversol in ascending phlebography—a clinical trial.
Scott H; Palmer FJ. Australas Radiol 1990; 34(1): 44–46.

In this controlled randomised double-blind parallel group study of the use of ioversol-240 and ioversol-320 in venography all studies were considered diagnostic with comparable quality in the two groups. Patient tolerance was high with mild heat observed in 7 patients in the ioversol-320 group and 1 patient in the ioversol-240 group. Assessment of pain was also comparable (2 patients in the ioversol-240 group and 1 in the ioversol-320 group). Both strengths of the contrast agent produced no clinically significant, drug related, changes in vital signs or laboratory parameters and there were no significant clinical adverse reactions.

Incompatibility of Hexabrix and papaverine in peripheral arteriography.
Shah SJ; Gerlock AJ Jr. Radiology 1987; 162(3): 619–620.

Bilateral blurring of vision after administration of contrast medium during i.v. digital subtraction angiography.
Sharma S; Rajani M. AJR 1989; 152(2): 429–430.

The influence of buscopan on adverse reactions to intravascular contrast media.
Sharma S; Rajani M; Khosla A; Misra N; Goulatia RK. Br J Radiol 1989; 62(744): 1056–1058.

We have analysed the ability of prior intravenous Buscopan (hyoscine butyl-bromide) injection to influence the incidence and severity of adverse reactions to intravascularly administered, iodinated, ionic contrast medium in 258 consecutive digital subtraction angiographic (DSA) examinations. Adverse reactions were seen in 7.9% of the intravenous and 2.4% of the intra-arterial DSA examinations. The incidence of adverse reactions with and without prior Buscopan injection during intravenous DSA examinations was 8.2% and 7.1%, respectively and during intra-arterial DSA examinations was 5.6% and 1.5%, respectively. This difference is not statistically significant (chi 2-test). We conclude that prior intravenous injection of Buscopan has no influence on the incidence or severity of adverse reactions to intravascular contrast media.

Double blind comparison of Iomeprol 350 and Iopamidol 340 in intravenous digital subtraction angiography for peripheral vascular disease.
Simmons MJ; Waite DW; Galland RB; Torrie EP. Clin Radiol 1992; 45(5): 338–339.

A randomized double blind study was undertaken to compare the diagnostic efficacy and side effects of a new non-ionic contrast medium Iomeprol with a commonly used one—Iopamidol. Visual land densitometric comparison was made of intravenous digital subtraction angiograms performed for peripheral vascular disease. The results show the two media to be similar both in imaging quality and in the incidence of associated side effects. Ninety-eight percent of the intravenous digital subtraction angiograms were assessed as adequate for clinical management by the vascular surgeon.

Viscosity of some contemporary contrast media before and after mixing with whole blood.
Smedby O. Acta Radiol 1992; 33(6): 600–605.

The viscosity of 7 contrast media was measured using a rotational viscometer. When solutions with similar iodine concentrations were compared, the highest viscosities were found for the nonionic dimers iodixanol and iotrolan, the lowest for diatrizoate, iopamidol, and iopromide, and intermediate values for iohexol land ioxaglate. The viscosity of iohexol and ioxaglate was found to vary linearly with temperature and quadratically with concentration. Whole-blood viscosity was measured for 5 subjects at high and low shear rates before and after mixing with contrast media in various proportions. Low-shear viscosity was found to decrease and high-shear viscosity to increase with contrast medium concentration. It is concluded that the contrast media currently used may affect blood rheology less than previous agents, despite their higher viscosity.

Three new low-osmolality contrast agents: a comparative study of patient discomfort.
Smith DC; Yahiku PY; Maloney MD; Hart KL. AJNR 1988; 9(1): 137–139.

Relative patient discomfort resulting from carotid injections of three new low-osmolality contrast agents was assessed in 78 patients. Omnipaque-300 (iohexol), Isovue-300 (iopamidol), and hexabrix (ioxaglate) were sequentially injected into both common carotid arteries of each patient. Patients were asked to rank the relative intensities of the three injections on each side. Mean patient rankings revealed that Hexabrix was preferred most often, Omnipaque-300 next, and Isovue-300 the least. The differences are statistically significant. We conclude that while patients usually tolerated all intracarotid low-osmolality contrast agents rather well, the agent preferred most often was Hexabrix.

Contrast agent nephrotoxicity: comparison of ionic and nonionic contrast agents.
Stacul F; Carraro M; Magnaldi S; Faccini L; Guarnieri G; Dalla Palma L. AJR 1987; 149(6): 1287–1289.

The effects on glomerular and proximal tubular function of an ionic contrast agent (sodium meglumine diatrizoate) and a nonionic agent (iopamidol) were compared in 34 patients with normal renal function. The patients received large doses (2.5 ml/kg body weight) of contrast material for IV digital subtraction angiography. Urine samples, collected before, immediately after, and on the first and third days after digital subtraction angiography, were analyzed for albumin, alanil-aminopeptidase, alpha-glucosidase, and beta-2-microglobulin. The changes noted were mild and of short duration with both contrast agents, despite the high dose given. These results suggest that, at least as far as renal toxicity is measured by these tests is concerned, ionic monomers can be safely used instead of more expensive nonionic media in procedures, such as digital subtraction angiography, that require high doses of contrast material.

Iohexol and ioxaglate in peripheral angiography.
Stiris MG; Laerum F. Acta Radiol 1987; 28(6): 767–770.

A double-blind, cross-over trial of the non-ionic, low-osmolar contrast medium iohexol (Omnipaque) and the ionic, low-osmolar medium ioxaglate (Hexabrix) at concentrations of 300 mg I/ml was carried out in 107 consecutive patients with arterial insufficiency of the lower limbs. The purpose of the study was to observe possible 'carry-over' effects from any of the contrast media, and to evaluate patient discomfort such as pain, adverse reactions, or effect on peripheral blood pressure. No carry-over effect was seen. Ioxaglate caused less injection pain and heat sensations than iohexol, and showed less effect on the systemic blood pressure.

Present state of contrast media as related to thromboembolic complications.
Stormorken H. Semin Hematol 1991; 28(4 Suppl 7): 60–72.

Human pharmacokinetics of iodixanol.
Svaland MG; Haider T; Langseth Manrique K; Andrew E; Hals PA. Invest Radiol 1992; 27(2): 130–133.

The pharmacokinetic properties of the x-ray contrast medium, iodixanol, a new nonionic dimer, were investigated in a phase I study including 40 healthy male volunteers. Iodixanol (300 mg I/mL) was administered intravenously (i.v.) at four dose levels—0.3, 0.6, 0.9, and 1.2 g iodine (I)/kg body weight—and saline was given as a control. 51Cr-EDTA was given concomitantly with iodixanol at all dose levels to study renal excretion of iodixanol. Mean half-lives were 26 and 131 minutes in the distribution and elimination phase, respectively. Apparent volume of distribution was 0.28 1/kg body weight, indicating distribution to extracellular fluid only. Within 24 hours after injection, 97% of the dose was excreted unmetabolized in the urine via glomerular filtration. The excretion in feces was 1.2% of the dose. The parameters calculated were independent of the given dose. The pharmacokinetics of iodixanol are comparable with those reported for other intravascular contrast media.

Peripheral MR angiography with variable velocity encoding. Work in progress.
Swan JS; Weber DM; Grist TM; Wojtowycz MM; Korosec FR; Mistretta CA. Radiology 1992; 184(3): 813–817.

An electrocardiographically triggered two-dimensional phase-contrast (PC) magnetic resonance angiographic pulse sequence was developed in which velocity encoding (VENC) was varied throughout an acquisition in response to changes in blood velocity during the cardiac cycle. This was done to better capture signal in the peripheral vasculature, where pulsatile flow degrades images. After reconstruction, a matched filter addition technique was applied to the cardiac phase images to obtain a single high-quality static image. Images were obtained of six healthy volunteers—with and without varying VENC—and contrast-to-noise ratio (C/N) calculations were performed for the added images. Varying VENC significantly improved vascular signal from small and large vessels (P less than .02), but it was most helpful for small vessels, for which the C/N increased by as much as 260% (average increase, 149%). These preliminary findings suggest that variable VENC can enhance the signal from the small and large peripheral blood vessels in cardiac-gated PC acquisitions.

The dose-response relationship in the use of hexabrix in angiography.
Tatochenko KV; Kondrashin SA. Vestn Rentgenol Radiol 1991; Sept-Oct (5): 18–20.

The authors present the results of a clinical trial of Hexabrix, a new radiopaque low osmolar agent, to be used in visceral catheterization translumbar angiography. Hexabrix was shown to reduce the frequency of side-effects by 40% as compared to triiodinated agents. The new agent causes no marked reactions in intraarterial administration even at a dose over 2 ml/kg. Hexabrix is an agent of choice to be used for patients at risk of angiographic investigation (allergy, advanced age, a severe general condition).

[Ambulatory angiography] Ambulante Angiographie.
Teifke A; Thelen M. Fortschr Med 1991; 109(17): 357–359; discussion 359–360.

Vasopressin release in response to intravenously injected contrast media (see comments).
Trewhella M; Dawson P; Forsling M; McCarthy P; O'Donnell C. Br J Radiol 1990; 63(746): 97–100.

We have previously reported that intravenously administered contrast media produce a rise in plasma vasopressin (antidiuretic hormone) concentrations. We have now shown that this occurs both when contrast medium is injected into a peripheral vein and when it is centrally injected into the right atrium. The peak vasopressin concentration recorded varies with the osmolality of the contrast medium. The vasopressin response was greater when contrast agent was centrally injected.

Frequencies of reactions to iohexol versus ioxaglate.
Vacek JL; Gersema L; Woods M; Bower C; Beauchamp GD. Am J Cardiol 1990; 66(17): 1277–1278.

[The side effects of phlebography of the lower extremities using iohexol. A prospective study] Effetti collaterali della flebografia degli arti inferiori con ioexolo. Studio prospettico.
Vigo M; Prandoni P; Casara D; Corbetti F; Biondetti PR; Coga A; Breda F; Tomasella G; Carta M. Radiol Med (Torino) 1989; 78(1–2): 53–56.

In this prospective study 463 consecutive outpatients, who had undergone phlebography because of clinically suspected deep venous thrombosis (DVT) were examined with clinical follow-up and impedance plethysmography to evaluate the rate of contrast media complications. Seventy-nine patients had immediate and mild side effects, and one had moderate side effects (bronchospasm); no patient suffered from severe life-threatening conditions. There was only one case of DVT which occurred after an initially negative phlebography. In a subgroup of 40 patients, who underwent iodine-125-fibrinogen scanning after phlebography, the study was positive in 9 cases. None of them presented with any evidence of DVT at follow-up phlebography. Contrast phlebography with iohexol is a safe and comfortable procedure. Low-osmolality nonionic contrast media are well tolerated by the patient.

The adverse effects of angiographic radiocontrast media.
Westhoff Bleck M; Bleck JS; Jost S. Drug Saf 1991; 6(1): 28–36.

Radiographic procedures which require the intravascular administration of water-soluble radiocontrast media are performed with increasing frequency. Each examination carries risks that are related either to the technique itself or to the opaque medium chosen. The pathogenesis of radiocontrast media-related adverse effects cannot be explained by a unique theory. The major factors implicated are direct chemotoxic effects and the physicochemical properties of contrast media, the latter being the basis for development of new contrast agents. With nonionic opaque media cardiovascular adverse effects, heat sensation and local pain are observed less frequently. However, it remains unclear whether the incidence of organ dysfunction or anaphylactic reactions with nonionic contrast media currently used can be reduced. This review compares ionic and nonionic contrast media, and current thoughts on the pathophysiology and treatment of adverse reactions are presented.

Ascending lower limb phlebography: comparison of ioversol and iothalamate meglumine.
Wilson AJ; Murphy WA; Destouet JM; Gilula LA; Hardy DC; Monsees B; Totty WG. Can Assoc Radiol J 1989; 40(3): 142–144.

Fifty patients undergoing ascending phlebography of a lower limb were evaluated, in a randomized double-blind fashion, to compare the efficacy, patient tolerance, and safety of two different contrast agents. Ioversol-240 (MP-238), a new nonionic agent, and iothalamate-202 (Conray 43), an established ionic agent, were the contrast agents used. Twenty-five patients were injected with iothalamate and 25 with ioversol. The phlebograms were evaluated for diagnostic quality and the patients for symptoms, with special reference to complaints of heat and pain. No significant difference was demonstrated between the two agents in either examination quality or patient tolerance. No major contrast-related reactions were recorded. We conclude that ioversol-240 appears to be a safe and acceptable alternative to iothalamate-202.

Recommended precautions when using low-osmolality or nonionic contrast agents with vasodilators.
Zagoria RJ; D'Souza VJ; Baker AL. Invest Radiol 1987; 22(6): 513–514.

Low-osmolality contrast agents were tested for potential chemical incompatibility with vasodilators commonly used in angiography. A mixture of Hexabrix and papaverine produced a white crystalline precipitate. Hexabrix and tolazoline exhibited transient immiscibility. Injection of a flush solution between vasodilator and contrast agent is recommended as a precaution.

Section 4

Thrombolytic Agents

I. Bibliography

A symposium: Interventional cardiology at a crossroad—diagnostics and therapeutics. March 26, 1988, Atlanta, Georgia. Am J Cardiol 62: 1K–29K.

Abel H (1992) Thrombolysis: the logical approach for the treatment of vascular occlusions (editorial). Acta Cardiol 47(4): 287–295.

Abu-Nema T, Ayyash K, Wafaii IK, Al-Hassan J, Thulesius O (1988) Jellyfish sting resulting in severe hand ischaemia successfully treated with intra-arterial urokinase. Injury 19: 294–296.

AbuRahma AF, Sadler D, Stuart P, Khan MZ, Boland JP (1991) Conventional versus thrombolytic therapy in spontaneous (effort) axillary-subclavian vein thrombosis. Am J Surg 161: 459–465.

Adler J, Ibrahim IM, Goldman M, Thomashow DF (1983) Combined thrombolysis with low-dose streptokinase and angioplasty in the treatment of renal artery occlusion. Urol Radiol. 5: 113–116.

Allen DR, Smallwood J, Johnson CD (1992) Intra-arterial thrombolysis should be the initial treatment of the acutely ischaemic lower limb. Ann R Coll Surg Engl 74(2): 106–110; discussion 111.

Anderson BJ, Keeley SR, Johnson ND (1991) Caval thrombolysis in neonates using low doses of recombinant human tissue-type plasminogen activator. Anaesth Intensive Care 19: 22–27.

Anderson JL (1991) Update: current role of thrombolytic therapy. Compr Ther 17: 51–58.

Anderson K (1992) Thrombolytic therapy for treatment of acute peripheral arterial occlusion. J Vasc Nurs 10(3): 20–24.

Andrews JC, Griggs TJ, Ensminger WD, Gyves JW, Cho KJ (1987) Local thrombolytic therapy for hepatic artery thrombosis following chemotherapy infusion catheter placement. Invest Radiol 22: 467–471

Annonier P, Benichou C, Flament J, Bronner A (1988) (Role of fibrinolysis in the treatment of retinal arterial occlusion. Discussion of 5 cases.) Bull Soc Ophtalmol Fr 88: 1167–1171.

Anonymous (1991) Domiciliary thrombolytic treatment [letter]. BMJ 303: 120.

Anonymous (1991) Postscript: fibrinolysis after acute myocardial infarction. Drug Ther Bull 29: 16.

Anonymous (1991) Thrombolytic therapy in cardiopulmonary disease. Chest 99 (4 Suppl): 95S–179S.

Atkinson JB, Bagnall HA, Gomperts E (1990) Investigational use of tissue plasminogen activator (t-PA) for occluded central venous catheters. JPEN 14: 310–311.

Avellone G, Mandala V, Pinto A, Martino A, Strano A (1986) Clinical evaluation of short-term defibrotide treatment of patients with atherosclerosis obliterans of the lower limbs. Haemostasis 16 (Suppl 1): 55–58.

Backeljauw PF, Moodie DS, Murphy DJ Jr (1991) High-dose urokinase therapy for the lysis of a central venous catheter-related thrombus in a young patient with Hodgkin's disease. Clin Pedia 30: 274–277.

Bahr, RD (1991) Trial design in the thrombolytic age [letter]. Lancet 337: 610–611.

Balkuv-Ulutin S (1986) Fibrinolytic system in atherosclerosis. Semin Thromb Hemost 12: 91–101.

Barbano EF, Newman GE, McCann RL, Hackel DB, Stack RS, Palmos LE, Mikat EM (1989) Correlation of clinical history with quantitative histology of lower extremity atheroma biopsies obtained with the Simpson atherectomy catheter. Atherosclerosis 78: 183–196.

Barnwell SL, Higashida RT, Halbach VV, Dowd CF, Hieshima GB (1991) Direct endovascular thrombolytic therapy for dural sinus thrombosis. Neurosurg 28: 135–142.

Battery PM, Fulenwider JT, Smith RB 3d, Martin LG, Stewart MT, Perdue GD (1987) Intra-arterial thrombolysis for acute limb ischemia: a three-year experience. South Med J 80: 479–482.

Bauriedel G, Dartsch PC, Voisard R, Roth D, Simpson JB, Hofling B, Betz E (1989) Selective percutaneous "biopsy" of atheromatous plaque tissue for cell culture. Basic Res Cardiol 84: 326–331.

Beard JD, Nyamekye I, Earnshaw JJ, Scott DJ, Thompson JF (1993) Intraoperative streptokinase: a useful adjunct to balloon-catheter embolectomy. Br J Surg 80(1): 21–24.

Beck A, Egheoni GC, Milic S, Spagnoli AM (1989) The long-term effects of percutaneous transluminal angioplasty, local catheter-lysis and stent-implantation. Clin Ter 131: 149–164.

Beck AH, Muhe A, Ostheim W, Heiss W, Hasler K (1989) Long-term results of percutaneous transluminal angioplasty: a study of 4750 dilatations and local lyses. Eur J Vasc Surg 3: 245–252.

Becker RC (1991) Seminars in thrombosis, thrombolysis, and vascular biology. Part 2: Coagulation and thrombosis. Cardiology 78: 257–266.

Belfiglio A, Traietti P, Bologna E, Salvo G (1989) Effects of oral and intravenous defibrotide on blood viscosity in patients with peripheral obliterative arterial disease. Clin Ther 11: 479–484.

Belkin M, Belkin B, Bucknam CA, Straub JJ, Lowe R (1986) Intra-arteria, fibrinolytic therapy. Efficacy of streptokinase vs urokinase. Arch Surg 121: 769–773.

Benedetti-Valentini F, Irace L, Gattuso R, Ciocca F, Aracu A, Intrieri F, Marini P, Massa R, Gossetti B (1988) Arterial repair of the lower limbs: prevention of prosthetic grafts occlusion by LMW-heparin. Int Angiol 7: 29–32.

Bennett KA, Grines CL (1990) Current controversies in patient selection for thrombolytic therapy. J Emerg Nurs 16 (3 Pt 2): 191–194.

Berkman WA, White RI Jr, Parandian BB (1983) Lysis of a chronic arterial occlusion with streptokinase. AJR 141: 403–404.

Berliner PJ, Grun B, Koppers B, Roth FJ (1988) A complication and angioplasty: successful catheter lysis of an occlusion of the external iliac artery. ROFO 149: 101–102.

Berridge DC (1989) Use of recombinant tissue plasminogen activator before balloon angioplasty [letter; comment]. Lancet 2: 390–391.

Berridge DC, Earnshaw JJ, Westby JC, Makin GS, Hopkinson BR (1989) Fibrinolytic profiles in local low-dose thrombolysis with streptokinase and recombinant tissue plasminogen activator. Thromb Haemost 61: 275–278.

Berridge DC, Gregson RH (1989) Acute lower limb ischemia (letter). Br J Surg 76: 651.

Berridge DC, Gregson RH, Hopkinson BR, Makin GS (1989) Intra-arterial thrombolysis using recombinant tissue plasminogen activator (r-TPA): the optimal agent, at the optimal dose? Eur J Vasc Surg 3: 327–332.

Berridge DC, Gregson RH, Hopkinson BR, Makin GS (1989) Repeated successful thrombolysis of an acute peripheral arterial thrombosis with tissue plasminogen activator. J R Coll Surg Edinb 34: 49–51.

Bertele V, Mussoni L, Del Rosso G, Pintucci G, Carriero MR, Merati MG, Libretti A, De Gaetano G (1988) Defective fibrinolytic response in atherosclerotic patients: effect of iloprost and its possible mechanism of action. Thromb Haemost 60: 141–144.

Bilbao JI, Rodriguez-Cabello J, Longo J, Zornoza G, Paramo J, Lecumberri FJ (1989) Portal thronmbosis: percutanaous transhepatic treatment with urokinase: a case report. Gastrointest Radiol 14: 326–328.

Bisig CJ Jr, Kerstein MD (1983) Successful thrombolytic therapy for acute and chronic occlusion of polytef vascular grafts. Arch Surg 118: 1218–1220.

Bizollon T, Bissuel F, Detry L, Trepo C (1991) Fibrinolytic therapy for portal vein thrombosis [letter]. Lancet 337: 1416.

Blanck Z, Cheirif J, Blick DR, Harris SL, Heibig J (1990) Thrombolysis with recombinant tissue plasminogen activator in late saphenous vein graft thrombosis. Am Heart J 119: 952–953.

Blankenship J, Indeck M (1991) Splenic hemorrhage after tissue plasminogen activator for acute myocardial infarction [letter]. New Engl J Med 325: 969.

Bode C, Kubler W (1989) (Antibody mediated thrombolysis. A new therapeutic principle). Klin Wochenschr 67: 651–658.

Bode C, Runge MS, Haber E (1990) Future directions in plasminogen activator therapy. Clin Cardiol 13: 375–381.

Boissel JP (1986) ICTH (International Committee on Haemostasis and Thrombosis)—- Sub committee on Clinical Trials. Registry of Multicenter Clinical Trials. Seventy Report—- 1985. Thromb Haemost 55: 282–291.

Bonnet J, Brottier L, Colle JP, Bricaud H (1986) Fibrinolytic treatment of severe arterial disease of the legs. Haemostasis 16 (Suppl 3): 86–89.

Bonnet J, Brottier L, Colle JP, Bricaud H (1986) (Fibrinolytic treatment of severe arteriopathies of the lower limbs). Traitement fibronolytique des arteriopathies severes des membres inferieurs. Haemostasis 16 (Suppl 4): 90–93.

Bookstein JJ, Fellmeth B, Roberts A, Valji K, Davis G, Machado T (1989) Pulsed-spray pharmacomechanical thrombolysis: preliminary clinical results. AJR 152: 1097–1100

Bounameaux H (1987) (Selective thrombolysis of clots: effect of tissue-type plasminogen activator in the treatment of thromboembolic diseases). Rev Med Suisse Romande 107: 267–272.

Bounameaux H, Prins TR, Schmitt HE, Schneider PA (1992) Venography of the lower limbs. Pitfalls of the diagnostic standard: The ETTT Trial Investigators. Investig Radiol 27(12): 1009–1011.

Braun AE (1991) Drugs that dissolve clots. RN 54: 52–57.

Brenot F, Pacouret G, Meyer G, Sors H, Charbonnier B, Simonneau G (1991) Adverse reactions with anistreplase [letter]. Lancet 338: 114–115.

Breslau PJ, Van der Linden CJ, Janovski B, Jorning PJ (1984) Local low dose streptokinase in the treatment of acute peripheral arterial occlusion. Neth J Surg 36: 65–68.

Brock FE, Nobbe F (1986) Local longtime lysis in combination with percutaneous transluminal angioplasty (TPA). Int Angiol 5: 155–160.

Brott T (1991) Thrombolytic therapy for stroke. Cerebrovasc Brain Metab Rev 3: 91–113.

Brown WD, Goldhaber SZ (1989) How to select patients with deep vein thrombosis for tPA therapy. Chest 95 (5 Suppl): 276S–278S.

Bruckmann H, Ferbert A (1989) Putaminal hemorrhage after recanalization of an embolic MCA occlusion treated with tissue plasminogen activator. Neuroradiology 31: 95–97.

Bruckmann HJ, Ringelstein EB, Buchner H, Zeumer H (1987) Vascular recanalizing techniques in the hind brain circulation. Neurosurg Rev 10: 197–198, 200.

Buckenham TM, George CD, Chester JF, Taylor RS, Dormandy JA (1992)

Accelerated thrombolysis using pulsed intra-thrombus recombinant human tissue type plasminogen activator (rt-PA). Eur J Vasc Surg 6(3): 237–240.

Bucknall C, Darley C, Flax J, Vincent R, Chamberlain D (1988) Vasculitis complicating treatment with intravenous anisoylated plasminogen streptokinase activator complex in acute myocardial infarction. Br Heart J 59: 9–11.

Burns E, Dudley NJ (1991) New deal for old heart [letter]. Br Med J 303: 719.

Buteux G, Jubault V, Suisse A, Courtheoux P (1988) Local recombinant tissue plasminogen activator to clear cerebral artery thrombosis developing soon after surgery (letter). Lancet 2: 1143–1144.

Buth J (1988) The administration of thrombolytic agents in peripheral vascular occlusion. Ned Tijdschr Geneeskd 132: 1785–1789.

Cade JF (1989) Thrombolytic therapy. Blood Rev 3: 5–10.

Campieri C, Raimondi C, Fatone F, Mignani R, Di Luca M, Todeschini P, Stacchiotti L, Boccadoro R, Sanguinetti M, Cacciari M, et al (1989) Normalization of renal function and blood pressure after dissolution with intra-arterial fibrinolytics of a massive renal artery embolism to a solitary functioning kidney. Nephron 51: 399–401.

Cange S, Laberge LC, Rivard GE, Garel L (1987) Streptokinase in the management of limb arterial thrombosis following free-flap surgery. Plast Reconstr Surg 79: 974–976

Carter BL (1991) Therapy of acute thromboembolism with heparin and warfarin. Clin Pharm 10: 503–518.

Chiu AS, Landsberg DN (1991) Successful treatment of acute transplant renal vein thrombosis with selective streptokinase infusion. Transplant Proc 23: 2297–2300.

Chop WM Jr, Evans PJ, Felty K (1991) Thrombolytic therapy during active menstruation: a case report. J Fam Pract 33: 79–81.

Cilliers PH (1986) Arterial embolism and fibrinolysis. A case report. S Afr Med J 69: 447–450.

Cizmeci G (1986) In vivo effects of defibrotide on platelet c-AMP and blood prostanoid levels. Haemostasis 16 (Suppl 1): 31–35.

Clagett GP (1992) Antithrombotic therapy for lower extremity bypass. J Vasc Surg 15(5): 873–875.

Clagett GP, Graor RA, Salzman EW (1992) Antithrombotic therapy in peripheral arterial occlusive disease. Chest 102(4 Suppl): 516S–528S.

Cohen LH, Kaplan M, Bernhard VM (1986) Intraoperative streptokinase. An adjunct to mechanical thrombectomy in the management of acute ischemia. Arch Surg 121: 708–715.

Cole PL (1991) Thrombolytic therapy: then and now. Heart & Lung 20: 542–551.

Collen D, Lijnen HR (1991) Thrombolytic therapy. Ann NY Acad Sci 614: 259–269.

Collen D, Lijnen HR, Gold HK (1991) Towards better thrombolytic therapy. Prog Cardiovasc Dis 34: 101–112.

Come PC, Kim D, Parker JA, Goldhaber SZ, Braunwald E, Markis JE (1987) Early reversal of right ventricular dysfunction in patients with acute pulmonary embolism after treatment with intravenous tissue plasminogen activator. JACC 10: 971–978.

Comerota AJ (1991) Safety and efficacy of thrombolytic therapy for superior vena caval syndrome [editorial; comment]. Chest 99: 3–4.

Comerota AJ, Rubin RN, Tyson RR, White JV, Williams FF, Soulen RL, Sherry S (1987) Intra-arterial thrombolytic therapy in peripheral vascular disease. Surg Gynecol Obstet 165: 1–8.

Comerota AJ, White JV, Grosh JD (1989) Intraoperative intra-arterial thrombolytic therapy for salvage of limbs in patients with distal arterial thrombosis. Surg Gynecol Obstet 169: 283–289.

Connors ML (1987) Thrombolytic therapy. J Cardiovascul Nurs 1: 59–64.

Conti CR (1991) Brief overview of the end points of thrombolytic therapy. Am J Cardiol 68: 8E–10E.

Cooper G, Timms J, Nashef SA, Smith GH (1991) Streptokinase through the pressure lumen of the intraaortic balloon [letter; comment]. J Thorac Cardiovasc Surg 101: 748–749.

Corser G, Masey S, Jacob G, Kernoff P, Browne D (1985) Ischaemia following self administered intra-arterial injection of methylphenidate and diamorphine. A case report of treatment with intra-arterial urokinase and review. Anaesthesia 40: 51–54.

Courtheoux P, Theron J, Derlon JM, Alachkar F, Casasco A (1986) In situ fibrinolysis in supra-aortic main vessels. A preliminary study. J Neuroradiol 13: 111–124.

Crabbe SJ, Cloninger CC (1987) Tissue plasminogen activator: a new thrombolytic agent (published erratum appears in Clin Pharm 1987 Dec, 6 (12):925). Clin Pharm 6: 373–386.

Cragg AH, Smith TP, Corson JD, Nakagawa N, Castaneda F, Kresowik TF, Sharp WJ, Shamma A, Berbaum KS (1991) Two urokinase dose regimens in native arterial and graft occlusions: initial results of a prospective, randomized clinical trial. Radiology 178: 681–686.

Cruickshank MK, Levine MN, Hirsh J, Roberts R, Siguenza M (1991) A standard heparin nomogram for the management of heparin therapy. Arch Intern Med 151: 333–337.

Cunningham MW, May S, Tucker WY, Gerlock AJ Jr (1983) Response of an abdominal aortic thrombotic occlusion to local low-dose streptokinase therapy. Surgery 93: 541–544.

Dacey LJ, Dow RW, McDaniel MD, Walsh DB, Zwolak RM, Cronenwett JL (1988) Cost-effectiveness of intra-arterial thrombolytic therapy. Arch Surg 123: 1218–1223.

Daily EK (1991) Clinical management of patients receiving thrombolytic therapy. Heart & Lung 20: 552–565.

Dake MD, Zemel G, Dolmatch BL, Katzen BT (1990) The cause of superior vena cava syndrome: diagnosis with percutaneous atherectomy. Radiology 174: 957–959.

Davidson A, Luhmer I, Kallfelz HC (1989) Aortic arch thrombosis in the neonate (letter). J Thorac Cardiovasc Surg 97: 152–153.

Dawson K, Stansby G, Hamilton G (1990) Non-coronary thrombolysis [letter; comment]. Lancet 336: 250–251.

Dawson KJ, Hamilton G (1991) Recombinant tissue-type plasminogen activator versus urokinase in peripheral arterial occlusions [letter; comment]. Radiology 178: 283–284.

Dawson KJ, Reddy K, Platts AD, Hamilton G (1991) Results of a recently instituted programme of thrombolytic therapy in acute lower limb ischaemia. Br J Surg 78: 409–411.

Del Zoppo GJ, Hacle W (1987) (Febrinolytic therapy in ischemic brain infarct). Dtsch Med Wochenschr 112: 603–608.

Dembski JC, Zeitler E (1978) Selective arterial clot lysis with angiography catheter. In: Zeitler E et al. (eds) Percutaneous Vascular Recanalization. Berlin Heidelberg New York, Springer, pp 157–159.

Dieck JA, Benrey J (1991) High-dose thrombolytic therapy and angioplasty for thrombosis in a subacute femoropopliteal bypass graft. Tex Med 87(11): 80–82.

Diskin CJ, Thomas CE, Lock S, Campagna KD (1990) Subclavian vein thrombosis treated with recombinant tissue plasminogen activator [letter]. Nephrol Dial Transplant 5: 400.

Dobrin PB (1981) Balloon embolectomy catheters in small arteries: I. Lateral wall pressures and shear forces. Surgery 90: 177–185.

Dorros G, Jamnadas P, Lewin RF, Sachdev N (1989) Percutaneous aspiration of a thromboembolus. Cathet Cardiovasc Diagn 17: 202–206.

Doyle JE (1986) Treatment modalities in peripheral vascular disease. Nurs Clin North Am 21: 241–253.

Drobinski G, Quininha J, Metzger JP, Canny M, Moussallem N, Artigou JY, Grosgogeat Y (1988) Treatment by redilatation and thrombolysis of occlusion occurring during percutaneous coronary angioplasty. Arch Mal Coeur 81: 745–752.

Duckert F (1984) Thrombolytic therapy. Semin Thromb Hemost 10: 87–103.

Durham JD, Geller SC, Abbott WM, Shapiro H, Waltman AC, Walker TG, Brewster DC, Athanasoulis CA (1989) Regional infusion of urokinase into occluded lower-extremity bypass grafts: long-term clinical results. Radiology 172: 83–87.

Earnshaw JJ (1991) Thrombolytic therapy in the management of acute limb ischaemia. Br J Surg 78: 261–269.

Earnshaw JJ, Gregson RH, Makin GS, Hopkinson BR (1989) Acute peripheral arterial ischemia: a prospective evaluation of differential management with surgery or thrombolysis. Ann Vasc Surg 3: 374–379.

Earnshaw JJ, Gregson RH, Makin GS, Hopkinson BR (1987) Early results of low dose intra-arterial streptokinase therapy in acute and subacute lower limb arterial ischaemia. Br J Surg 74: 504–507.

Earnshaw JJ, Hopkinson BR, Makin GS (1987) Intraoperative fibrinolytic therapy (letter). J Vasc Surg 6: 98.

Earnshaw JJ, Scott DJ, Horrocks M, Baird RN (1993) Choice of agent for peripheral thrombolysis. Br J Surg 80(1): 25–27.

Earnshaw JJ, Westby JC, Gregson RH, Makin GS, Hopkinson BR (1988) Local thrombolytic therapy of acute peripheral arterial ischaemia with tissue plasminogen activator: a dose-ranging study. Br J Surg 75: 1196–1200.

Earnshaw JJ, Westby JC, Makin GS, Hopkinson BR (1987) Low dose intra-arterial streptokinase and acylated plasminogen-streptokinase activator complex: a retrospective review of two thrombolytic regimes in recent peripheral arterial ischaemia. Eur J Vasc Surg 1: 151–158.

Earnshaw JJ, Westby JC, Makin GS, Hopkinson BR (1986) The systemic fibrinolytic effect of BRL 26921 during the treatment of acute peripheral arterial occlusions. Thromb Haemost 55: 259–262.

Eaton DL, Fless GM, Kohr WJ, McLean JW, Xu QT, Miller CG, Lawn RM, Scanu AM (1987) Partal amino acid sequence of apolipoprotein(a) shows that it is homologous to plasminogen. Proc Natl Acad Sci U S A 84: 3224–3228.

Ehringer H, Minar E (1987) (Therapy of acute ilio-femoral vein thrombosis). Internist (Berlin) 28: 317–335.

Eisenbud DE, Brener BJ, Shoenfeld R, Creighton D, Goldenkranz RJ, Brief DK, Alpert J, Huston J, Novick A, Krishnan UR (1990) Treatment of acute vascular occlusions with intra-arterial urokinase. Am J Surg 160: 160–164; discussion 164–165.

Emami A, Saldanha R, Knupp C, Kodroff M (1987) Failure of systemic thrombolyic and heparin therapy in the treatment of neonatal aortc thrombosis. Pediatrics 79: 773–777.

Endoarterial treatment of acute ischemia of the limbs with urokinase. (1989) Italian Cooperative Study "Bologna." Int Angiol 8: 53–56.

Enge I (1990) The limits of vascular interventional radiology. Acta Chir Scand 555 Suppl: 21–24.

Esente P, Giambartolomei A (1989) On percutaneous aspiration of a coronary thrombus (letter; comment). Comment on: Cathet Cardiovasc Diagn 1989 Jun;17(2): 97–98. Cathet Cardiovasc Diagn. 18: 199.

Fareed J, Walenga JM, Leya F, Bacher P, Hoppensteadt D, Messmore H, Pifarre R (1991) Some objective considerations for the use of heparins and recombinant hirudin in percutaneous transluminal coronary angioplasty. Semin Thromb Hemost 17(4): 455–470.

Faris I (1987) Thrombolytic therapy (editorial). Aust NZ J Surg 57: 283–284.

Fava C, Grosso M, Malara D, Barile C (1987) (Treatment of acute arterial embolism of the kidney) Sul trattamento dell'embolia arteriosa acuta del rene. Istituto di Radiologia dell'Universita. Ospedale S Giovanni, Torino. Radiol Med 74: 18–22.

Feldman M, Goldfarb IW, Slater H, Hafeez M, Long ET (1985) Streptokinase treatment of acute arterial occlusions in burn patients (case report). J Burn Care Rehabil 6: 102–104.

Fiessinger JN, Vitoux JF, Pernes JM, Roncato M, Aiach M, Gaux JG (1986) Complications of intraarterial urokinase-lys-plasminogen infusion therapy in arterial ischemia of lower limbs. AJR 146: 157–159.

Fiessinger JN, Vitoux JF, Pernes JM, Roncato M, Aiach M, Gaux JG (1987) Peripheral artery thrombolysis with urokinase-lys-plasminogen. A disappointing experience. Int Angiol 6: 183–186.

Findlay JM, Weir BK, Stollery DE (1991) Lysis of intraventricular hematoma with tissue plasminogen activator. Case report. J Neurosurg 74: 803–807.

Foessinger JN, Aiach M, Vitoux JF, Pernes JM, Roncato M, Gaux JC (1986) (Thrombolytic treatment of arteriopathies. Do thrombolytics compete with surgery?) Traitement thrombolytique des arteriopathies. Les thrombolytiques concurrencent-ils la chirurgie? Haemostasis 16 (Suppl 4): 87–89.

Fox KA (1991) Comparative analysis of long-term mortality after thrombolytic therapy. Am J Cardiol 68: 38E–44E.

Francis CW, Marder VJ (1991) Fibronolytic therapy for venous thrombosis. Prog Cardiovasc Dis 34: 193–204.

Frey FJ, Stirnemann P, Fritschi P, Mahler F (1986) Renal artery embolism treated with intra-arterial streptokinase infusion results in patent but small renal arteries. Am J Nephrol 6: 214–216.

Fudem GM, Walton RL (1989) Microvascular thrombolysis to salvage a free flap using human recombinant tissue plasminogen activator. J Reconstr Microsurg 5: 231–234.

Gagnon RF, Horosko F, Herba MJ (1984) Local infusion of low-dose streptokinase for renal artery thromboembolism. Can Med Assoc J 131: 1089–1091.

Gagnon RM, Goudreau E, Joyal F, Morissette M, Roussin A (1985) The role of intravenous streptokinase in acute arterial occlusions after cardiac catheterization. Cathet Cardiovasc Diagn 11: 409–412.

Galichia JP, Bajaj AK, Milfeld DJ (1984) Angioplasty with streptokinase infusion of a totally occluded Dacron femoropopliteal graft. Cardiovasc Intervent Radiol 7: 18–20.

Gallus AS (1986) The use of antithrombotic drugs in artery disease. Clin Haematol 15: 509–559.

Garcia R, Saroyan RM, Senkowsky J, Smith F, Kerstein M (1990) Intraoperative intra-arterial urokinase infusion as an adjunct to Fogarty catheter embolectomy in acute arterial occlusion. Surg Gynecol Obstet 171: 201–205.

Gardiner GA Jr, Harrington DP, Koltun W, Whittemore A, Mannick JA, Levin DC (1989) Salvage of occluded arterial bypass grafts by means of thrombolysis. J Vasc Surg 9: 426–431.

Gardiner GA Jr, Koltun W, Kandarpa K, Whittemore A, Meyerovitz MF, Bettmann MA, Levin DC, Harrington DP (1986) Thrombolysis of occluded femoropopliteal grafts. AJR 147: 621–626.

Gaston JG, Sensarma PK, Sadiq S (1991) Urokinase infusion in total occlusion of peripheral vascular disease. Kan Med 92: 73–75.

Genton E, Clagett GP, Salzman EW (1986) Antithrombotic therapy in peripheral vascular disease. Chest 89 (2 Suppl): 75S–81S. (55 Refs.)

Gertz SD, Kurgan A (1988) Tissue plasminogen activator and selective coronary vasodilation (letter). Am J Cardiol 62: 173.

Gibbons KJ, Guterman LR, Ahuja A, Hopkins LN (1992) Thrombolytic therapy for vascular occlusions [letter]. J Neurosurg 76: 168–169.

Gibson SP, Mosquera DA, O'Donnell MJ, Odurny A (1991) Streptokinase in the treatment of innominate-vein thrombosis in association with haemodialysis catheter. Preservation of a precious arteriovenous fistula. Nephrol Dial Transplant 6: 206–208.

Giddings AE, Walker WJ (1992) Intra-arterial thrombolysis should be the initial treatment of the acutely ischaemic lower limb (letter; comment). Ann Royal Coll Surg 74(4): 301.

Giorgetti PL, Lovaria A, Saccheri S, Arpesani A, Rignano A, Bortolani EM, Galimberti M (1991) Locoregional fibrinolysis using tissue plasminogen activator in 2 cases of acute thromosis of the renal artery. Panminerva Med 33(4): 180–184.

Girard P, Hauuy MP, Musset D, Simonneau G, Petitpretz P (1989) Acute inferior vena cava thrombosis. Early results of heparin therapy. Chest 95: 284–291.

Giraud C, Joffre F, Puel P, Cerene A (1986) Is a combination of urokinase and LYs-plasminogen by regional infusion indicated in ischaemia due to popliteal or infra-popliteal thrombosis? Haemostasis 16 (Suppl 3): 79–82.

Giraud C, Joffre F, Puel P, Cerene A (1986) (Is it permissible to use the combination urokinase-plasminogen by local administration in ischemias caused by popliteal or sub-popliteal thrombosis?) Est-il licite d'utiliser l'association urokinase-plasminogene par voie locale dans les ischemies par thrombose poplitees ou sous-poplitees? Haemostasis 16 (Suppl 4): 83–86.

Goffette P, Kurdziel JC, Dondelinger RF (1989) Local urokinase infusion for total occlusion of the lower abdominal aorta. Report of two cases and a review of the literature. Eur J Radiol 9: 121–124.

Goffette P, Kurdziel JC, Dondelinger RF (1991) Percutaneous local arterial thrombolytic infusion. Therapeutic effects and complications. Acta Radiol 32: 305–310.

Goldberg RE, Cohen AM, Bryan PJ, Olsen M, Martin RJ (1989) Neonatal aortic thrombosis treated with intra-arterial urokinase therapy. Can Assoc Radiol J 40: 55–56.

Goldhaber SZ, Kessler CM, Heit JA, Elliott CG, Friedenberg WR, Heiselman DE, Wilson DB, Parker JA, Bennett D, Feldstein ML, et al (1992) Recombinant tissue-type plasminogen activator versus a novel dosing regimen of urokinase in acute pulmonary embolism: a randomized controlled multicenter trial. Am J Coll Cardiol 20(1): 24–30.

Goldhaber SZ, Kim J, Loscalzo J (1987) Recombinant tissue plasminogen activator in patients with pulmonary embolism: correlation of fibrinolytic specificity and ef. Circulation 75: 1200–1203.

Gossetti B, Irace L, Gattuso R, Intrieri F, Aracu A, Ciocca F, Marini P, Massa R, Benedetti-Valentini F (1988) Prevention of deep venous thrombosis in vascular surgical procedures by LMW-heparin. Int Angiol 7: 25–27.

Graor RA, Risius B, Denny KM, Young JR, Beven EG, Hertzer NR, Ruschhaupt WF 3d, O'Hara PJ, Geisinger MA, Zelch MG (1985) Local thrombolysis in the treatment of thrombosed arteries, bypass grafts, and arteriovenous fistulas. J Vasc Surg 2: 406–414.

Graor RA, Risius B, Young JR, Lucas FV, Beven EG, Hertzer NR, Krajewski LP, O'Hara PJ, Olin J, Ruschhaupt WF (1988) Thrombolysis of peripheral arterial bypass grafts: surgical thrombectomy compared with thrombolysis. A preliminary report. J Vasc Surg 7: 347–355.

Gray BH, Olin JW, Graor RA, Young JR, Bartholomew JR, Ruschhaupt WF (1991) Safety and efficacy of thrombolytic therapy for superior vena cava syndrome [see comments]. Chest 99: 54–59.

Greenberg S, Kosinski R, Daniels J (1991) Treatment of superior vena cava thrombosis with recombinant tissue type plasminogen activator. Chest 99: 1298–1301.

Greene R, Lind S, Jantsch H, Wilson R, Lynch K, Jones R, Carvalho A, Reid L, Waltman AC, Zapol W (1987) Pulmonary vascular obstruction in severe ARDS: angiographic alterations after i.v. fibrinolytic therapy. AJR 148: 501–508.

Gregson RH (1991) Thrombolysis for peripheral arterial occlusion [editorial]. Br J Hosp Med 46: 79.

Grill HP, Brinker JA (1989) Nonacute thrombolytic therapy: an adjunct to coronary angloplasty in patients with large intravascular thrombi. Am Heart J 118: 662–667.

Gross-Fengels W, Neufang KF, Lechler E, Schmitz-Rixen T (1988) Treatment of arterial occlusions of the lower extremities using 2-stage local applicaiton of urokinase. ROFO 148: 269–274.

Gussenhoven EJ, Essed CE, Frietman P, van Egmond F, Lancee CT, van Kappellen WH, Roelandt J, Serruys PW, Gerritsen GP, van Urk H, et al (1989) Intravascular ultrasonic imaging: histologic and echographic correlation. Eur J Vasc Surg 3: 571–576.

Haapanen A, Leinonen A, Seppanen S (1984) Preangioplasty fibrinolytic therapy using SP-54 including acute and subacute occlusions. Ann Radiol 27: 340.

Hacke W, Zeumer H, Ferbert A, Bruckmann H, del Zoppo GJ (1988) Intraarterial thrombolytic therapy improves outcome in patients with acute vertebrobasilar occlusive disease. Stroke 19: 1216–1222.

Halfman-Franey M, Coburn C (1990) Techniques in cardiac care: lasers, stents, and atherectomy devices. REVIEW ARTICLE: 128 REFS. AACN Clin Issues Crit Care Nurs 1: 87–109.

Hallett JW Jr, Yrizarry JM, Greenwood LH (1983) Regional low dosage thrombolytic therapy for peripheral arterial occlusions. Surg Gynecol Obstet 156: 148–154.

Handa K, Sasaki Y, Kiyonaga A, Fujino M, Hiroki T, Arakawa K (1988) Acute pulmonary thromboembolism treated successfully by balloon angioplasty: a case report. Angiology 39: 775–778.

Hansen DD, Auth D, Vracko R, Ritchie JL (1986) Mechanical thrombolysis in acute canine coronary thrombosis. JACC 7: 207A.

Hansen DD, Auth DC, Vracko R, Ritchie JL (1985) In vivo mechanical thrombolysis in subacute canine arterial occlusion. Circulation 72(Part II): III–469.

Hartl D, Tiso E, Anderle K, Philapitsch A, Anger G (1988) Reduced fibrinolytic potential in patients with arterial occlusive disease (AOD) in compariton with normal subjects. Haemostasis 18 (Suppl): 93–98.

Hartmann J, McKeever L, Teran J, Bufalino V, Marek J, Brown A, Goodwin M, Amirparviz F, Motarjeme A (1987) Prolonged infusion of urokinase for recanalization of chronically occluded aortocoronary bypass grafts. Am J Cardiol 6: 183–186

Henze T, Boeer A, Tebbe U, Romatonski J (1987) Lysis of basilar artery occluson with tissue plasminogen activator (letter). Lancet 1: 1391.

Hess H, Mietaschk A, Becker-Lienau C (1988) Fibrinolysis with rt-PA in peripheral arterial occlusions. Klin Wochanschr 66 (Suppl 12): 135–136.

Hess H, Mietaschk A, Bruckl R (1987) Peripheral arterial occlusions: a 6-year experience with local low-dose thrombolytic therapy. Privatklinik Josefinum, Munich, Federal Republic of Germany. Radiology 163: 753–758.

Hicks ME, Picus D, Darcy MD, Kleinhoffer MA (1991) Multilevel infusion catheter for use with thrombolytic agents. J Vasc Intervent Radiol 2(1): 73–75.

Hill LN (1991) Streptokinase therapy and breakaway pulmonary embolism [letter; comment]. Am J Med 90: 411–413.

Hoffmann JJ, Bonnier JJ (1991) Histidine-rich glycoprotein in thrombolytic therapy: has it clinical relevance? Blood Coag Fibrino 2: 237–241.

Honigl K, Pilger E, Stark G, Bertuch H (1988) Fibrinolytic therapy: plasminogen activator inhibitors. Vasc Suppl 26 103–106.

Horvath L, Radnay B, Mark B, Kollar L, Hazafi K, Balogh E, Losonczy H (1987) (Selective catheter—thrombolysis in arterial occlusion) Veroerelzarodasban alkalmazott szelektiv kateteres verrogoldas. Orv Hetil 128: 63–69.

Hu CK, Chen CY, Chen CL, Wang PY (1987) Postoperative pulmonary embolism: an analysis of eight cases. Kao Hsiung I Hsueh Ko Hsueh Tsa Chih 3: 393–399.

Hurley JJ, Burrell MJ, Auer AI, Woods JJ Jr, Binnington HB, Hershey FB (1984) Surgical implications of fibrinolytic therapy. Am J Surg 148: 830–835.

Hurwitz RL, Gelabert H (1989) Thrombosed iliac venous aneurysm: a rare cause of left lower extremity venous obstruction. J Vasc Surg 9: 822–824.

Ilgenfritz FM, Fanelli RD (1991) The role of streptokinase in treating complicated popliteal entrapment syndrome [letter]. J Vasc Surg 13: 563–564.

Ino T, Benson LN, Freedom RM, Barker GA, Aipursky A, Rowe RD (1988) Thrombolytic therapy for femoral artery thrombosis after pediatric cardiac catheterization. Am Heart J 115: 633–639.

Inoue Y, Shichijo Y, Ibukuro K (1986) (Arterial infusion therapy in mesenteric artery embolisms. A report of two cases treated by infusion therapy using only urokinase) Rinsho Hoshasen 31: 377–388.

Ishiguchi T, Fakatsu H, Itoh S, Shimamoto K, Sakuma S (1992) Budd-Chiari syndrome with long segmental inferior vena cava obstruction: treatment with thrombolysis, angioplasty, and intravascular stents. J Vasc Intervent Radiol 3(2): 421–425.

Jafar JJ, Tan WS, Crowell RM (1991) Tissue plasminogen activator thrombolysis of a middle cerebral artery embolus in a patient with an arteriovenous malformation. Case report. J Neurosurg 74: 808–812.

Janosik JE, Bettmann MA, Kaul AF, Souney PF (1991) Therapeutic alternatives for subacute peripheral arterial occlusion. Comparison by outcome, length of stay, and hospital charges. Invest Radiol 26: 921–925.

Jelalian C, Mehrhof A, Cohen IK, Richdrdson J, Merritt WH (1985) Streptokinase in the treatment of acute arterial occlusion of the hand. J Hand Surg 10: 534–538.

Jorgensen B, Nielson JD (1992) Intra-arterial thrombin activity produced by percutaneous transluminal angioplasty eliminated by segmentally enclosed thrombolysis. Eur J Vasc Surg 6(2): 153–157.

Jorgensen B, Tonnesen KH, Bulow J, Nielsen JD, Jorgensen M, Holstein P, Andersen E (1989) Femoral artery recanalization with percutaneous angioplasty and segmentally enclosed plasminogen activator (see comments). Comment in: Lancet 2: 390–391. Lancet 1: 1106–1108.

Jorgensen B, Tonnesen KH, Nielsen JD, Holstein P, Bulow J, Jorgensen M, Andersen E (1991) Segmentally enclosed thrombolysis in percutaneous transluminal angioplasty for femoropopliteal occlusions: a report from a pilot study. Cardiovasc Intervent Radiol 14: 293–298.

Kadir S, Watson A, Burrow C (1987) Percutaneous transcatheter recanalization in the management of acute renal failure due to sudden occlusion of the renal artery to a solitary kidney. Am J Nephrol 7: 445–449.

Kakkasseril JS, Cranley JJ, Arbaugh JJ, Roedersheimer LR, Welling RE (1985) Efficacy of low-dose streptokinase in acute arterial occluson and graft thrombosis. Arch Surg 120: 427–429.

Kamiya T, Sakaguchi S (1985) Hemodynamic effects of the antithrombotic drug cilostazol in chronic arterial occlusion in the extremities. Arzneimittelforschung 35: 1201–1203.

Karnik R, Perneczky G, Ammerer HP, Brenner H, Slany J (1984) (Regional lysis of acute basilar artery occlusion : case report) Regionale Lyse eines akuten Basilarisarterienverschlusses—ein Fallbericht. Wien Klin Wochenschr 96: 26–30.

Karsch KR, Haase KK, Mauser M, Voelker W (1989) Initial angiographic results in ablation of atherosclerotic plaque by percutaneous coronary excimer laser angioplasty without subsequent balloon dilatation. Am J Cardiol 64: 1253–1257.

Katzen BT (1988) Technique and results of "low-dose" infusion. Cardiovasc Intervent Radiol 11 (Suppl): 41–47.

Katzen BT, Edwards KC, Albert AS, van Breda A (1984) Low-dose direct fibrinolysis in peripheral vascular disease. J Vasc Surg 1: 718–722.

Khan B (1991) Coronary thrombolysis—a Pakistani perspective. JPMA 41: 113–116.

Kim SW (1988) Axillo-subclavian deep venous thrombosis in quadriplegia: a case report. J Am Paraplegia Soc 11: 13–15.

Kirk CR, Bhrolchain CN, Qureshi SA (1988) Streptokinase for aortic thrombosis. Arch Dis Child 63: 1086–1087.

Kirk CR, Qureshi SA (1989) Streptokinase in the management of arterial thrombosis in infancy. Int J Cardiol 25: 15–20.

Klatte EC, Becker GJ, Holden RE, Yune HY (1986) Fibrinolytic therapy. Radiology 159: 619–624.

Kleiman NS (1991) Goals of thrombolytic therapy. Am J Cardiol 68: 67C–71C.

Klimiuk PS, Kay EA, Illingworth KJ, Gush RJ, Taylor LJ, Baker RD, Perkins C, Jayson MI (1992) A double blind placebo controlled trial of recombinant tissue plasminogen activator in the treatment of digital ischemia in systemic sclerosis. J Rheumatol 19(5): 716–720.

Kohler M, Kramann B, Hellstern P, Fess W, Walter P, Woerner H, Kiehl R, Wenzel E (1985) (Successful treatment of superior mesenteric artery thrombosis with local high-dose urokinase therapy) Erfolgreiche Behandlung einer Thrombose der Arteria mesenterica superior durch lokale, hochdosierte Urokinasetherapie. Klin Wochenschr 63: 722–727.

Kolts RL, Kuehner ME, Swanson MK, Carlson RD, Myers WO, Friedenberg WR (1985) Local intra-arterial streptokinase therapy for acute peripheral arterial occlusions. Should thrombolytic therapy replace embolectomy? Am Surg 51: 381–387.

Koot HW, Veen HF (1991) Local thrombolytic therapy for axillary-subclavian vein thrombosis. Neth J Surg 43: 71–74.

Koppensteiner R, Minar E, Ahmadi R, Jung M, Ehringer H (1988) Low doses of recombinat human tissue-type plasminogen activator for local thrombolysis in peripheral arteries (letter). Radiology 168: 877–878.

Krahenbuhl B (1987) (Medical treatment of peripheral arterial diseases) Le traitement medical des affections arterielles peripheriques. Ther Umsch 44: 637–640.

Krawczyk W (1987) (Use of streptokinase in the treatment of thrombotic complications of Climino-Brescia arteriovenous fistulas in patients on long-term hemodialysis). Wiad Led 40: 1014–1019.

Krings W, Roth FJ, Cappius G, Schmidtke I (1985) Catheter-lysis: indications and primary results. Int Angiol 4: 117–123.

Krupski WC, Feldman RK, Rapp JH (1989) Recombinant human tissue-type plasminogin activator is an effective agent for thrombolysis of peripheral arteries and bypass grafts: preliminary report. J Vasc Surg 10: 491–498, discussion 499–500.

Kunkel JM, Machleder HI (1989) Spontaneous subclavain vein thrombosis: a successful combined approach of local thrombolytic therapy followed by first rib resection (letter). Surgery 106: 114.

Lambiase RE, Paolella LP, Haas RA, Dorfman GS (1991) Extensive thromboembolic disease of the hand and forearm: treatment with thrombolytic therapy. J Vasc Intervent Radiol 2(2): 201–208.

Lammer J, Pilger E, Justich E, Neumayer K, Schreyer H (1985) Fibrinolysis in chronic atherosclerotic occlusions: intrathrombotic injections of streptokinase. Work in Progress. Radiology 157: 45–50

Lammer J, Pilger E, Neumayer K, SchreyerH (1986) Intraarterial fibrinolysis: long-term results. Radiology 161: 159–163.

Lammle B, Noll G, Christe M, Fritschi J, Czendlik C, Marbet GA, Biland L, Da Silva A, Huber P, Widmer LK, et al (1983) (Systemic thrombolysis of arterial occlusions of the lower extremities. Comparison of various treatment schedules) Systemische thrombolyse arterieller verschlusse der unteren extremitaten vergleich verschiedener behandlungsschemata. Schweiz Med Wochenschr 113: 1570–1576.

Lancashire MJ, Williams BW, Torrie EP, Galland RB (1989) Acute lower limb ischemia (letter). Br J Surg 76: 526.

Lang EV, Bookstein JJ (1989) Accelerated thrombolysis and angioplasty for hand ischemia in Buerger's disease. Cardiovasc Intervent Radiol 12: 95–97.

Lawrence PF, Goodman GR (1992) Thrombolytic therapy. Surg Clin North Am 72(4): 899–918.

LeBolt SA, Tisnado J, Cho SR (1988) Treatment of peripheral arterial obstruction with streptokinase: results in arterial vs graft occlusions. AJR 151: 589–592.

Lederer W, Dingler WH (1989) (Subclavlan occlusion and an anomaly of the vertabral artery with subclavian steal syndrome. Fibrinolysis and PTA therapy). ROFO 150: 477–479.

Levy M, Benson LN, Burrows PE, Bentur Y, Strong DK, Smith J, Johnson D, Jacobson S, Koren G (1991) Tissue plasminogen activator for the treatment of thromboembolism in infants and children. J Pediatr 118: 467–472.

LiMandri G, Dunn D, Burd C, Gregory J (1991) Tissue plasminogen activator: hospital experience. NJ Med 88: 561–565.

Lipton HA, Jupiter JB (1987) Streptokinase salvage of a free-tissue transfer: case report and review of the literature. Plast Reconstr Surg 79: 977–981.

Lonsdale RJ (1991) Intra-arterial thrombolytic therapy in the management of acute and chronic limb ischaemia (letter). Br J Surg 78: 1020.

Lonsdale RJ (1991) Results of a recently instituted programme of thrombolytic therapy in acute lower limb ischemia (letter). Br J Surg 78: 1273.

Lonsdale RJ, Berridge DC, Makin GS, Hopkinson BR, Wenham PW (1992) Detection of left heart thrombus by echocardiography is not essential before peripheral arterial thrombolysis. J R Coll Surg Edinburg 37(1): 19–22.

Lonsdale RJ, Makin GS, Wenham PW, Hopkinson BR (1991) Thrombolysis in critical ischaemia [letter] Eur J Vas Surg 5: 361.

Lund F, Ekestrom S, Frisch EP, Magaard F (1975) Thrombolytic treatment with i.v. brinase of advanced arterial obliterative disease of the limbs. Angiology 26: 534–556.

Lupattelli L, Barzi F, Corneli P, Lemmi A, Mosca S (1988) Selective thrombolysis with low-dose urokinase in chronic arteriosclerotic obstructions. Cardiovasc Intervent Radial 11: 123–126

Mahony L, Nikaidoh H, Fixler DE (1988) Thrombolytic treatment with streptokinase for late intraatrial thrombosis after modified Fontan procedure. Am J Cardiol 62: 343–344.

Marcon JL, Annweiler M, Bonijoly S, Favre E (1989) (Local thrombolysis using a combination of RTPA and Lys-plasminogen in ischemia due to a previous thrombosis). J Mal Vasc 14: 265–266.

Mark DB, Hlatky MA, O'Connor CM, Pryor DB, Wall TC, Honan MB, Phillips HR, 3d, Califf RM (1988) Administration of thrombolytic therapy in the community hospital: established principles and unresolved issues. J Am Coll Cardiol (6 Suppl A)12: 32A–43A.

Martin M, Fiebach BJ (1991) Short-term ultrahigh streptokinase treatment of chronic arterial occlusions and acute deep vein thromboses. Semin Thromb Hemost 17: 21–28.

Martin M, Zeitler E (1978) Percutaneous transluminal recanalization (PTR) and fibrinolysis: fibrinolytic treatment of femoral reocclusions subsequent to PTR procedures. In: Zeitler E et al. (eds) Percutaneous Vascular Recanalization. Berlin Heidelberg New York, Springer, pp 152–156.

Mathias K (1991) Local thrombolysis for salvage of occluded bypass grafts. Semin Thromb Hemost 17: 14–20.

Matsumoto AH, Sarosi MG, Selby JB Jr, Tegtmeyer CJ (1992) Thromboembolectomy with the transluminal extraction catheter (TEC) as an adjunct to thrombolysis. J Vasc Intervent Radiol 3(3): 491–495.

Matsuo O, Mihara H, Motomatsu K (1984) Discrepancy in the thrombolytic effect of UK between angiography and circulatory evaluations. Angiology 35: 523–527.

May JW Jr, Rothkopf DM (1989) Salvage of a failing microvascular free muscle flap by direct continuous intravascular infusion of heparin: a case report. Plast Reconstr Surg 83: 1045–1048.

McCall J, Gleeson FV, McGann G, Dawson K, Platts AD, Hamilton G (1992) Thrombolysis in high risk patients. Clin Radiol 45(5): 298–301.

McFadden PM, Ochsner JL, Mills N (1983) Management of thrombotic complications of invasive arterial monitoring of the upper extremity. J Cardiovasc Surg 24: 35–39.

McKeever L, Hartmann J, Bufalino V, Marek J, Brown A, Goodwin M, Stamato N, Cahill J, Colandrea M, Amirparviz F (1988) Prolonged selective urokinase infusion in totally occluded coronary arteries and bypass grafts: two case reports. Cathet Cardiovasc Diagn 15: 247–251.

McKendall GR, Woolard RH, Williams DO (1991) Prehospital administration of thrombolytic therapy: current status in Rhode Island—results of the Prehospital Administration of t-PA Study (PATS). RI Med J 74: 405–408.

McNamara T (1988) Technique and results of "higher-dose" infusion. Cardiovasc Intervent Radiol 11 (Suppl): 48–57.

McNamara TO (1987) Role of thrombolysis in peripheral arterial occlusion. Am J Med 83: 6–10.

McNamara TO, Bomberger RA, Merchant RF (1991) Intra-arterial urokinase as the initial therapy for acutely ischemic lower limbs [see comments]. Circulation 83 (2 Suppl): I106–119.

McNamara TO, Fischer JR (1985) Thrombolysis of peripheral arterial and graft occlusions: improved results using high-dose urokinase. AJR 144: 769–775.

Mehta J, Roy L (1984) Platelet-suppressive therapy in cardiovascular disease. Cardiovasc Clin 14: 211–234.

Messmer BJ, Uebis R, Rieger C, Mingle C, Hofstadter F, Effert S (1989) Late results after intracoronary thrombolysis and early bypass grafting for acute myocardial infarction. J Thorac Cardiovasc Surg 97: 10–18.

Mies S, Alfieri Jr F, Chamone DF, Raia S (1991) Portal vein thrombosis repermeabilization with rt-PA [letter]. Thromb Haemost 65: 108.

Mingoli A, Di Marzo L, Sciacca V, Castrucci M, Pavone P, Farina C, Tamburelli A, Cavallaro A (1989) Thrombolysis of graft occlusion using high dose urokinase. An alternative to surgical treatment? Ital J Surg Sci 19: 79–84.

Mohadjer M, Eggert R, May J, Mayfrank L (1990) CT-guided stereotactic fibrinolysis of spontaneous and hypertensive cerebellar hemorrhage: long-term results. J Neurosurg 73: 217–222.

Monturo CA, Dickerson RN, Mullen JL (1990) Efficacy of thrombolytic therapy for occlusion of long-term catheters. JPEN 14: 312–314.

Mori E, Tabuchi M, Yoshida T, Yamadori A (1988) Intracarotid urokinase with thromboembolic occlusion of the middle cerebral artery. Stroke 19: 802–812.

Mugge A, Gulba DC, Frei U, Wagenbreth I, Grote R, Daniel WG, Lichtlen PR (1990) Renal artery embolism: thrombolysis with recombinant tissue-type plasminogen activator. J Intern Med 228: 279–286.

Nand S, Robinson JA (1988) Plasmapheresis in the management of heparin-associated thrombocytopenia with thrombosis. Am J Hematol 28: 204–206.

Nayak PR, Bhaktaram V, Shetty PK, Sivaraman S, Narayanan GR, Pais P (1991) Third World profile of racial differences in thrombolytic effects of streptokinase [letter]. Circulation 84: 2205–2207.

Neglen P, Al-Hassan HK, Endrys J, Nazzal MM, Christenson JT, Eklof B (1991) Iliofemoral venous thrombectomy followed by percutaneous closure of the temporary arteriovenous fistula. Surgery 110: 493–499.

Newman GE, Miner DG, Sussman SK, Phillips HR, Mikat EM, McCann RL (1988) Peripheral artery atherectomy: description of technique and report of initial results. Radiology 169: 677–680.

Noll G, Lammle B, Duckert F (1985) Treatment with stanozolol before thrombolysis in patients with arterial occlusions. Thromb Res 37: 529–532.

Norem RF 2d, Short DH, Kerstein MD (1988) Role of intraoperative fibrinolytic therapy in acute arterial occlusion. Surg Gynecol Obstet 167: 87–91.

Norgren L (1991) The limited applicability of thrombolysis [letter]. Eur J Vasc Surg 5: 361.

O'Donnell M (1991) Battle of the clotbusters. Br Med J 302: 1259–1261.

Oglesby JT, Martin SE, Goldenberg EM (1984) Medical grand rounds: regional streptokinase therapy for arterial occlusion. Del Med J 56: 271–9.

Ohashi S, Iwatoni M, Hyakuna Y, Morioka Y (1985) Thermographic evaluation of the hemodynamic effect of the antithrombotic drug cilostazol in peripheral artetial occlusion. Arzneimittelforschung 35: 1203–1208.

Okamura T, Nanno S, Sueishi K, Tanaka K (1984) Inhibitor of plasminogen activator in human arterial wall. I. Histochemical study. Acta Pathol Jpn 34: 743–747.

Okamura T, Nanno S, Sueishi K, Tanaka K (1984) Inhibitor of plasminogen activator in human arterial wall. II. Biochemical characterization. Acta Pathol Jpn 34: 749–757.

Okrent D, Messersmith R, Buckman J (1991) Transcatheter fibrinolytic therapy and angioplasty for left iliofemoral venous thrombosis. J Vasc Intervent Radiol 2(2): 195–197; discussion 198–200.

Olin JW, Graor RA (1988) Thrombolytic therapy in the treatment of peripheral arterial occlusions. Ann Emerg Med 17: 1210–1215.

Ostrow CL (1992) Thrombolytics. Aacn Clin Issues Crit Care Nursing 3(2): 423–436.

Overgaard K, Pedersen H, Boesen J, Waldemar G, Knudsen JB, Boysen G (1990) Thrombolytic therapy of cerebral arterial occlusion with recombinant tissue plasminogen activator. Neurol Res 12: 78–80.

Overgaard K, Pedersen H, Knudsen JB, Boysen G (1990) Fatal ischaemic brain edema after unsuccessful thrombolysis. Neurol Res 12: 81–82.

Palmieri G, Ambrosi G, Agrati AM, Ferraro G, Marcozzi S (1988) A new low molecular weight heparin in the treatment of peripheral arterial disease. In Angiol 7: 41–47.

Pan JY (1988) (107 patients with thromboangiitis obliterans treated by traditional Chinese medicine combined with Western medicine therapy). Chung Hsi I Chieh Ho Tsa Chih 8: 665—667, 646.

Parent FN 3d, Bernhard VM, Pabst TS 3d, McIntyre KE, Hunter GC, Malone JM (1989) Fibrinolytic treatment of residual thrombus after catheter embolectomy for severe lower limb ischemia. J Vasc Surg 9: 153–160.

Parent FN 3d, Piotrowski J, Bernhard VM, Pond GD, Pabst TS 3d, Bull DA, Hunter GC McIntyre KE (1991) Outcome of intraarterial urokinase for acute vascular occlusion. J Cardiovasc Surg 32: 680–689.

Parker BC, Morano JU, Huckabee RE (1990) Radiological seminar CCXLV: Use of the Simpson atherectomy catheter in a lesion resistant to percutaneous transluminal angioplasty. J Miss State Med Assoc 31: 71–74.

Parkhouse N, Smith PJ (1991) The use of streptokinase in replant salvage. J Hand Surg 16: 53–55.

Paulson EK, Miller FJ (1988) Embolization of cardiac mural thrombus: complication of intraarterial fibrinolysis. Radiology 166: 95–96.

Pell AC, Stuart PC, Stewart MJ, Fraser DM (1990) Thrombolysis and the general practitioner [letter]. Br Med J 300: 1196–1197.

Perler BA, Kinnison M, Halden WJ (1986) Transgraft hemorrhage: a serious complication of low-dose thrombolytic therapy. J Vasc Surg 3: 936–938.

Perler BA, White RI Jr, Ernst CB, Williams GM (1985) Low dose thrombolytic therapy for infrainguinal graft occlusions: an idea whose time has passed? J Vasc Surg 2: 799–805.

Permiakov NK, Galankina IE (1988) Morphologic manifestations of the medicinal lysis of a coronary artery thrombus. Kardiologiia 28: 33–36.

Pernes JM, de Almeida Augusto M, Vitoux JF, Raynaud A, Fiessinger JN, Brenot P, Fabiani JN, Murday A, Gaux JC (1987) Local thrombolysis in peripheral arteries and bypass grafts. Department of Cardiovascular Radiology, Hopital Broussais, Paris, France. J Vasc Surg 6: 372–378.

Pernes JM, Vitoux JF, Brenoit P, Raynaud A, Parola JL, Roth JP, Angel CY, Fiessinger JN, Roncato M, Gaux JC (1986) Acute peripheral arterial and graft occlusion: treatment with selective infusion of urokinase and lysyl plasminogen. Radiology 158: 481–485.

Peruzzi G, Tallarida G, Baldoni F, Raimondi G, Grimaldi I, Sangiorgi M (1985) (Current trends in medical therapy of chronic peripheral obliterating arteriopathies) Prospettive attuali della terapia medica delle arteriopatie obliteranti croniche periferiche. Clin Ter 114: 3–26.

Pilger E, Lammer J, Bertuch H, Steiner H (1986) Intraarterial fibrinolysis: in vitro and prospective clinical evaluation of three thrombolytic agents. Radiology 161: 597–599.

Poeck K (1988) Intraarterial thrombolytic therapy in acute stroke. Acta Neurol Belg 88: 35–45

Pola P, Flore R, Tondi P (1986) Blood and plasma viscosity in experimentally induced hyper- and hypo-fibrinogenaemia. Int J Tissue React 8: 333–336.

Poliwoda H, Avenarius HJ (1986) Antiplatelet drugs or dicoumarol: what is the most effective prophylaxis in occlusive arterial disease? Int Angiol 5: 169–180.

Poredos P, Keber D, Videcnik V (1989) Late results of local thrombolytic treatment of peripheral arterial occlusions. Angiology 40: 941–947.

Price C, Jacocks MA, Tytle T (1988) Thrombolytic therapy in acute arterial thrombosis. Am J Surg 156: 488–491

Pritchard SL, Culham JA, Rogers PC (1985) Low-dose fibrinolytic therapy in infants. J Pediatr 106: 594–598.

Proano M, Oh JK, Frye RL, Johnson CM, Tajik AJ, Taliercio CP (1988) Successful treatment of pulmonary embolism and associated mobile right atrial thrombus with use of a centera thrombolytic infusion. Mayo Clin Proc 63: 1181–1185.

Quinones-Baldrich WJ, Baker JD, Busuttil RW, Machleder HI, Moore WS (1989) Intraoperative infusion of lytic drugs for thrombotic complications of revascularization. J Vasc Surg 10: 408–417.

Quinones-Baldrich WJ, Rutherford RB (1991) Thrombolytic therapy. Adv Surg 24: 103–137.

Quinones-Baldrich WJ, Zierler RE, Hiatt JC (1985) Intraoperative fibrinolytic therapy: an adjunct to catheter thromboembolectomy. J Vasc Surg 2: 319–326.

Rapaport E (1991) Thrombolysis, anticoagulation, and reocclusion. Am J Cardiol 68: 17E–22E.

Rees M, Gehani AA, Richens D (1988) Percutaneous dynamic removal of atheroma [letter] Lancet 1: 174.

Reiner AP, Bell WR (1984) The fibrinolytic system in man. CRC Crit Rev Oncol Hematol 2: 33–81.

Reznik VM, Anderson J, Griswold WR, Segall ML, Murphy JL, Mendoza

SA (1989) Successful fibrinolytic treatment of arterial thrombosis and hypertension in a cocaine-exposed neonate. Pediatrics 84: 735–738.

Ricotta J (1991) Intra-arterial thrombolysis. A surgical view [comment]. Circulation 83 (2 Suppl): I120–121.

Ricotta JJ, Green RM, DeWeese JA (1987) Use and limitations of thrombolytic therapy in the treatment of peripheral arterial ischemia: results of a multi-institutional questionnaire. J Vasc Surg 6: 45–50.

Riess H, Hiller E, Reinhardt B, Brauning C (1984) Effects of BM 13.177, a new antiplatelet drug in patients with atherosclerotic disease. Thromb Res 35: 371–378.

Rinast E, Weiss HD (1991) Regional angiotherapy by application of recombinant tissue-type plasminogen activator, followed by PTA and vascular endoprosthesis. Acta Radiol Suppl (Stockh) 377: 29–34.

Risius B, Graor RA, Geisinger MA, Zelch MG, Lucas FV, Young JR, Grossbard EB (1986) Recombinant human tissue-type plasminogin activator for thrombolysis in peripheral areries and bypass grafts. Radiology 160: 183–188.

Ritchie JL, Hansen DD, Hall M, Intlekofer MJ, Vracko R, Auth D (1987) Thrombolysis—combined rotational catheter thrombectomy followed by intra-arterial streptokinase: evaluation by angioscopy and angiography. JACC 9: 82A.

Ritchie JL, Hansen DD, Intlekofer MJ, Vracko R, Auth D (1987) Thrombolysis—A new rotational thrombectomy catheter and evaluation by angioscopy. Lasers Surg Med 7:85.

Ritchie JL, Hansen DD, Vracko R, Auth D (1986) In vivo rotational thrombectomy—evaluation by angioscopy. Circulation 74(Suppl II): II–362.

Ritchie JL, Hansen DD, Vracko R, Auth DC (1986) Mechanical thrombolysis: A new rotational catheter approach for acute thrombi. Circulation 73: 1006–1012.

Ritchie JL, Hansen DD, Vracko R, Auth DC (1985) Rotational guidewire thrombectomy: in vivo canine thrombus disruption and removal. JACC 5: 440.

Robison JG, Elliott BM (1991) Venous thromboembolism: anticoagulation, lysis, or filter?. JSC Med Assoc 87: 413–417.

Rodriguez RL, Short DH, Kerstein MD (1986) Selective management of arterial occlusion with low-dose streptokinase. Curr Surg 43: 40–42.

Rosenthal D, Evans RD, Borrero E, Lamis PA, Clark MD, Daniel WW (1989) Massive pulmonary embolism: triple-armed therapy. J Vasc Surg 9: 261–270.

Rossique Delmas P, Moreno Rico MJ, Martinex Lagares FJ, Toledo Gonzalez A, Checa Andres MD, Diaz Cremades JM (1988) Local fibrinolysis and percutaneous transluminal angioplasty in embolism of the renal artery. Med Clin 91: 267–269.

Roth FJ, Krings W, Cappius G, Schmidtke I, Kohler M (1984) (Local low dosage, fibrinolytic therapy: indications, technic and results) Die lokale, niedrig dosierte, fibrinolytische therapie: indikationen, technik und resultate. Vasa (Suppl 12): 52–58.

Roth FJ, Rieser R, Scheffler A, Krings W (1991) Intra-arterial fibrinolytic therapy of chronic arterial occlusions. Semin Thromb Hemost 17: 39–47.

Routh WD, Tatum CM, Barton RE, Gross GM, McDowell HA, Keller FS (1991) Urokinase infusion: feasibility of monitoring for complications in a non-intensive care setting. J Vasc Intervent Radiol 2(1): 69–72.

Rubin JR, Pond GD, Bernhard VM (1988) Combined thrombolytic therapy and percutaneous transluminal angioplasty for treatment of complex arterial graft thrombosis—a case report. Angiology 39: 169–173.

Ruckley CV, Boulton FE, Redhead D (1987) The treatment of venous thrombosis of the upper and lower limbs with "APSAC" (p-anisoylated striptokinase-plasminogen complex). Eur J Vasc Surg 1: 107–112.

Rudofsky G (1989) (Current therapeutic aspects in arterial and vebiys vascular occlusion). Krankenpfl J 27: 33–35.

Sabba C, Zupo V, Dina F, Nazzari M, Albano O (1988) A pilot evaluation of the effect of defibrotide in patients affected by peripheral arterial occlusive disease. Int J Clin Pharmacol Ther Toxicol 26: 249–252.

Safian RD, Gelbfish JS, Erny RE, Schnitt SJ, Schmidt DA, Baim DS (1990) Coronary atherectomy. Clinical, angiographic, and histological findings and observations regarding potential mechanisms [see comments]. Comment in: Circulation 82: 305–307. Circulation 82: 69–79.

Sakurai J, Egashira T, Yamada Y, Nomura N (1991) Lysis of middle-cerebral-artery occlusion with alteplase [letter]. Lancet 338: 1206–1207.

Salem DN, Pauker SG (1991) The need to identify patients who have received streptokinase therapy [letter]. New Engl J Med 324: 1742.

Samara EN, Voss BL, Pederson JA (1988) Renal artery thrombosis associated with elevated cyclosporine levels: a case report and review of the literature. Transplant Proc 20: 119–123.

Sanborn TA (1988) Laser angioplasty. What has been learned from experimental studies and clinical trials? Circulation 78: 769–774.

Sane DC, Stump DC, Topol EJ, Sigmon KN, Clair WK, Kereiakes DJ, George BS, Stoddard MF, Bates ER, Stack RS et al (1991) Racial differences in responses to thrombolytic therapy with recombinant tissue-type plasminogen activator. Increased fibrin(ogen)olysis in blacks. The Thrombolysis and Angioplasty in Myocardial Infarction Study Group. Circulation 83: 170–175.

Schild H, Schuster CJ, Gronniger J, Schmied W, Weilemann L, Lindner P, Wagner P, Brunier A, Thelen M, Meyer J (1987) (Local fibrinolytic therapy of vascular occlusions in the pelvec-leg area and the upper extremity) Lokale Fibrinolysetherapie von Gefassverschlussen im Becken-Bein-Bereich und der oberen Extremitat. ROFO 146: 57–62.

Schmidt C, Schmitt J, Scheffmann M (1987) Hemodynamics of the postphlebitic syndrome. Int Angiol 6: 187–192.

Schneeman NJ, Stein EM (1991) Thrombolytic therapy and gastrointestinal bleeding [letter]. Am Fam Physician 43: 53–56.

Schneider E (1989) (Percutaneous transluminal angioplasty, local thrombolysis and percutaneous thrombus extraction in the treatment of arterial occlusions of the extremities). Internist 30: 440–446.

Schroeder J (1989) Catheter lysis and percutaneous transluminal angioplasty below the knee via the popliteal artery in a patient with femoral artery obstruction: technical note. Cardiovasc Intervent Radiol 12: 344–345.

Schubert W, Hunter DW, Guzman-Stein G, Ahrenholz DH, Solem LD, Dressel TD, Cunningham BL (1987) Use of streptokinase for the salvage of a free flap: case report and review of the use of thrombolytic therapy. Microsurgery 8: 117–121.

Schwartz MW, McDonald GB (1987) Cholesterol embolization syndrome. Occurrence after intravenous streptokinase therapy for myocardial infarction. JAMA 258: 1934–1935.

Schweitzer DH, van der Wall EE, Bosker HA, Scheffer E, Macfarlane JD (1991) Serum-sickness-like illness as a complication after streptokinase therapy for acute myocardial infarction. Cardiology 78: 68–71.

Scott DJ, Wyatt MG, Wilson YG, Murphy P, Baird RN, Horrocks M (1991) Intra-arterial streptokinase infusion in acute lower limb ischaemia. Br J Surg 78: 732–734.

Seabrook GR, Mewissen MW, Schmitt DD, Reifsnyder T, Bandyk DF, Lipchik EO, Towne JB (1991) Percutaneous intraarterial thrombolysis in the treatment of thrombosis of lower extremity arterial reconstructions. J Vasc Surg 13: 646–651.

Segasothy M, Parameswaran V (1991) Thrombolytic therapy in a patient with chronic renal vein thrombosis [letter]. Nephron 59: 168–169.

Seifert KB, Blackshear WM Jr, Cruse CW, Schwartz JA, Suslavitch F (1988) Bilateral upper extremity ischemia after administration of dihydroergotamine-heparin for prophylaxis of deep venous thrombosis. J Vasc Surg 8: 410–414.

Seifried E, Tanswell P, Rijken DC, Kluft C, Hoegee E, Nieuwenhuizen W (1987) Fibrin degradation products are not specific markers for thrombolysis in myocardial infarction (letter). Lancet 2: 333–334.

Shackford SR, Davis JW (1988) Refractory vasospasm occurring in a trauma patient receiving dihydroergotamine and heparin. Crit Care Med 16: 909–910.

Sharma S, Loya YS, Daxini BV (1992) Percutaneous balloon membranotomy combined with prolonged streptokinase infusion for management of inferior vena cava obstruction. Am Heart J 123(2): 515–518.

Sheehan FH, Doerr R, Schmidt WG, Bolson EL, Uebis R, von Essen R, Effert S, Dodge HT (1988) Early recovery of left ventricular function after thrombolytic therapy for acute myocardial infarction: an important determinant of survival. JACC 12: 289–300.

Sherry S (1991) Thrombolytic therapy for noncoronary diseases. Ann Emerg Med 20: 396–404.

Shinoya S, Yamada I, Sakurai T, Ohta T, Matsubara J (1989) Thrombectomy for acute deep vein thrombosis: prevention of postthrombotic syndrome. J Cardiovasc Surg (Torino) 30: 484–489.

Sicard GA, Schier JJ, Totty WG, Gilula LA, Walker WB, Etheredge EE, Anderson CB (1985) Thrombolytic therapy for acute arterial occlusion. J Vasc Surg 2: 65–78.

Simpson JB, Selmon MR, Robertson GC, Cipriano PR, Hayden WG, Johnson DE, Fogarty TJ (1988) Transluminal atherectomy for occlusive peripheral vascular disease. Am J Cardiol 61: 96G–101G.

Skinner RE, Hefty T, Long TD, Rosch J, Forsyth M (1989) Recovery of function in a solitary kidney after intra-arterial thrombolytic therapy. J Urol 141: 108–110.

Slany J, Enzenhofer V, Karnik R (1984) Local thrombolysis in arterial occlusive disease. Angiology 35: 231–237.

Smith PK, Miller DA, Lail S, Mehta AV (1991) Urokinase treatment of neonatal aortoiliac thrombosis caused by umbilical artery catheterization: a case report. J Vasc Surg 14: 684–687.

Smokovitis A, Kokolis N, Alexaki-Tzivanidou E (1988) Fatty streaks and fibrous plaques in human aorta show increased plasminogen activator activity. Haemostasis 18: 146–153.

Sniderman KW, Kalman PG, Odurny A, Shewchun J, Glynn MF (1989) Low-dose fibrinolytic therapy for recent lower extremity thromboembolism. Can Assoc Radiol J 40: 98–103.

Sniderman KW, Kalman PG, Shewchun J, Goldberg RE (1989) Lower-extremity in situ saphenous vein grafts: angiographic interventions. Radiology 179: 1023–1027.

Sorensen K, Hegedus V (1986) Selective streptokinase fibrinolysis in femoro-iliac arterial obstruction. Acta Radiol (Diagn) 27: 279–283.

Sorrentino MJ (1991) Thrombolytic therapy [letter; comment]. Ann Intern Med 114: 521.

Stack RS (1989) New interventional technologies in cardiology. (1989) Mayo Clin Proc 64: 867–870.

Steckel A, Johnston J, Fraley DS, Bruns FJ, Segel DP, Adler S (1984) The use of streptokinase to treat renal artery thromboembolism. Am J Kidney Dis 4: 166–170.

Stewart JH, Olin JW, Graor RA (1989) Thrombolytic therapy. A review (Part 1 of 2). Clev Clin J Med 56: 189–196.

Stiegler H, Hess H, Mietaschk A, von Bilderling P, Ingrisch H (1986) Long-term results of local low dose thrombolytic therapy of arterial embolism of the lower limb. Vasa 15: 71–76.

Stiegler H, Lander T, Standl E, Steckmeier B (1986) (Local thrombolysis in acute occlusion of a femoropopliteal Gore-Tex bypass) Lokale Thrombolyse bei akut verschlossenem femoro-poplitealem Gore-Tex-Bypass. Dtsch Med Wochenschr 111: 99–101.

Stirnemann P, Z'Brun AP, Mahler F (1988) Clinical aspects and treatment of acute arterial occlusion. Schweiz Med Wochenschr 118: 1767–1772.

Strife JL, Ball WS Jr, Towbin R, Keller MS, Dillon T (1988) Arterial occlusions in neonates: use of fibrinolytic therapy. Radiolgoy 166: 395–400.

Sullivan KL, Gardiner GA Jr, Kandarpa K, Bonn J, Shapiro MJ, Carabasi RA, Smullens S, Levin DC (1991) Efficacy of thrombolysis in infrainguinal bypass grafts. Circulation 83 (2 Suppl): I99–105.

Sullivan KL, Gardiner GA Jr, Shapiro MJ, Bonn J, Levin DC (1989) Acceleration of thrombolysis with a high dose transthrombus bolus technique. Radiology 173: 805–808.

Sullivan KL, Minken SL, White RI Jr (1988) Treatment of a case of thromboembolism resulting from thoracic outlet syndrome with intra-arterial urokinase infusion. J Vasc Surg 7: 568–571.

Sultan Y, Harris A, Strauch G, Venot A, De Lauture D (1988) A dynamic test to investigate potential tissue plasminogen activator activity. Comparison of deamino-8-D-argininevasopressin with venous occlusion in normal subjects and patients. J Lab Clin Med 111: 645–653.

Sussman B, Dardik H, Ibrahim IM, Fox R, Mendes D, Kahn M (1984) Improved patient selection for enzymatic lysis of peripheral arterial and graft occlusion. Am J Surg 148: 244–248.

Szczeklik A (1991) Fibrinolytic activity and response to t-PA in blacks and whites [letter]. Circulation 84: 2205–2207.

Tan AC, Van Loenhout TT, Tan HS, Kloppenborg PW, Benraad TJ (1989) Reciprocal changes in atrial natriuretic peptide levels and plasma renin activity during treatment of pulmonary embolism. Am J Hypertens 2: 570–572.

Taniguchi T, Hashimoto K, Ogawa O, Nagagawa T (1988) A case of renal artery embolism treated with urokinase. Hinyokika Kiyo 34: 318–321.

Tesi M, Bronchi GF, Carini A, Karavassili M (1985) Therapy of atherosclerotic arteriopathy of lower limbs. Aspects and results. Angiology 36: 720–735.

Theron J, Courtheoux P, Casasco A, Alachkar F, Notari F, Ganem F, Maiza D (1989) Local intraarterial fibrinolysis in the carotid territory. AJNR 10: 753–765.

Thomas SH, Shepherd SM, Allison EJ Jr (1993) Thrombolytic therapy in review (see comments). J Emerg Med 11(1): 83–89.

Tilsner V, Witte G (1988) Effectiveness of intraarterial plasminogen application in combination with percutaneous transluminal angioplasty (PTA) or catheter assisted lysis (CL) in patients with chronic peripheral occlusive disease of the lower limbs (POL). Haemostasis 18(Suppl 1): 139–156.

Todo T, Usui M, Takakura K (1991) Treatment of severe intraventricular hemorrhage by intraventricular infusion of urokinase. J Neurosurg 74: 81–86.

Tomaru T, Uchida Y, Sonoki H, Tsukamoto M, Sugimoto T (1989) The thrombolytic effects of native tissue-type plasminogen activator (AK-124) on experimental canine coronary thrombosis. Angiology 40: 429–435.

Tonnesen KH, Holstein P, Andersen E (1991) Femoro-popliteal artery occlusions treated by percutaneous transluminal angioplasty and enclosed thrombolysis: results in 55 patients. Eur J Vasc Surg 5: 429–434.

Topol EJ (1991) Which thrombolytic agent should one choose?. Prog Cardiovasc Dis 34: 165–178.

Topol EJ, George BS, Kereiakes DJ, Candela RJ, Abbottsmith CW, Stump DC, Boswick JM, Stack RS, Califf RM (1988) Comparison of two dose regimens of intravenous tissue plasminogen activator for acute myocardial infarction. Am J Cardiol 61: 723–728.

Towne JB, Bandyk DF (1987) Application of thrombolytic therapy in vascular occlusive disease. A surgical view. Am J Surg 154: 548–559.

Towne JB, Hussey CV, Bandyk DF (1988) Abnormalities of the fibrinolytic system as a cause of upper extremity ischemia: a preliminary report. J Vasc Surg 7: 661–666.

Traughber PD, Cook PS, Micklos TJ, Miller FJ (1987) Intraarterial fibrinolytic therapy for popliteal and tibial artery obstruction: comparison of streptokinase and urokinase. AJR 149: 453–456.

Troop B, Peterson GJ, Pilla T (1983) Treatment of advanced vascular disease with intra-arterial thrombolytic therapy followed by arterial dilatation. Angiology 34: 527–534.

Tsuji M, Ohtaki M, Kuribayashi Y, Koide S, Shoutsu A (1985) Intraarterial urokinase infusion in the treatment of lower limbs arterial occlusions) Rinsho Hoshasen 30: 1513–1516.

Turnipseed WD, Starck EE, McDermott JC, Crummy AB, Acher CW, Jensen SR, Voegeli DR (1986) Percutaneous aspiration thromboembolectomy

(PAT): an alternative to surgical balloon techniques for clot retrieval. J Vasc Surg 3: 437–441

Uchida Y, Masuo M, Tomaru T, Kato A, Sugimoto T (1986) Fiberoptic observation of thrombosis and thrombolysis in isolated human coronary arteries. Am Heart J 112: 691–696.

Uchino A, Onomura K, Ohno M, Tokuhisa G (1988) (Short-term intraarterial urokinase infusion in the treatment of traumatic peripheral arterial occlusion, a case report). Rinsho Hoshasen 33: 1609–1611.

Uglietta JP, O'Connor CM, Boyko OB, Aldrich H, Massey EW, Heinz ER (1991) CT patterns of intracranial hemorrhage complicating thrombolytic therapy for acute myocardial infarction. Radiology 181: 555–559.

Ulutin ON (1986) Atherosclerosis and hemostasis. Semin Thromb Hemost 12: 156–174.

Ulutin ON, Ilhan-Berkel N, Tunali H, Ozer M, Balkuv-Ulutin S, Onsel C, Urgancioglu I (1986) Effects of difibrotide on peripheral obliterative vascular disease. Haemostasis 16 (Suppl 1) 59–62.

Urano T, Sakaguchi S, Kamiya T, Ishii K, Takada Y, Takada A (1984) (Arterial and venous thrombolis of the extremities) Rinsho Ketsueki 25: 1036–1042.

Valji K, Bookstein JJ, Roberts AC, Davis GB (1991) Pharmacomechanical thrombolysis and angioplasty in the management of clotted hemodialysis grafts: early and late clinical results. Radiology 178: 243–247.

Valji K, Roberts AC, Davis GB, Bookstein JJ (1991) Pulsed-spray thrombolysis of arterial and bypass graft occlusions. AJR 156: 617–621.

Van Breda A, Graor RA, Katzen BT, Risius B, Gillings D (1991) Relative cost-effectiveness of urokinase versus streptokinase in the treatment of peripheral vascular disease. J Vasc Intervent Radiol 2(1): 77–87.

Van Breda A, Katzen BT, Deutsch AS (1987) Urokinase versus streptokinase in local thrombolysis. Radiology 165: 109–111.

Van Woert JH, Thompson RC, Cangemi JR, Metzger PP, Blackshear JL, Fleming CR (1990) Streptokinase therapy for extensive venous thromboses in a patient with severe ulcerative colitis [see comments]. Mayo Clin Proc 65: 1144–1149.

Vannini P, Ciavarella A, Mustacchio A, Rossi C (1991) Intra-arterial urokinase infusion in diabetic patients with rapidly progressive ischemic foot lesions. Diabetes Care 14(10): 925–927.

Verhaeghe R (1983) (Antithrombotic drugs in peripheral arterial diseases) Medications antithrombotiques dans les arteriopathies peripheriques. J Mal Vasc 8: 23–27.

Verhaeghe R, Wilms G, Vermylen J (1987) Local low-dose thrombolysis in arterial disease of the limbs. Semin Thromb Hemost 13: 206–211.

Vermilya SK (1989) Future indications for thrombolytic therapy with tissue plasminogen activator. JEN 15 (2(Pt2) 204–207.

Verstraete M, Hess H, Mahler F, Mietaschk A, Roth FJ, Schneider E, Baert AL, Verhaeghe R (1988) Femoro-popliteal artery thrombolysis with intra-arterial infusion of recombinant tissue-type plasminogen activator—report of a pilot trial. Eur J Vasc Surg 2: 155–159.

Vitoux JF, Pernes JM, Roncato M, Aiach M, Fiessinger JN, Gaux JC, Housset E (1984) (Intra-arterial thrombolysis with the combination of urokinase and lysyl-plasminogen. 27 cases of acute arterial obliteration of the lower limbs) Thrombolyse intra-arterielle par l'association urokinase-lysyl-plasminogene. Rev Med Interne 5: 255–261.

Vitoux JF, Roncato M, Pernes JM, Fiessinger JN, Aiach M, Gaux JC (1986) (Treatment with the urokinase-lysyl plasminogen combination of developmental outbreaks of arteriopathies) Traitement par l'association urokinase-lysyl-plasminogene des poussees evolutives des arteriopathies. Ann Med Interne (Paris) 137: 105–107.

Vogelzang RL, Moel DI, Cohn RA, Donaldson JS, Langman CB, Nemcek AA Jr (1988) Acute renal vein thrombosis: successful treatment with intraarterial urokinase. Radiology 169: 681–682.

Von Polnitz A, Hofling B (1989) Percutaneous atherectomy of a recurrent renal transplant artery stenosis. Transplantation 48: 880–883.

Von Polnitz A, Nerlich A, Berger H, Hofling B (1990) Percutaneous peripheral atherectomy: angiographic and clinical follow-up of 60 patients [see comments]. Comment in: J Am Coll Cardiol 1: 689–690. J Am Coll Cardiol 1: 682–688.

Von Romatowski HJ, Henze T, Tebbe U (1988) Recanalization of basilar artery occlusion with tissue-type plasminogen activator (letter). Dtsch Med Wochenschr 113: 616.

Vorwerk D, Guenther RW (1990) Removal of intimal hyperplasia in vascular endoprostheses by atherectomy and balloon dilatation. AJR Am J Roentgenol 154: 617–619.

Vreeken J (1985) (Fibrinolytic therapy) Fibrinolytische therapie. Ned Tijdschr Geneeskd 129: 1720–1721.

Walker A, Plant G, Rees M (1990) New hope for claudicants. Practitioner 234: 328.

Walker WJ, Giddings AE (1988) A protocol for the safe treatment of acute lower limb ischaemia with intra-arterial streptokinase and surgery. Br J Surg 75: 1189–1192.

Waller BF (1990) Topography of atherosclerotic coronary artery disease. Clin Cardiol 13: 435–442. (Review).

Walter LM (1989) Alternative therapy in atherosclerotic heart disease. Heart Lung 18: 316–320.

Weisman ID, Stanchfield WR Jr, Herzog CA, Ney AL, Blake DP (1988) Left ventricular thromboembolic occlusion of the popliteal artery treated nonoperatively with local urokinase infusion—a case report. Angiology 39: 179–186.

Welzel D, Wolf H, Koppenhagen K (1988) Antithrombotic defense during the postoperative period. Clinical documentation of low molecular weight heparin. Arzneimittelforschung 38: 120–123.

Wessel DL, Keane JF, Fellows KE, Robichaud H, Lock JE (1986) Fibrinolytic therapy for femoral arterial thrombosis after cardiac catheterization in infants and children. Am J Cardiol 58: 347–351.

White HD (1991) Thrombolytic therapy. Introduction. Am J Cardiol 68: 1E–2E.

Wholey MH, Smith JA, Godlewski P, Nagurka M (1989) Recanalization of total arterial occlusions with the Kensey dynamic angioplasty catheter. Radiology 172: 95–98.

Willis BK (1991) Timing of anticoagulant therapy for thromboembolic complications after craniotomy for brain tumors [letter; comment]. Neurosurgery 28: 929–930.

Wilms G, Vermylen J, Baert A (1987) Intraarterial low-dose streptokinase infusion in the treatment of acute renal thromboembolism. Eur J Radiol 7: 72–74.

Wu KK (1985) New pharmacologic approaches to thromboembolic disorders. Hosp Pract 20: 101–104, 107–108, 117–120.

Wyffels PL, DeBord JR, Marshall JS, Thors G, Marshall WH (1992) Increased limb salvage with intraoperative and postoperative ankle level urokinase infusion in acute lower extremity ischemia. J Vasc Surg 15(5): 771–778; discussion 778–779.

Yankes JR, Uglietta JP, Grant J, Braun SD (1988) Percutaneous transhepatic recanalization and thrombolysis of the superior mesenteric vein. AJR 151: 289–290.

Yin AC, Ming TT (1991) Misuse of streptokinase in dissecting aortic aneurysm. New Zeal Med J 104: 257–258.

Young JW, Vujic I, Gobien RP (1984) Low dose topical streptokinase in the treatment of arterial embolization. Ann Radiol 27: 324–326.

Zajko AB, McLean GK, Grossman RA, Barker CF, Freiman DB, Ring EJ, Alavi A, Perloff LJ (1982) Percutaneous transluminal angioplasty and fibrinolytic therapy for renal allograft arterial stenosis and thrombosis. Transplantation 33: 447–450.

Zeumer H (1985) Vascular recanalizing techniques in interventional neuroradiology. J Neurol 231: 287–294.

Zeumer H, Hundgen R, Ferbert A, Ringelstein EB (1984) Local intraarterial fibrinolytic therapy in inaccessible internal carotid occlusion. Neuroradiology 26: 315–317.

II. Synopses of Pertinent Articles

A. Chronic/Acute Ischemia of Lower Leg

Intra-arterial thrombolysis should be the initial treatment of the acutely ischaemic lower limb.
Allen DR; Smallwood J; Johnson CD. Ann R Coll Surg Engl 1992; 74(2): 106–110; discussion 111.

We review and discuss the initial management of acute arterial occlusion. Thrombolytic therapy has been available for over 25 years but has failed to gain universal acceptance in the initial management of this condition. Support for the use of initial thrombolytic therapy in all patients is based on the following arguments. It may be difficult to distinguish clinically between an embolic or a thrombotic occlusion, and inappropriate surgery in the latter may have disastrous consequences. Therefore, arteriography should be performed in all patients. It is then easy to place a catheter for thrombolytic therapy. This therapy allows treatment of associated medical problems before definitive surgery, and it may enable a more accurate assessment of the obstruction and better planning of surgery after dissolution of some of the occluding thrombus. Recanalisation may make reconstructive surgery easier and, finally, the results with initial thrombolysis are better than with surgery alone. The case against the motion is that expeditious surgery is in the patient's best interest, particularly in embolus, and when there is ischaemic damage to the limb. Furthermore, the reports of thrombolysis currently available are uncontrolled and do not demonstrate convincingly that the results of thrombolytic therapy are superior to surgery alone. (35 Refs.)

Clinical evaluation of short-term defibrotide treatment of patients with atherosclerosis obliterans of the lower limbs.
Avellone G; Mandala V; Pinto A; Martino A; Strano A. Haemostasis 1986; 16(Suppl 1): 55–58.

Ten patients with atherosclerosis obliterans of the lower limbs (Fontaine stage IV) were studied under basal conditions during and after short-term administration of defibrotide (800 mg/day intravenously from day 1 to 10 and then 400 mg/day intramuscularly from day 11 to 30). The clinical effectiveness of defibrotide was evaluated not only clinically (subjective and objective symptomatology) but also by Doppler velocimetry (Windsor's Index [WI] and primary antiplasmin activity. Seven patients (70%) showed improvement in subjective and objective symptomatology. There were increases in WI at the end of intravenous treatment in 6 patients (60%). In the remaining 40%, WI did not change from basal values. All patients showed normalization of primary antiplasmin activity versus basal values (55.62%, 17.75 SD) at the end of both intravenous and intramuscular treatment (101.37%, 15.71 SD and 102.5%, 13.86 SD, respectively). Therefore, we think that defibrotide may be useful for therapy of atherosclerosis obliterans of the lower limbs.

Intra-arterial thrombolysis for acute limb ischemia: a three-year experience.
Battery PM; Fulenwider JT; Smith RB 3d; Martin LG; Stewart MT; Perdue GD. South Med J 1987; 80: 479–482.

Peripheral arterial thromboembolism and thrombosis of arterial grafts continue to threaten viability of extremities. Percutaneous intra-arterial thrombolysis (IAT) and angiodilatation have afforded limb salvage in some of these patients. Proper patient selection appears to be the hallmark of success with IAT. During a recent three-year period. we used IAT in 32 extremities in 28 patients who had acute arterial insufficiency. Before IAT, 16 extremities were painful at rest, and 16 had incapacitating claudication. The overall success rate was 38%, but some degree of thrombolysis occurred in 88%. Limb salvage was achieved in 27 of 32 extremities (84%). Only five of 17 limbs (29%) with arterial graft thrombosis required no operation or an operation of lesser magnitude than predicted before IAT. Of six extremities with native arterial embolism, four (67%) were completely cleared with IAT. Major complications occurred in eight cases (25%), with two IAT-related deaths (6%). This study suggests that IAT is best reserved for individuals with acute limb ischemia caused by arterial embolus, those whose degree of ischemia would tolerate a 24-hour trial of IAT, and those whose femoral or tibial runoff is not likely to require remedial operation.

Long-term results of percutaneous transluminal angioplasty: a study of 4750 dilatations and local lyses.
Beck AH; Muhe A; Ostheim W; Heiss W; Hasler K. Eur J Vasc Surg 1989; 3: 245–252.

During a period of 8 years, 4750 percutaneous transluminal angioplasties and local lyses have been performed in the Department of Radiology of the University of Freiburg and the Hochrheinklinik Bad Sackingen. From 1984 to 1987 all patients have been assessed clinically and in 320 cases angiographically. Lesions were localized mainly to the pelvic and the femoropopliteal regions. The short and long term results have been compared, i.e. 2–8 years after PTA. Patients with occlusive disease from stage IIa to stage IV were treated. Long-term success of PTA (2–8 years after the intervention) reached 85% in stage IIa, 73% in stage IIb, 68% in stage III and 36% in stage IV, when all treated lesions were included.

Local low dose streptokinase in the treatment of acute peripheral arterial occlusion.
Breslau PJ; Van der Linden CJ; Janovski B; Jorning PJ. Neth J Surg 1984; 36: 65–68.

Case report of local low dose streptokinase therapy in a patient with acute occlusion of the left branch of an aortobifurcation graft. Objective evidence of complete thrombolysis was demonstrated both by arteriography and hemodynamic perimeters. In carefully selected cases this thrombolytic therapy is a promising alternative to surgery.

Transluminal catheter treatment in arteriovenous leg ulcers.
Brock FE; Hesse G. Hautarzt 1987; 38: 142–145.

Early diagnosis of possible atherosclerosis as a cause of ulcers in the lower leg is necessary for adequate therapy whether it is conservative, invasive, or operative. Percutaneous transluminal treatment of arteriosclerotic obstructions offer good and long-lasting results, particularly for the inoperable patient. Sometimes it is the prerequisite for the necessary venous treatment.

Intraoperative streptokinase: an adjunct to mechanical thrombectomy in the management of acute ischemia.
Cohen LH; Kaplan M; Bernhard VM. Arch Surg 1986; 121: 708–715.

Streptokinase was injected directly into the arterial tree following balloon-catheter embolectomy on 13 occasions to remove residual thrombus that could not be mechanically retrieved in 12 patients with imminent limb (ten patients) or kidney (two patients) necrosis. Effective lysis, confirmed by arteriography, pulse return, and increased ankle pressures, was achieved in 11 trials (85%). Bleeding complications, minor in three patients and severe in two patients, were ascribed to systemic lysis although other factors were contributory. One of five deaths was related to therapy. Six limbs were salvaged. The average total dose of streptokinase used, 110,000 units, was given in intermittent boluses of 25,000 to 50,000 units injected below a clamp placed to temporarily occlude distal circulation. Safe application of this technique requires intraoperative monitoring of coagulation parameters, aggressive replacement therapy, and prudent patient selection. This preliminary experience suggests that intraoperative lytic therapy (1) is an effective method for clearing thrombus not amenable to mechanical extraction and (2) may improve patency and tissue salvage.

Intraoperative, intra-arterial thrombolytic therapy as an adjunct to revascularization in patients with residual and distal arterial thrombus.
Comerota AJ; White JV. Semin Vasc Surg (USA) 1992; 5/2: 110–117.

Intraoperative intra-arterial thrombolytic therapy for salvage of limbs in patients with distal arterial thrombosis.
Comerota AJ; White JV; Grosh JD. Surg Gynecol Obstet 1989; 169: 283–289.

Acute arterial embolic or thrombotic occlusion of the runoff vessels is associated with an incomplete operative thromboembolectomy and an unacceptably high rate of amputation. This report presents a six year analysis of the use of intraoperative intra-arterial thrombolytic therapy, evaluating 38 patients who presented with impending loss of limb because of an acute occlusion of the runoff vessels. All of the patients had extensive thrombosis of a distal vessel and a complete distal thromboembolectomy was not possible. Fourteen patients received infusion of streptokinase, maximum dose of 50,000 units; 26 received urokinase (UK), maximum dose of 150,000 units, and two underwent an isolated limb perfusion technique using one million units of UK. Thirty-four lower and four upper extremities were treated. Twenty-eight of 38 patients had successful revascularization procedures that resulted in salvage of the limbs, and ten of the 38 underwent an extensive amputation. In 18 of the 28 who were successfully revascularized, lysis was clearly obtained, which contributed to the ultimate success; in ten of the 28, it was unclear whether or not lysis significantly contributed to salvage of the limbs. Although four of the 38 died within 30 days postoperatively and one patient had a hemorrhagic complication, neither the deaths nor the complication could be attributed to a lytic agent. There was no evidence of systemic thrombolysis in these patients. Intraoperative intra-arterial thrombolytic therapy administered by the slow bolus injection technique is safe. It can be an important adjunct to mechanical thromboembolectomy and bypass procedures in patients with limb-threatening ischemia caused by thrombosis of the distal part of the vessel. The isolated limb perfusion technique using high dose UK is particularly valuable in acute, small vessel, multiarterial occlusion. Intraoperative intra-arterial infusion of thrombolytic agents may make the difference between salvage or amputation of the limb without causing additional risk for the patient.

Assessment of long-term efficacy of fibrinolytic therapy in the ischemic extremity.
Durham JD; Rutherford RB. Semin Intervent Radiol (USA) 1992; 9/3: 166–173.

Acute peripheral arterial ischemia: a prospective evaluation of differential management with surgery or thrombolysis.
Earnshaw JJ; Gregson RH; Makin GS; Hopkinson BR. Ann Vasc Surg 1989; 3: 374–379.

In this three-year prospective study of 177 patients with acute peripheral arterial ischemia those subjects with acute iliofemoral emboli or ischemia with a neurosensory deficit had urgent operations. The remainder included patients less likely to have limb salvage after surgery and who therefore were treated with thrombolytic therapy. This was done in three open studies of intravenous, acylated, plasminogen-streptokinase activator complex, low dose intraarterial streptokinase and intraarterial tissue-plasminogen activator (t-PA). The overall outcome after 30 days of thrombolytic therapy was limb salvage (55%), amputation (15%), and death (30%). The severity of the presenting ischemia was the most important prognostic indicator. In patients with a neurosensory deficit, limb salvage after either embolectomy or surgical reconstruction (59%) was more likely than after thrombolysis (31%). In patients without a neurosensory deficit, limb salvage after thrombolysis (68%) was better, though not significantly, than after surgery (53%) Local intraarterial thrombolysis with either streptokinase or t-PA produced an encouraging 66% limb salvage in 59 cases. In management of acute peripheral arterial occlusions an approach based on the severity of ischemia is optimal, with urgent surgery for patients with a neurosensory deficit and intraarterial thrombolytic therapy reserved as an alternative in selected cases with stable ischemia.

Early results of low dose intra-arterial streptokinase therapy in acute and subacute lower limb arterial ischaemia.
Earnshaw JJ; Gregson RH; Makin GS; Hopkinson BR. Br J Surg 1987; 74: 504–507.

Thirty-two patients with acute and subacute limb-threatening peripheral arterial ischaemia were treated with low dose intra-arterial streptokinase infusions. The mean duration of infusion was 38 h. Six patients developed pericatheter thrombosis and two had distal embolization of fragments of thrombus but in all cases these responded to repositioning the catheter and continuing the infusion. Five patients developed groin haematomata and in three of these there was evidence of a systemic fibrinolytic effect from the streptokinase with plasma fibrinogen reduced below 1 g/l. The most serious complication was perforation of the popliteal and tibial arteries which occurred on two occasions and required cessation of the infusion. Twenty-two patients (69 per cent) achieved limb salvage, eight (25 per cent) suffered a major amputation and two (6 per cent) died. The outcome was not related to the site, nature or duration of the arterial occlusion but patients with loss of sensation or paralysis of the affected limb were significantly less likely to obtain limb salvage (P = 0.001). For occlusions greater than 30 cm in length a new technique was used where the thrombus was lysed from distal to proximal in short lengths by gradual catheter withdrawal. This was successful in five out of six cases. Low dose intra-arterial streptokinase has been confirmed as an effective, relatively safe method of treatment in recent arterial ischaemia and can be recommended in situations where the results of surgery may not be favourable. In particular, patients with arterial thromboses and no distal run-off, distal and late arterial emboli, thrombosed popliteal aneurysms and patients after a failed embolectomy, have all been shown to respond to thrombolytic therapy with intra-arterial streptokinase.

Local thrombolytic therapy of acute peripheral arterial ischaemia with tissue plasminogen activator: a dose-ranging study.
Earnshaw JJ; Westby JC; Gregson RH; Makin GS; Hopkinson BR. Br J Surg 1988; 75: 1196–1200.

Low-dose streptokinase has been established as an alternative to surgery in selected patients with acute peripheral arterial ischaemia. Tissue plasminogen activator (t-PA) is responsible for normal plasma fibrinolytic activity and has recently become available for clinical use owing to recombinant DNA technology. It has the theoretical advantage of fibrin specificity, which may result in enhanced thrombolytic effects with greater safety. Twenty-three patients with recent lower limb arterial occlusions received t-PA over a tenfold range of concentrations and five patients received low-dose streptokinase. One month after treatment with t-PA or streptokinase 19 (68 per cent) patients had limb salvage, five (18 per cent) had required amputations and four (14 per cent) had died. Systemic fibrinolytic effects were variable but basically dose related Haemorrhage occurred most frequently at the highest t-PA concentration and was major in four (17 per cent) cases, including a fatal stroke. Plasma fibrinogen concentration fell below 1.2 gl-1 in five (22 per cent) patients who received t-PA and was found to be a significant risk factor for haemorrhage, t-PA was an effective thrombolytic agent at all concentrations studied. The dose currently used in clinical studies at this institution is 0.5 mg h-1.

The systemic fibrinolytic effect of BRL 26921 during the treatment of acute peripheral arterial occlusions.
Earnshaw JJ; Westby JC; Makin GS; Hopkinson BR. Thromb Haemost 1986; 55: 259–262.

BRL 26921 is a new acylated streptokinase-plasminogen complex which may have a more specific local thrombolytic effect than streptokinase or urokinase. 34 patients with acute peripheral arterial occlusions were given eight hourly bolus injections of 5 mg BRL 26921 for up to 72 h. Systemic fibrinolysis was observed in all patients yet in only 24% was the occluding thrombus lysed 44% of the patients had haemorrhagic complications and 24% suffered further thrombotic events during or soon after treatment. There was no correlation between the degree of systemic fibrinolysis produced and dissolution of the thrombi. The degree of systemic fibrinolysis did not affect the complication rate. There is no evidence from this study that BRL 26921 has a specific local thrombolytic effect.

Percutaneous transluminal angioplasty of crural arteries.
Flueckiger F; Lammer J; Klein GE; Hausegger K; Pilger E; Waltner F; Aschauer M. Acta Radiol 1992; 33(2): 152–155.

In 91 patients suffering from peripheral arterial occlusive disease (Fontaine stage IIb-IV) 125 percutaneous transluminal angioplasties (PTA) of crural arteries were performed. Eighty-six of the dilatations were done in combination with a recanalization procedure (PTA, laser angioplasty, fibrinolysis) of a femoropopliteal obstruction in order to improve outflow. PTA was performed with 5 F balloon catheters 2.5 to 4 mm in diameter in combination with steerable guide wires. A primary technical success was achieved in 41 of 42 (97.6%) vessels with a single stenosis, in 64 of 68 (94.1%) vessels with 2 or more stenoses, and 9 of 15 (60%) vessels with total occlusions (overall primary success rate 91.2%). Complications included spasm (n = 3), thrombosis (n = 2), peripheral embolization (n = 2), and dissection (n = 1). None of the complications required surgical intervention. After PTA, accumulative patency rate of 71% at 2 years and 64.2% at 3 years was achieved. These results demonstrated that PTA of crural arteries is a safe procedure with an excellent primary success rate and satisfying long-term results. Thus we believe that even arterial occlusive disease in the clinical stage Fontaine IIb should be accepted as an indication for crural PTA. Furthermore, crural PTA should be used to improve reduced peripheral outflow after femoropopliteal PTA.

Catheter-directed thrombolysis for the failed lower extremity bypass graft.
Gardiner GA Jr; Sullivan KL. Semin Vasc Surg (USA) 1992; 5/2: 99–103.

Percutaneous local arterial thrombolytic infusion. Therapeutic effects and complications.
Goffette P; Kurdziel JC; Dondelinger RF. Acta Radiol 1991; 32: 305–310.

All complications occurring in 55 local thrombolytic infusions performed for (sub)acute limb ischemia using streptokinase (SK) in 22 procedures and urokinase (UK) in 33 procedures were recorded. Success was achieved in 74.5% of the procedures. Major complications occurred in 31.8% of the procedures using SK, and in 12.1% of the procedures using UK (p = 0.07). Hemorrhage was the most common major complication and occurred in 27.2% of SK procedures and in 9.0% of UK procedures, a difference which was not significant. Overall, 30 day mortality was 16.3% and procedure-related death was 1.8%. Moderate complications necessitating only the adjustment of drug regimen and minor complications without consequence were observed in 45.5% and 45.5%, respectively, of the SK procedures, and in 57.6% and 66.7% of the UK procedures.

Treatment of arterial occlusions of the lower extremities using 2-stage local applicaiton of urokinase.
Gross-Fengels W; Neufang KF; Lechler E; Schmitz-Rixen T. ROFO 1988; 148: 269–274.

We report the results of a 2-phase urokinase protocol for treatment of 28 arterial occlusions of the lower extremities. 26 patients, aged 43–86, with up to 6 weeks old occlusions were treated. In Phase I (average duration 2.7 h) the urokinase solution was injected in intervals directly into the occlusion-material via a F-5 catheter (120,000 U/h). In the following phase II (average duration 26.1 h) 1000,000 U/h were given as a continuous arterial infusion and a full heparin regimen was started. In 86% of the treatments there was an improvement as shown by angiography. 75% of the patients could be released from the hospital without a further surgical revascularization. Alterations of the systemic coagulation-system and bleeding-complications at the puncture site must be expected.

Regional low dosage thrombolytic therapy for peripheral arterial occlusions.
Hallett JW Jr; Yrizarry JM; Greenwood LH. Surg Gynecol Obstet 1983; 156: 148–154.

This report describes successful management of recent peripheral arterial occlusions by intra-arterial low dosage thrombolytic drug infusions and percutaneous balloon angioplasty. An intra-arterial infusion of either streptokinase or urokinase at ½0 of the usual systemic dose was delivered through an angiographic catheter into the region of the thrombus. Clot lysis was achieved for arterial occlusions of the iliac artery, an old aortofemoral graft limb and femoropopliteal arteries. Arterial clots of several weeks duration were lysed. Recurrent thrombosis can be prevented by anticoagulation, balloon angioplasty or surgical repair of causative arterial lesions. Thrombolytic therapy for arterial occlusions is not a replacement for surgical management but an important adjunct to the over-all treatment. Low dosage regional thrombolytic therapy deserves wider application in the management of selected arterial occlusions.

Reduced fibrinolytic potential in patients with arterial occlusive disease (AOD) in comparison with normal subjects.
Hartl D; Tiso E; Anderle K; Philapitsch A; Anger G. Haemostasis 1988; 18(Suppl): 93–98.

When combining angioplasty and local lysis with urokinase (UK) in treatment of peripheral arterial occlusions we have observed marked differences in the individual patient's response irrespective of the age of the thrombus. The extensive arteriosclerotic changes revealed by angiography in some of these patients suggest a reduced fibrinolytic potential depending on the underlying disease. In the standard in vitro test system we measured the UK-dependent thrombolysis in blood samples from 10 normal controls at UK concentrations of 150,200, and 300 IU/ml of whole blood. In comparison we determined the whole blood thrombolysis time (WBTT) of 10 patients with AOD using UK concentrations of 150, 200, and 300 IU/ml of whole blood. The mean WBTT values for normal controls obtained at UK concentrations of 150 IU/ml, 200 IU/ml, and 300 IU/ml, respectively, amounted to 9.5, 5.5, and 3.5 minutes, respectively, while in patients mean values of 20.7, 8.1, and 5.5 minutes, respectively, were found. Studies on plasma samples had shown that the lysis time could be shortened in a dose-dependent manner by addition of lys-plasminogen (LYS-PLASMINOGEN Steam Treated) and to some extent also glu-plasminogen. Since lys-plasminogen gave clearly superior results we tried to improve the lytic potential in terms of a shortening of the WBTT by adding different doses lys-plasminogen (0.14–0.56 CU/ml whole blood) to each patient sample. Although the individual response varied, the addition of lys-plasminogen to the patient samples resulted in a clear dose-dependent improvement of pathologically prolonged lysis times. (ABSTRACT TRUNCATED AT 250 WORDS)

Fibrinolysis with rt-PA in peripheral arterial occlusions.
Hess H; Mietaschk A; Becker-Lienau C. Klin Wochenschr 1988; 66(Suppl 12): 135–136.

First experiences using rt-PA for the local lysis of peripheral arterial occlusions have shown thats a potent activator of the fibrinolytic system. 2 to 5 mg of rt-PA administered for 1 to 1 ½ hours are sufficient to completely dissolve even long occlusions. With doses up to 20 mg over 2 hours no systemic bleeding was observed. With 50 mg given within 5 hours and with an infusion of 2.5 mg per hour for 48 hours there were two cases of systemic haemorrhaging entirely due to the fibrinolysis. No appreciable defects in the coagulation system and no other side effects were observed.

Peripheral arterial occlusions: a 6-year experience with local low-dose thrombolytic therapy.
Hess H; Mietaschk A; Bruckl R. Radiology 1987; 163: 753–758.

Early and long-term resusts of treatment with local low-dose thrombolysis in 554 patients with 564 peripheral arterial occlusions are reported. Of 92 embolic occlusions present for 2 months or more, 59 (64.1%) were recanalized with a cumulative patency of 89.5% after 5 years. Of 472 thrombotic occlusions present for up to 6 months and more, 254 (53.8%) were successfully treated with a cumulative patency of 58 8% after 5 years. The hospital mortality and amputation rate were 1.6% and 1.95%, respectively. The average age of the patients was 69.1 years and more than half of those treated had stage III or IV disease. A 6-year experience with local low-dose thrombolytic therapy has completely confirmed its efficacy and has led to improvements in technique, which were described. The doses of streptokinase and urokinase needed for a successful result have been substantially reduced and the duration of treatment shortened. The number of complications has also been reduced. Differential therapeutic considerations compared to vascular surgery are mentioned. The results should motivate a reconsideration of the diagnostic and therapeutic measures to be used in the treatment of peripheral arterial occlusions.

Therapeutic alternatives for subacute peripheral arterial occlusion. Comparison by outcome, length of stay, and hospital charges.
Janosik JE; Bettmann MA; Kaul AF; Souney PF. Invest Radiol 1991; 26: 921–925.

Thrombolytic therapy using streptokinase or urokinase has been shown to be a viable alternative to surgical thrombectomy in patients with subacute peripheral arterial occlusion. Urokinase is associated with higher success and lower complication rates than streptokinase, but the cost of urokinase is at least seven times higher. To address questions of utility and effectiveness in the treatment of subacute peripheral arterial occlusions, the authors designed a retrospective study of patients treated either by surgical thrombectomy (n = 70), thrombolysis with streptokinase (n = 19), or thrombolysis with urokinase (n = 22). Outcome of therapy, length of hospital stay, and total hospital charges in the three groups were examined. Treatment successes in the three groups, defined as complete clearing of the occluded segment with patency maintained for 60 days, were 76% for thrombectomy, 32% for streptokinase, and 64% for urokinase. Total duration of hospitalization was 21.1, 21.3, and 11.5 days (P less than .05), respectively. Mean charges for thrombolytic agents were $690 for streptokinase and $6429 for urokinase. Mean total hospital charges, however, were $25,978 for streptokinase, $22,203 for urokinase, and $25,336 for thrombectomy (P = NS). The higher cost of urokinase, then, accounted for the similar total charges, despite the shortened length of stay. These results suggest that urokinase is cost-effective compared to streptokinase for subacute peripheral arterial occlusion. Compared to thrombectomy, thrombolysis with urokinase has a marginally lower patency rate at 60 days, but a significantly shorter length of hospital stay.

Femoral artery recanalisation with percutaneous angioplasty and segmentally enclosed plasminogen activator.
Jorgensen B; Tonnesen KH; Bulow J; Nielsen JD; Jorgensen M; Holstein P; Andersen E. Lancet 1989; 1: 1106–1108.

To establish whether re-occlusion of the femoral artery could be prevented, in 6 consecutive patients undergoing percutaneous transluminal angioplasty (PTA) for superficial femoral artery occlusion the recanalised segment was isolated, with a 7-French double-balloon catheter. 5 mg recombined human tissue-type plasminogen activator (rt-PA) and 1000 IU heparin were then infused into the enclosed space for 30 minutes, followed by intravenous heparin for 24 hours. At 10 and 30 days all 6 patients had evidence of recanalisation and remission of symptoms. Mean ankle-arm pressure index improved by 72% at 24 hours, by 118% at 10 days, and by 103% at 30 days after the procedure. No patients had major complications. Treatment of superficial femoral artery occlusions by PTA with rt-PA and intravenous heparin seems to prevent rethrombosis.

[Intra-arterial thrombolytic therapy for lower limb ischemia] Traitement thrombolytique intra-arteriel des ischemies des membres inferieurs.
Juhan C; Haupert S; Miltgen G; Dulac P; Girard N; Barthelemy P; Raybaud C. Bull Acad Natl Med (Paris) 1990; 174: 197–209.

Between 1984 and 1989, 35 patients with recent arterial or graft occlusions have been treated with intra-arterial infusion using sequential association of Urokinase (U.K.) and Lys-Plasminogen. Occlusion was thrombotic in 68.5% of the cases and embolic in 31.5%, involving 28 native arteries and 7 bypass grafts. The mean duration was 16 days (2 to 90). Continuous infusion of U.K.: 84,000 U.I./H and bolus of Lys-Plasminogen 15 microKatals every 30 minutes were delivered through a catheter embedded into the clot. Intra-venous heparin was always associated. The mean duration of lytic drug infusion was 8 H. Complementary arterial reconstruction by vascular surgery of percutaneous transluminal angioplasty was performed in 23% of the patients. Patients with recent alimentary tract bleeding, hemorrhagic stroke in the last six months or severe high blood pressures were contraindicated. Complete lysis was obtained in 23 cases (66%), partial lysis in 7 (20%) and no lysis in 5 (14%). The clinical result was excellent in 24 cases (68.5%), good in 3 (8.5%) and bad in 8 (23%) in which amputation was always necessary. 5 local hematoma (14%) treated by surgery or transfusion and one death (3%) due to neurological complication occurring 24 hours after the end of the procedure were observed. The literature survey has shown that the results of low doses of Streptokinase (S.K.) local infusions were not better, and that higher doses of S.K. of U.K. delivered during a shorter infusion time increased the efficacy of lysis and decreased the rate of hemorrhagic complications. We have proposed the local thrombolytic treatment to the limb threatening ischemic cases when the traditional medical or surgical techniques where thought to be associated to a high risk of failure or complication. The specific indications are the acute or sub-acute ischemic situation due to atheromatous artery thrombosis, distal or old embolism where the Fogarty catheter is inefficient, and graft thrombosis. Severe acute ischemia with neurologic involvement are not good indications. Local thrombolysis can be successful on arterial occlusion even after one month duration.

Technique and results of "low-dose" infusion.
Katzen BT. Cardiovasc Intervent Radiol 1988; 11 (Suppl): 41–47.

The results or 125 urokinase (UK) infusions in 108 patients were analyzed. Results showed total clot lysis in 61% of patients, partial lysis in 24%, and no lysis in 15%. Predictably, patients with acute occlusions had the highest incidence of complete clot lysis. However, clots older than 3 weeks had a surprisingly high lysis rate of 57%. None of the patients had a fibrinogen level below 100 mg/dL. Overall incidence of bleeding (major and minor) was 15%; patients having the most severe bleeding were on concomitant anticoagulation. We conclude that UK is a safe and effective therapeutic option in patients with acute and chronic obstruction. Significant bleeding episodes are uncommon during UK therapy and are related primarily to ongoing anticoagulation.

Low-dose direct fibrinolysis in peripheral vascular disease.
Katzen BT; Edwards KC; Albert AS; Van Breda A. J Vasc Surg 1984; 1: 718–722.

One hundred thirty patients underwent low-dose, catheter-directed fibrinolytic therapy for arterial and graft occlusions present for various periods of time. In 65 consecutive patients the therapeutic parameters were identical, and a careful hematologic evaluation was performed. In the subsequent 65 patients, varying doses of fibrinolytic agents were employed. Fibrinolytic therapy was found to be beneficial in a diverse group of clinical situations and in patients whose occlusions had occurred at varying lengths of time. Early study demonstrated that effective fibrinolysis can be achieved at approximately one-twentieth of the systemic level and that systemic effects could be avoided in all patients during 24-hour infusions and in many patients infused up to 96 hours. Bleeding complications occurred only in patients in whom concomitant heparinization was employed, and this was thought to be the causative factor. Therapeutic success and avoiding complications are strongly dependent on close monitoring of patients and joint decision making by the vascular surgeon and radiologist.

Intraarterial urokinase infusion therapy for arterial occlusive disease of the pelvis and extremities with special reference to short-term high dose infusion.
Kichikawa K; Nishimine K; Uchida H; Kubota Y; Yoshioka T; Honda N; Hirai T; Tamada T; Nishimura Y; Maeda M; et al. Nippon Igaku Hoshasen Gakkai Zasshi 1990; 50: 229–239.

Thirty-five complete arterial occlusions of pelvis and extremity in 29 patients were treated with intraarterial urokinase infusion therapy. In 28 limbs, the occlusions were due to arteriosclerotic change and in 7 lesions, the occlusions were due to Burger's disease. The patients with arteriosclerotic change ranged in age from 52 to 84 years with a mean age of 68 years, and the patients with Burger's disease ranged in age from 35 to 47 years with a mean age of 43 years. There were 24 men and 5 women. The estimated duration of the occlusion was from 5 days to 5 years with a mean duration of 11 months. The length of the occluded segments ranged from 1 to 45 cm with a mean length of 13.9 cm. The occlusion was located in the iliac artery in 13 patients, the femoral artery in 11 patients, both the iliac and the femoral artery in 2 patients, the popliteal artery in 5 patients, the femoropopliteal artery in 1 patient, the brachial artery in 2 patients and the radial artery in 1 patient. The infusion catheter was gently advanced into the proximal portion of the clot over a flexible guide wire, and urokinase was infused at a rate of 5000–10000 IU/min, as a short term high dose infusion (SHI), until antegrade blood flow was reestablished. The catheter was then withdrawn to a point proximal to all of the remaining clot, and the infusion rate was reduced to 10000–20000 IU/h as a continuous low dose infusion (CLI). After thrombolytic recanalization, a percutaneous transluminal angioplasty (PTA) was performed in those cases which demonstrated a residual narrowing of the lumen. The initial success rate was 86%. Reocclusions were observed in 5 lesions (17%) and a second recanalization was successful in 2 of 3 patients. The 1-year cumulative patency rate following recanalization was 88.4% and the 2-year patency rate was 78.6%. No significant complications directly related to the procedure were observed. SHI combined with CLI and PTA appears to be an effective and safe therapy for chronic long segmental arterial occlusion.

Fibrinolysis in chronic arteriosclerotic occlusions: intrathrombotic injections of streptokinase. Work in progress.
Lammer J; Pilger E; Justich E; Neumayer K; Schreyer H. Radiology 1985; 157: 45–50.

Forty-seven patients with chronic arteriosclerotic occlusions of iliac and femoropopliteal arteries were treated by intrathrombotic fibrinolysis. The occlusions were 10–65 cm (mean, 22 cm) long and 6 weeks to 2 years (mean, 4.5 months) old. By means of consistent intrathrombotic injections of 2,500 units of streptokinase every 5 minutes, the thrombi were recanalized within 1–7 hours (mean, 2.5 hours). The primary recanalization rate was 75% (35/47), the patency rate after 2 weeks, 68%. In 29 patients (62%), a residual stenosis had to be dilated by balloon angioplasty. Because of the low total dose of streptokinase (mean, 70,000 units), the thrombin time was elevated up to twice the normal value in only one patient. Bleeding that required transfusions was observed in only two patients (4%). Advantages of intrathrombotic fibrinolysis include higher recanalization rate, lower total dose of streptokinase, fewer bleeding complications, and shorter therapy time than previously reported with other treatments.

Intraarterial fibrinolysis: long-term results.
Lammer J; Pilger E; Neumayer K; Schreyer H. Radiology 1986; 161: 159–163.

Intraarterial fibrinolytic therapy was performed in 136 patients suffering from arteriosclerotic thrombosis of the iliac and femoropopliteal arteries. The initial success rate was 78%. Despite anticoagulation therapy, early recurrent thrombosis was observed in 10% of the patients. The 2-year cumulative patency rate after recanalization was 81%. These results are competitive with those of reconstructive vascular surgery. Therefore, intraarterial fibrinolysis has become a viable alternative to surgery in treating segmental peripheral occlusions more than 4 cm in length that are less than 6–9 months in duration.

Low-dose urokinase regimen for the treatment of lower extremity arterial and graft occlusions: experience in 132 cases.
LeBlang SD; Becker GJ; Benenati JF; Zemel G; Katzen BT; Sallee SS. J Vasc Intervn Radiol 1992; 3(3): 475–483.

In a retrospective review, a low-dose urokinase (UK) infusion regimen (mean, 87,000 U of UK per hour and 100 U of heparin per hour) was evaluated for lower extremity arterial and graft occlusions. Results of 132 infusions in 111 patients were analyzed to determine efficacy, limb salvage, and complications. Angiographic success was achieved with 126 infusions (95%), and amelioration of presenting signs and symptoms was achieved after 116 infusions (88%). Patients who underwent additional percutaneous procedures were more likely to have a successful outcome. There was no significant difference in success rates for patients receiving low-dose heparin through the arterial sheath (n = 29) versus those receiving concomitant systemic heparinization (n = 101), (P = .08). Of 88 threatened extremities (with rest pain, cold, ulcers, or gangrene), nine were amputated (limb salvage = 90%), accounting for 82% (nine of 11) of amputations in the overall study. Patients with zero- or one-vessel runoff before infusion were more likely to require limb amputation compared with the group with two- or three-vessel runoff before infusion (P less than .01). Major periprocedural complications occurred in nine of 132 (7%) infusions, five of which necessitated specific surgery and/or transfusion for bleeding. Pericatheter thrombosis was not encountered in either subgroup. This standard local low-dose infusion represents a safe and effective treatment for lower extremity arterial and graft occlusions. (19 Refs.)

Treatment of peripheral arterial obstruction with streptokinase: results in arterial vs graft occlusions.
LeBolt SA; Tisnado J; Cho SR. AJR 1988: 151: 589–592.

A retrospective study of the efficacy of local low-dose intraarterial streptokinase for the treatment of peripheral arterial occlusion was performed in 60 cases. The results of treatment of occlusion of native arterial and arterial graft occlusions were compared. Twenty-two (73%) of 30 cases of arterial occlusion showed complete or partial angiographic resolution, compared with 16 (53%) of 30 cases of arterial graft occlusion. Ten (71%) of 14 patients with venous arterial grafts were successfully treated vs only six (38%) of 16 patients with prosthetic arterial grafts. These results suggest that streptokinase is an effective fibrinolytic agent for the treatment of arterial occlusion and arterial graft occlusion. Its effectiveness in arterial graft obstruction is comparatively low, although patients with venous grafts respond much more favorably than those with synthetic conduits.

Selective thrombolysis with low-dose urokinase in chronic arteriosclerotic obstructions.
Lupattelli L; Barzi F; Corneli P; Lemmi A; Mosca S. Cardiovasc Intervent Radiol 1988; 11: 123–126.

Twenty-one patients, 15 males and 6 females aged 52–75 years, with angiographically demonstrated occlusions of the superficial femoral or popliteal arteries, were treated by low-dose urokinase intraarterial infusion. The obstructions were 2–12 months old and from 7 to 18 cm in length. Urokinase was infused at 50,000 U/h; heparin was simultaneously administered by intravenous route in doses of 800 U/h. The average duration of treatment was 18 h. Effective clot lysis was accomplished in 18 cases (85%); 15 patients had underlying stenoses treated by balloon dilatation to prevent rethrombosis. Of the primarily recanalized arteries, two reoccluted within 4 weeks.

Thromboembolectomy with the transluminal extraction catheter (TEC) as an adjunct to thrombolysis.
Matsumoto AH; Sarosi MG; Selby JB Jr; Tegtmeyer CJ. J Vasc Intervn Radiol 1992; 3(3): 491–495.

Multiple surgical and percutaneous interventional radiologic techniques have been used to restore blood flow in an acutely ischemic extremity. The transluminal extraction catheter (TEC) system was used as a mechanical thromboembolectomy device to supplement pharmacologic thrombolysis in one patient. In this case, 40 hours of direct intraarterial infusion of urokinase into the occluded vascular segments of a threatened lower extremity resulted in incomplete thrombolysis. Therefore, a 7-F TEC system was advanced percutaneously through the occluded vessels with restoration of luminal patency in all vessels treated. No distal embolization occurred. The TEC system facilitated prompt recanalization of vessels occluded by acute thrombus superimposed on atherosclerotic disease.

Thrombolysis as an alternative initial therapy for the acutely ischemic lower limb.
McNamara TO. Semin Vasc Surg (USA) 1992; 5/2: 89–98.

Intra–arterial urokinase as the initial therapy for acutely ischemic lower limbs [see comments].
McNamara TO; Bomberger RA; Merchant RF. Circulation 1991; 83(2 Suppl): I106–119. Comment in Circulation 1991 Feb; 83 (2 Suppl): I120–1.

Acute ischemia of the lower limb remains a significant risk to both life and limb. Mortality rates of approximately 10–30% and amputation rates of the same magnitude in the survivors are repeatedly reported despite advances in medical and surgical techniques. Our experience, which utilized percutaneous intra-arterial thrombolysis as the initial treatment in 72 instances (63 patients), has resulted in a markedly lower mortality rate of 1.6% and a lower amputation rate of 8.5% in the survivors. Careful categorization by clinical degree of ischemia indicates that 82% of the cases were either threatened or irreversible limb ischemia. The initial treatment with thrombolysis did not preclude subsequent prompt surgical treatment when necessary; in these cases thrombolysis promoted improved surgical results (100%) when it was successful. It markedly reduced the need for urgent surgery, usually simplified the subsequent surgical approach, diminished the overall need for surgery, and often accomplished a successful outcome alone (31%). Significant bleeding was not noted during subsequent surgical procedures and was noted in only 2.8% of the cases. Confirmation of these results and further improvements in technique might justify the use of an initially high-dose urokinase transcatheter infusion regimen as the initial treatment of choice for acute lower-limb ischemia.

Thrombolysis of peripheral arterial and graft occlusions: improved results using high-dose urokinase.

McNamara TO; Fischer JR. AJR 1985; 144: 769–775.

Ninety-three thromboembolic occlusiona of peripheral arteries or grafts in 85 patients were treated with high-dose urokinase by direct intraarterial infusion. Urokinase was infused at 4000 IU/min until antegrade blood flow was reestablished and then at 1000 or 2000 IU/min until clot lysis was completed. Of the 93 infusions, 75 (81%) resulted in clinical improvement. The infusion therapy was incomplete in nine patients. The mean duration of the 84 completed infusions was 18 ± 20 hr, the incidence of complete clot lysis was 83%, and the incidence of clinical improvement was 89%. Significant bleeding, requiring transfusion, occurred during or after four of the urokinase infusions (4%). Other complications included distad clot migration, thrombus formation on the catheter, revascularization phenomena, oliguria, skin rash, pseudoaneurysm, balloon rupture during angioplasty, and vascular spasm. There were no instances of drug resistance or adverse drug reactions. These results indicate that an initially high-dose urokinase regimen accomplishes more rapid recanalization, a higher incidence of total clot lysis, and produces fweer complications than the standard low-dose streptokinase regimen.

Recombinant tissue-type plasminogen activator versus urokinase in peripheral arterial and graft occlusions: a randomized trial [see comments].

Meyerovitz MF; Goldhaber SZ; Reagan K; Polak JF; Kandarpa K; Grassi CJ; Donovan BC; Bettmann MA; Harrington DP. Radiology 1990; 175: 75–78.

A randomized prospective trial was undertaken to compare intraarterial administration of recombinant human tissue-type plasminogen activator (rt-PA) with urokinase (UK) in 32 patients with peripheral arterial or bypass graft occlusions. Sixteen patients were randomized to receive rt-PA and 16 to receive UK. The rt-PA dose was administered as a 10-mg bolus into the thrombus, followed by 5 mg/h for up to 24 hours. The UK dose was administered as a 60,000 IU bolus into the thrombus, followed by 240,000 IU/h for 2 hours, 120,000 IU/h for 2 hours, and 60,000 IU/h for up to 20 hours. Serial arteriograms were obtained at baseline and at 4, 8 or 16, and 24 hours. The endpoint was defined as 95% of greater clot lysis. The cumulative numbers of patients with successful thrombolysis (rt-PA vs UK) were four vs none at 4 hours, seven vs one at 8 hours, seven vs three at 16 hours, and eight vs six at 24 hours. Lysis occurred more rapidly in the rt-PA group (P = .04). Major bleeding complications occurred in five rt-PA patients and two UK patients (P = .39). At 24 hours, fibrinogen levels were significantly lower in the rt-PA group than in the UK group (P = .01). There was no apparent difference in 30-day clinical success.

Surgical treatment versus thrombolysis in acute arterial occlusion: a randomised conrolled study.
Nilsson L; Albrechtsson U; Jonung T; Ribbe E; Thorvinger B; Thorne J; Astedt B; Norgren L. Eur J Vasc Surg 1992; 6(2): 189–193.

Thrombolytic treatment has been tried in various forms for acute limb ischaemia with varying degrees of success but is also often accompanied by bleeding problems. The present investigation compares the effect of surgical thrombectomy (TE) and thrombolysis (TL) using recombinant tissue plasminogen activator (rt-PA). Twenty patients with a need for intervention owing to ischaemia lasting more than 24 h but less than 14 days were included. Patients randomised to TE were operated under epidural anaesthesia and patients in the TL group received 30 mg rt-PA during a 3 h period through a catheter placed into the thrombus and advanced as lysis was achieved. Thrombectomy resulted in an immediate restitution of blood flow in six out of nine cases, in three cases a bypass procedure was performed, and one of these failed with a resultant amputation. Thrombolysis gave a good primary result in six cases which lasted in four of them. Three had a subsequent percutaneous transluminal angioplasty. Partial lysis was seen in two cases and a further two failed. Five went to surgery with three bypass and two fogarty procedures being necessary. There was no hospital mortality and there were no bleeding complications due to the rt-PA treatment in this series. In 19 out of 20 patients the circulation was re-established. Appropriate handing of acute ischaemic conditions implies the use of both thrombolysis and appropriate surgical procedures, including distal bypass grafts.

Role of intraoperative fibrinolytic therapy in acute arterial occlusion.
Norem RF 2d; Short DH; Kerstein MD. Surg Gynecol Obstet 1988; 167: 87–91.

Nineteen patients with acute onset of ischemia affecting the lower extremities were studied from January 1985 to March 1987. Patients with preoperative Doppler and angiographic studies consistant with arterial occlusions subsequently underwent a thromboembolectomy using a Fogarty catheter. All patients were given a bolus injection of 5,000 units of heparin intravenously at the start of the surgical procedure. In all patients studied, a clot was retrieved on the first pass, but after two additional passes, total distal blood flow was not shown to be restored on angiogram. Intraoperative angiograms showed distal emboli. All patients underwent intraoperative fibrinolytic therapy by local bolus infusion. Streptokinase, ranging from 50,000 to 200,000 units, was administered in 50,000 unit injections in ten to 15 minute intervals. Repeat attempts at thromboembolectomy with the Fogarty catheter resulted in an additional clot retrieved in all 19 patients with intraoperative angiographic, Doppler and clinical improvement. No perioperative or postoperative complications were observed, including anaphylactic reactions, uncontrollable bleeding or amputation. Four patients had nonacute femoropopliteal bypass operations within the next six months. Intraoperative fibrinolytic therapy can be a safe and effective adjunct in acute arterial embolic occlusion requiring balloon catheter thromboembolectomy.

Outcome of intraarterial urokinase for acute vascular occlusion.
Parent FN 3d; Piotrowski J; Bernhard VM; Pond GD; Pabst TS 3d; Bull DA; Hunter GC; McIntyre KE. J Cardiovasc Surg 1991; 32: 680–689.

Intraarterial urokinase (IAUK) was administered to 33 patients on 40 occasions for the treatment of acute extremity ischemia and long-term patency was assessed. Lysis was successful in 39 of the 40 cases (95%). Occlusive thrombus was cleared in 12 of 13 patients with native artery occlusion (7 complete, 5 partial), 8 of 9 with autologous vein grafts (5 complete, 3 partial), and in all 18 patients with synthetic grafts (17 complete, 1 partial). The primary cumulative patency following successful IAUK was 100% for native arteries and 47% for synthetic grafts at 12 months, and 23% for autologous grafts at 9 months. The difference in rethrombosis rate between autologous vein (67%) and native artery (0%) was significant (p = 0.02) as was the difference betwen infrainguinal prosthetic grafts (63%) and native artery (p = 0.025). IAUK is most effective for the treatment of native artery occlusion, but is significantly less effective for thrombosed infrainguinal autologous vein or synthetic grafts due to the likelihood of reocclusion, despite the high immediate success rate. For autologous vein grafts, lysis is frequently incomplete and patency rapidly deteriorates regardless of adjunctive therapy to relieve the underlying obstruction.

Immediate post-operative urokinase infusion: extending the limits of limb salvage surgery.
Perler BA; Osterman FA. J Cardiovasc Surg (Torino) 1990; 31: 184–188.

We report the case of a 74-year-old woman with multi-level arterial occlusive disease and severe ischemia of the right lower extremity who underwent a re-operative femoro-femoral and a right femoro-popliteal bypass graft. Her right foot remained non-viable post-operatively despite patent grafts. She then underwent a 12-hour infusion of urokinase through a percutaneously placed popliteal artery catheter during that first post-operative day, with salvage of the right leg.

[Results of in situ arterial thrombolysis by the combination of urokinase and lysyl plasminogen in acute arterial occlusive disease of the lower limbs] Resultats de la thrombolyse arterielle in situ par association urokinase-lysyl plasminogene dans les obliterations arterielles aigues des membres inferieurs.
Pernes JM; Brenot P; Raynaud A; Parola JL; Roth JP; Angel CY; Vitoux JF; Fiessinger JN; Roncato M; Gaux JC. J Radiol 1985; 66: 385–391.

35 patients with acute arterial occlusions [27] and graft thromboses [8], responsible for severe and recent ischemia, were treated by fibrinolytic therapy (Urokinase: 1,000 units/kg/hour, and Lys Plasminogen). These drugs were delivered at the site of occlusions using a 5 French catheter. Angiographically, initial success was obtained in 30 patients (85%) and a significant clinical benefit persisted 5 months later, in 20 patients (57%). 4 distal embolisms during the treatment were noted, and one woman died a few hours after the withdrawal of an axillary catheter of a cerebellar infarction. Only two minor (6%) and one severe (3%) groin hematoma were encoun-

tered. No patient had at any moment a fibrinogen concentration lower than 1 g/l. Thus, the thrombolytic treatment used in the study appears as effective as locally administered Streptokinase but better tolerated.

Local thrombolysis in peripheral arteries and bypass grafts.
Pernes JM; de Almeida Augusto M; Vitoux JF; Raynaud A; Fiessinger JN; Brenot P; Fabiani JN; Murday A; Gaux JC. J Vasc Surg 1987; 6: 372–378.

Sixty-two patients hospitalized for recent angiographically documented arterial occlusion in the legs (46 femoropopliteal arteries and i6 grafts) benefited from local fibrinolytic therapy delivered at the site of the occlusion with a No. 4F or No. 5F catheter. This therapy combined a continuous urokinase (UK) infusion of 1000 U/kg/hr and a lysyl plasminogen (LYS-PLG) infusion of 15 mukat every 30 minutes. Angiographically confirmed lysis was obtained in 77% of the cases. Five percent of the patients had major and 8% had minor groin hematomas. Only two patients had concentrations of fibrinogen as low as 100 mg/dl. Intravascular infusion of UK and LYS-PLG is as effective as streptokinase but produces lower systemic fibrinolysis. However, local fibrinolysis remains a potentially hazardous procedure (10% suffered major complications) and must only be applied to patients with severe ischemia and little or no possibility of surgical intervention.

Acute peripheral arterial and graft occlusion: treatment with selective infusion of urokinase and lysyl plasminogen.
Pernes JM; Vitoux JF; Brenoit P; Raynaud A; Parola JL; Roth JP; Angel CY; Fiessinger JN; Roncato M; Gaux JC. Radiology 1986; 158: 481–485.

Thirty-five patients hospitalized for recent angiographically documented arterial occlusion in the legs (27 femoropopliteal arteries and eight grafts) benefited from local fibrinolytic therapy delivered at the site of the occlusion with a 4- or 5-F catheter. This therapy combined a continuous urokinase (UK) infusion of 1,000 U/kg/hour and a lysyl plasminogen (LYS-PLG) infusion pf 15 microkatals every 30 minutes. Angiographically confirmed lysis was obtained in 85% of the cases. Only 3% of the patients had major and 6% had minor groin hematomas. Only two patients had concentrations of fibrinogen as low as 100 mg/dl. Intravascular infusion of UK-LYS-PLG is as effective as streptokinase. Its excellent tolerance makes it a good alternative in the treatment of acute ischemia in the lower limbs.

Late results of local thrombolytic treatment of peripheral arterial occlusions.
Poredos P; Keber D; Videcnik V. Angiology 1989; 40: 941–947.

One hundred thirty-four patients, in whom acute and subacute arterial occlusions of lower limbs were treated with low dose intraarterial streptokinase, were observed for periods of up to five years. Primary recanalization of occluded vessels was achieved in 66 patients, but in the remaining 68 patients recanalization was not observed. In 45% of the patients with successful thrombolytic treatment, percutaneous dilatation (PTA) of remnant stenosis was performed. In patients with successful recanalization the reocclusion rate was greatest in the first year (17.4%); the first two weeks after therapy were most critical in this respect. The reocclusion rate during the succeeding years ranged from 4% to 9% per year. The cumulative patency rate after five years was 63.4%. Late results were better in patients in whom more proximal vascular segments were affected. The preservation of vessel patency was highly dependent on the severity and extent of the previous atherosclerotic process and especially on the state of peripheral (runoff) arteries. Presence of diabetes mellitus increased the reocclusion rate of recanalized vessels. Of the patients with unsuccessful recanalization, only 5 reported some symptomatic improvement during the observation period, 39 (57%) needed immediate amputation, and an additional 8 (4.7%) were amputated later on. Considering the fact that all patients were previously refused for bypass surgery owing to unsuitable runoff vessels or bad general condition, the long-term results were surprisingly good, suggesting that thrombolytic treatment, combined in remnant stenosis with PTA, was an efficient method in patients with acute or subacute arterial occlusions.

Thrombolytic therapy in acute arterial thrombosis.
Price C; Jacocks MA; Tytle T. Am J Surg 1988; 156: 488–491.

The courses of 17 patients who underwent 20 separate attempts at thrombolysis for acute arterial thrombosis are reviewed to clarify the safety and efficacy of this therapy. Seventeen of 20 thrombolyses were angiographically successful. Patients who had correctable lesions identified and reconstructive procedures performed tended to do better than those who did not, and patients who had successful thrombolysis tended to have fewer and less radical amputations. Complications can be reduced by careful, close monitoring of patients undergoing therapy.

Use and limitations of thrombolytic therapy in the treatment of peripheral arterial ischemia: results of a multi-institutional questionnaire.
Ricotta JJ; Green RM; DeWeese JA. J Vasc Surg 1987; 6: 45–50.

In an attempt to assess the efficacy of thrombolytic infusions for arterial ischemia, a questionnaire was distributed to 142 vascular surgeons. Data from 45 respondents who had experience with thrombolytic infusion in 623 patients were reviewed. A successful outcome was obtained in 313 of 623 patients (50.2%). Morbidity was significant. with hemorrhage requiring transfusion or operation in 125 cases (20.1%) and major amputation in 103 cases (16.5%). There were nine strokes associated with thrombolytic infusion (1.4%), six of which were fatal. Sixteen deaths were associated with thrombolytic therapy, for a mortality rate of 2.5% (16 of 623 patients). Analysis of results by grouping centers according to numbers of lytic infusions failed to show significant correlation with center experience. Furthermore, morbidity and mortality were seen in centers with both limited and extensive experience with thrombolytic infusion. The initial enthusiasm for thrombolytic infusion to treat arterial ischemia is not substantiated by our data. Carefully controlled prospective trials are needed before this method can be offered as an alternative to arterial reconstruction.

Recombinant human tissue-type plasminogin activator for thrombolysis in peripheral arteries and bypass grafts.
Risius B; Graor RA; Geisinger MA; Zelch MG; Lucas FV; Young JR; Grossbard EB. Radiology 1986; 160: 183–188.

Recombinant human tissue-type plasminogen activator (rt-PA) was infused intraarterially at 0.1 mg/kg/h for 1–6 ½ hours in 25 patients with lower extremity thromboembolic occlusions (13 thrombosed arteries, 12 thrombosed bypass grafts). Occlusion duration ranged from 1 hour to 21 days. Thrombolysis occurred in 23 of 25 patients (92%). Time to lysis varied from 1 to 6.5 hours, with an average time of 3.6 hours. Twenty of 23 patients (87%) in whom thrombolysis was successful benefited clinically from thrombolytic therapy. Twelve of 23 patients (52%) required secondary procedures to maintain arterial segment patency. In 15 of 25 patients (60%) fibrinogen levels were maintained above 50% of baseline values. No major complications directly attributable to rt-PA infusions occurred. rt-PA is a potent, relatively fibrin-specific thrombolytic agent that can achieve rapid thrombolysis while usually avoiding the profound systemic fibrinogenolysis associated with currently available thrombolytic agents.

[Interventional radiologic procedures in complete occlusions of long stretches of the iliac artery] Interventionell-radiologisches Vorgehen bei langer-streckigen kompletten Beckenarterienverschlussen.
Rominger MB; Rauber K; Matthes B; Schulz A; Rau WS. ROFO 1991; 154: 310–314.

15 completely occluded iliac arteries (five cases of 10 cm, 8 cases between 5 and 10 cm and two cases below 5 cm) were reviewed for their interventional management, technical results and complications. The procedure was successful in 14 of 15 cases (93%). In six cases we performed local thrombolysis before PTA. In the patient group with "only PTA" the treatment had to be abandoned in one case because of the risk of embolism. Two patients suffered from a distal embolism of the same side and one patient from an ipsi- and contralateral embolism. A stent implantation was necessary in one patient. In the group of patients with prior local thrombolysis there was no complication nor was there an indication for a stent-implantation. Hence, we conclude that a primary local lysis with a consecutive PTA is an appropriate treatment of complete long occlusions of the iliac artery.

[Local lysis therapy in acute arterial thrombosis] Lokale Lysetherapie bei akuter arterieller Thrombose.
Roth FJ; Rieser R; Scheffler A. Langenbecks Arch Chir 1990; 427–434.

Acute thrombotic arterial occlusion is a complication of chronic vascular arterial disease. The arteriogram usually reveals a sudden occlusion and the collateral vessels. Treatment with low-dose fibrinolytic therapy is widely accepted. A combination of low-dose fibrinolysis, aspiration embolectomy and angioplasty yields the best primary success rate. In cases of sudden popliteal occlusion and dilating arteriopathy ultrasound sonography should be used to exclude the presence aneurysm which is a contraindication for fibrinolysis. There is a high risk of peripheral embolisation, in the presence of an aneurysm and this may cause severe deterioration of the arterial blood supply. (17 Refs.)

[Fibrinolytic therapy of peripheral arterial occlusive disease] Die fibrinolytische Therapie bei peripherer arterieller Verschlu sskrankheit.
Sailer S; Pilger E Wien Med Wochenschr 1985; 135: 393–399.

Occluded arterial segments can be recanalized by fibrinolytic drugs. In addition to systemic fibrinolysis another method of thrombolytic therapy has been established: Local thrombolytic therapy is carried out by infiltration of low dose of streptokinase into the thrombotic occlusion. According to the low dose streptokinase used and the short duration of therapy local thrombolysis is applicable in patients with high risks too. Therefore the range of indications to non-surgical recanalisations could be extended. The differential therapy depends on location, pathogenesis and clinical stage of the arterial occlusion.

Popliteal artery occlusion caused by cystic adventitial disease: successful treatment by urokinase followed by nonresectional cystotomy.
Samson RH; Willis PD. J Vasc Surg 1990; 12: 591–593.

Preoperative diagnosis of an occluded popliteal artery caused by cystic adventitial disease allowed use of urokinase to successfully dissolve secondary thrombosis. Subsequent non-resectional adventitial cystotomy and evacuation of cyst contents allowed lasting restoration of a patent arterial lumen and return of normal distal pulses. This nongrafting technique may serve as a model for future patients with occluded arteries caused by this condition.

Femoropopliteal stent placement: long-term results.
Sapoval MR; Slong AL; Raynaud AC; Beyssen BM; Fiessinger JN; Gaux JC. Radiology 1992; 184(3): 833–839.

Twenty-one patients who underwent percutaneous transluminal angioplasty (PTA) followed by attempted insertion of a self-expandable vascular endoprosthesis for femoropopliteal lesions were prospectively followed up for an average of 17.6 months with angiographic, Doppler ultrasound, and clinical examinations. Stents were placed bilaterally in one patient. Of the 22 lesions, 18 were total occlusions and four, stenoses. Stent placement was successful in 21 of 22 lesions. Nine occlusions occurred: for in the first 30 days and five 1–5 months after PTA. Three patients developed intrastent intimal hyperplasia that necessitated an additional percutaneous procedure. At 12 months, the patency rate without other interventions (the primary patency rate) was 49%. In patients who underwent secondary intervention (fibrinolysis, atherectomy, or PTA), the secondary patency rate was 67%, which fell to 56% after 18 months. At the end of the study, the overall rate of reocclusion was 43%. It is concluded that use of the self-expandable vascular endoprosthesis in the femoropopliteal region likely does not decrease the reocclusion rate after PTA alone. Its use is indicated for treatment of acute closures after femoropopliteal PTA.

[Local fibrinolytic therapy of vascular occlusions in the pelvic-leg area and the upper extremity] Lokale Fibrinolysetherapie von Gefassverschlussen im Becken-Bein-Bereich und der oberen Extremitat.
Schild H; Schuster CJ; Gronniger J; Schmied W; Weilemann L; Lindner P; Wagner P; Brunier A; Thelen M; Meyer J. ROFO 1987; 146: 57–62.

Seventy-three patients with vascular occlusions in the pelvis or lower limbs and three patients with upper limb lesions were treated by local low dose fibrinolysin, with strict control of any possible bleeding tendencies. Adequate recanalisation was obtained in 56 patients (73.6%). In ten patients, the occlusion recurred while the patient was still in hospital. After four to six months, 37 of the 56 (67%) of the vessels were still patent. In 18 patients, peripheral emboli resulted in some deterioration, but in 15 of these cases this could be treated successfully by operation. The methods and indications of local fibrinolysis therapy and the problems associated with it are discussed.

Thrombolytic therapy for acute arterial occlusion.
Sicard GA; Schier JJ; Totty WG; Gilula LA; Walker WB; Etheredge EE; Anderson CB. J Vasc Surg 1985; 2: 65–78.

To evaluate the role of selective intra-arterial low-dose thrombolytic therapy (SILDT) as an alternative to the surgical management of acute arterial occlusion, the hospital records of 40 patients who underwent 43 SILDT treatments with either streptokinase (36) or urokinase (7) between December 1979 and March 1984 were reviewed. Twenty-eight patients underwent 30 treatments (group 1) for native arterial occlusion and 12 patients underwent 13 treatments (group 2) for prosthetic or autogenous graft occlusions. Therapy was deemed successful if subsequent surgical therapy was obviated. In group 1, SILDT was successful in 13 of 28 (45%) patients with 12 of 25 lower extremity occlusions and one of three upper extremity occlusions. Successful lysis in the native artery occlusion group fell into three categories: five patients were successfully treated for arterial thrombosis complicating percutaneous transluminal angioplasty (PTA); four patients required PTA after complete lysis revealed an underlying arterial stenosis; and only three required no further therapy after SILDT. SILDT failed in all three patients with the aortoiliac occlusions. Eleven patients with femoral artery occlusions and unsuccessful SILDT required six bypass procedures, three amputations, one embolectomy, and one PTA. In group 2 only 3 of 14 treatments (21%) were successful. Bypass revision was not possible in 11 patients and all required amputation. Systemic fibrinolysis was seen in 20 (59%) of 34 patients with available data. Neither fibrinogen levels nor fibrin degradation products predicted the occurrence of complications. Minor complications occurred in 18 of 43 (43%) treatments; small hematomas at the catheter entry site were most common. Minor complications occurred in 20 of 43 treatments (44%) and included severe local hemorrhage (four), distant bleeding (three), pulmonary embolism (four), myocardial infarction (three), unmasking of an aortoduodenal fistula (one), and clot migration requiring emergency thrombectomy (four). SILDT is most effective in acute arterial thrombosis complicating arteriography or percutaneous angioplasty. It may play a role in the patient in whom thrombolysis can reveal an underlying stenosis amenable to percutaneous angioplasty. This experience shows SILDT to be of limited value in the management of prosthetic autogenous graft occlusions. Finally, thrombolytic therapy is associated with significant morbidity and mortality rates and requires cautious monitoring to detect arterial thrombus migration, worsening tissue ischemia, venous thromboembolism, intracerebral hemorrhage, and local or systemic bleeding.

Local thrombolysis in arterial occlusive disease.
Slany J; Enzenhofer V; Karnik R. Angiology 1984; 35: 231–237.

In a series of 38 subjects intra-arterial catheters were used to infuse streptokinase (SK) or urokinase (UK) just proximal to an acute thromboembolic occlusion in 20 limbs or to perfuse SK directly into the obstructing material in 23 extremities with subacute or chronic occlusions by stepwise advancing the catheter until the distal open segment of the artery was reached. Dosage of SK varied between 50.000 U and 400.000 U and was administered during 1 to 4 hours. Patency could be achieved in 16 out of 20 acute occlusions and in 16 out of 23 chronically obstructed vessels within same hours. A systemic hyperlytic state of 12 to 24 hours duration was observed when total dosage of SK exceeded 80.000 U. In 9 patients thrombolysis was immediately followed by angioplasty. Advantage of the described technique is its rapid effectiveness, low cost, high success rate even in chronic femoro-popliteal occlusions and its applicability to patients in whom systemic thrombolysis would be considered contraindicated on account of old age or other causes.

Low-dose fibrinolytic therapy for recent lower extremity thromboembolism.
Sniderman KW; Kalman PG; Odurny A; Shewchun J; Glynn MF. Can Assoc Radiol J 1989; 40: 98–103.

Low-dose catheter-directed fibrinolytic therapy (LDCF) using streptokinase (35) and urokinase (7) was performed on 42 separate occasions in 36 patients for recent lower extremity thromboembolic occlusion. Twenty-seven grafts and 15 native arteries were treated. Causes of occlusion were known in 32 instances: native artery proximal or distal occlusive disease or both (18 vessels); bypass graft stenosis (6); aneurysm (2); embolus (4); and postangiography thrombosis (2). Twenty-nine infusions were technically successful, and patients were clinically improved by 26 of the treatments. Twelve patients had unsuccessful infusions and six underwent subsequent amputation. In all patients, infusions longer than 12 hours resulted in prolonged thrombin times and lowered plasma fibrinogen concentrations; one infusion was discontinued due to a low fibrinogen concentration. Complications occurred on 17 occasions and included hemorrhage (6), distal embolization (3), compartment syndrome (1), retrograde thrombosis during infusion (5), hypotension (1), and systemic fibrinogenolysis (1). The cumulative success rate was 44% +/- 9% at 24 months. Late rethrombosis (five instances) was more common in patients who had inflow or outflow structural lesions not corrected following successful fibrinolysis. LDCF is a useful alternative to other methods of treatment for recent onset lower extremity thromboembolic occlusion. Structural vascular lesions uncovered by successful infusion should be corrected immediately after infusion to ensure long-term patency.

Selective streptokinase fibrinolysis in femoro-iliac arterial obstruction.
Sorensen K; Hegedus V. Acta Radiol 1986; 27: 279–283.

Percutaneous transluminal angioplasty of iliac and femoral arteries was in 17 patients combined with selective intra-arterial streptokinase treatment. The patients were divided into two groups, one given low dose long-term therapy and the other high dose short-term therapy. The experiences obtained during an observation period of over one year revealed greater benefit from high dose short-term therepy. It seems that the major cause of compllcations must be attributed to the development of a high level of streptokinase antibodies during low dose long-term therapy.

[Results of local thrombolysis with special reference to diabetic metabolism] Ergebnisse der lokalen Thrombolyse unter besonderer Berucksichtigung einer diabetischen Stoffwechsellage.
Stiegler H; Hufen V; Weichenhain B; Standl E; Mehnert H III. Med Klin 1990; 85: 171–175, 228.

The influence of diabetes on the primary and long-term success rate after 145 local thrombolyses in peripheral arterial disease stages III and IV was evaluated. 75 patients suffered from thrombotic, 62 patients from embolic occlusions, with eight patients suffering from thrombangitis obliterans. Regarding the localisation of vascular occlusion 0.6% suffered under an occlusion of the iliacal artery, 21% of the femoral artery, 16% of the popliteal artery, 7% of the vessel of the lower limb and 55.4% showed a combined occlusion of the femoral- and popliteal artery and the artery of the lower limb. In cases of embolic occlusions only marginal differences could be observed, while the primary success-rate of thrombotic occlusions showed greater differences between both groups (75% vs. 91%). During the follow-up, no differences between both groups could be established (patency-rate of 79% for both groups). The same applies to the prognostic factors: peripheral run off, length, duration of occlusion and the clinical stage (Fontaine IIb to IV). The remarkable differences between diabetic and non-diabetic patients in cases of occlusions of more than 16 cm (66% vs. 88% in primary and 55% vs. 77% in long-term success) can be explained by the high percentage of diabetic patients with poor run-off and microangiopathy. Regarding the above parameters, primary and long-term results seems to be less in diabetic patients, even though a long-term patency could be observed in 2/3 of diabetic patients in stages IIb and IV with primary success.

Clinical aspects and treatment of acute arterial occlusion.
Stirnemann P; Z'Brun AP; Mahler F Schweiz. Med Wochenschr 1988; 118: 1767–1772.

163 patients underwent surgery for acute ischemia of the lower extremity between 1982 and 1986. Thrombosis was present in 50 cases and embolism in 113. Half of the patients with thrombosis showed signs of chronic occlusive disease of the arteries (intermittent claudication); in the latter group 2/3 of the patients had atrial fibrillation and 1/4 coronary heart disease. For embolism Fogarty-catheter clot extraction was performed, mainly under

local anesthesia. This procedure is easy to perform even under emergency conditions (mortality 10%, amputation rate 8%). In contrast, the surgical procedure in thrombotic occlusion was more demanding (mortality 4%, amputation rate 16%) and in the case of severe ischemia had to be carried out on an emergency basis. In case of less severe ischemia the treatment consisted in initial heparinization and elective revascularization when the patient was stabilized. A new therapeutic approach involving local catheter thrombolysis, catheter clot aspiration and balloon dilatation is presented. The combined catheter intervention produces good results in 70% of patients, particularly those with femoral thrombosis

Improved patient selection for enzymatic lysis of peripheral arterial and graft occlusion.
Sussman B; Dardik H; Ibrahim IM; Fox R; Mendes D; Kahn M. Am J Surg 1984; 148: 244–248.

Intraarterial thrombolysis by remote intravenous or direct intraarterial infusion of streptokinase is possible. The latter may be more effective with a lesser potential for systemic hemorrhagic complications because of the smaller dose administered directly in the area. Fifty patients with prosthetic graft, embolic, and renal artery occlusions were evaluated. Embolic occlusion responded dramatically, particularly since lytic therapy was initiated at an early stage. Patients with severe ischemia or those with simple localized occlusion were best treated by surgical means. Successful thrombolysis was also obtained with renal artery occlusions combined with percutaneous transluminal angioplasty. The management of patients with prosthetic graft occlusion by lytic therapy is complex. Optimal results can be obtained in patients presenting with occluded grafts after the immediate postoperative period and in those in whom previous satisfactory runoff has been demonstrated. Failure of lysis in this group is associated with a high incidence of limb loss due to unreconstructable obliterative disease. Successful lysis of occluded prosthetic grafts will often require corrective angioplasty or surgical revision.

Short–term intrathrombotic injection of ultrahigh–dose urokinase for treatment of iliac and femoropopliteal artery occlusions.
Terada M; Satoh M; Mitsuzane K; Shioyoyama Y; Tsuda M; Kishi K; Maeda M; Momura S; Yamada R. Radiat Med 1990; 8: 79–87.

Thirty-two patients with iliac and femoropopliteal artery occlusions were treated with direct intrathrombotic injection of ultrahigh-dose urokinase (10,000 IU/min). Occlusions ranged from 3 to 25 cm (average 13.3 cm) in length and the total urokinase dose from 120,000 to 1,410,000 IU (average 688,000 IU). The procedure was usually followed by balloon angioplasty to dilate the underlying stenoses. The initial recanalization rate was 96.9%, the two week patency rate 81.3%, and the cumulative one-year patency rate 66.3%. Complications associated with this procedure included three episodes of minimal bleeding, two distal embolisms, one local hematoma, and one low-grade fever. All were well controlled by palliative treatment. Results indicate that this procedure can provide rapid recanalization at a higher success rate with fewer complications than previously reported.

Therapy of atherosclerotic arteriopathy of lower limbs. Aspects and results.

Tesi M; Bronchi GF; Carini A; Karavassili M. Angiology 1985; 36: 720–735.

As far as therapy is concerned, atherosclerotic arteriopathy may be divided into acute and chronic forms. In acute embolic forms, therapy should be surgical. Only in casee of peripheral embolism or polyembolism, and in rare cases for which vascular surgery cannot be adopted, can thrombolysis be carried out with UK. In acute thrombotic forms, therapy should be medical, because a thrombus of reccnt formation is rich in fibrin and may be lyzed by UK. Total recanalization takes place in 61% of cases treated, partial recanalization in 23%. Subsequently perviousness is maintained by adequate antithrombotic therapy. In chronic arteriopathy, the thrombus is lacking or almost lacking in fibrin and thrombolytic therapy is not indacated. Special therapeutic combinations are used containing platelet inhibitors (ticlopidine), antifibrin drugs (subcutaneous heparin), minor fibrinolytic agents (mesoglycan) and hemorheological drugs (pentoxyphylline). This therapy seams to give good results, as showed by the low percentage in amputation calculated on 2,565 patients treated and kept under observation for 5 years. Finally let us consider chronic progressive arteriopathy. This term indicates a very advanced stage, characterized by a gradual irreversible change for the worse leading towards gangrene. As a last resort, before amputating, a thrombolytic therapy with UK was tried to see if with strong fibrinolysis continued for 3 days amputation might be avoided. In a pilot study carried out on 12 patients, the angiographic data showed only partial lysis in small arteries or arterial branches. Clinical data showed reduction or disappearance of pain at rest in 80% of cases. In 70% of cases gangrene disappeared if it was initial and superficial, it was delimited if already in progress

Effectiveness of intraarterial plasminogen application in combination with percutaneous transluminal angioplasty (PTA) or catheter assisted lysis (CL) in patients with chronic peripheral occlusive disease of the lower limbs (POL).

Tilsner V; Witte G. Haemostasis 1988; 18(Suppl 1): 139–156.

The accepted correct procedure for treating occlusive arterial diseases includes surgical disobstruction, CL as well as PTA. Combined non-surgical strategies are effective in about 60% of these patients. However, a high risk of rethrombosis despite from the prophylaxis with anticoagulants like heparin or antiplatelet drugs like ASA is proven, especially in patients with multi-segmental stenosis as well as in patients with extensive narrowing of the arteries. In these cases primary lesions (endangitis obliterans) or secondary lesions of the endothelium cause local depletion of plasminogen in the endothelium. Independent of the method used for reopening the vessel in these patients, a significant progression of the vessel disease and a high rethrombosis rate during longterm follow-up is observed. These results lead us to apply plasminogen locally to decresse the rate of rethrombosis. In patients suffering from stage III-IV (La Fontaine) including patients with multi-segmental stenosis as well as extended narrowing of the artery, PTA in combination with CL was performed. The catheter was placed as near as possible to the thrombus. In some cases the 'fibrinolyticum' could be injected directly into the thrombus. In these cases a bolus of 4,000 U/ml was locally infused, otherwise 1.0–1.5 million U urokinase per 24 hrs. were locally infused with heparin. In 28% (22 patients) no sufficient clinical response occurred using this combined therapy and plasminogen was applied locally. The following criteria supported our decision to include the patients in this study: 1. Insufficient response occurring after 12–24 hrs. of local infusion. 2. Following 6 bolus injections no reopening of the vessel occured within 60 minutes or the clinical response was insufficient due to rethrombosis. 3. Insufficient effects of lysis therapy after 2 hours and contraindication for a systemic fibrinolytic therapy (e.g. hypertension, age, etc.). 1,000 U plasminogen per ml were infused locally or 2,000 U up to 5,000 U plasminogen (in 5 to 10 ml 0.9% saline) were infused slowly (2–4 minutes infusion time) into the catheter in these patients 10 minutes after unsuccessful treatment with local urokinase therapy. Five minutes after administering plasminogen local intraarterial fibrinolytic therapy with urokinase was continued. No severe side effects due to this therapy were observed, although some patients suffered from acute pains in the peripheral segments of the arteries occurring immediately after infusion of plasminogen. In 16 of 22 patients a complete recanalization occurred and in 3 patients a satisfying clinical improvement was observed. (ABSTRACT TRUNCATED AT 400 WORDS)

Femoro-popliteal artery occlusions treated by percutaneous transluminal angioplasty and enclosed thrombolysis: results in 55 patients.
Tonnesen KH; Holstein P; Andersen E. Eur J Vasc Surg 1991; 5: 429–434.

Removal of fibrin from the site of a newly dilated femoro-popliteal occlusion may be an attractive way of preventing rethrombosis. A double balloon catheter with a dilating tip balloon and an occlusive balloon 10, 15 or 20 cm approximately were introduced percutaneously. Following successful dilatation of femoro-popliteal occlusions, the balloons were inflated on both sides of the lesion. The dilated segment was then isolated from the circulation. Through a sideport between the balloons 5 mg of tissue type plasminogen activator and 1000 IU of heparin were installed within the segment for 30 min. The authors report the results of 53 technically successful dilatations of femoro-popliteal occlusions followed by enclosed thrombolysis. A 100% patency at 3 months was noted in 33 patients having one to three run-off arteries, and the one year patency was 90%. In 20 patients, with no infrapopliteal run-off artery, four rethrombosis occurred within 24 h, and the one year patency was 62%. This difference is significant. (Log rank test, Chi-square = 4.73, p less than 0.05). We conclude that enclosed thrombolysis prevents early reocclusion following PTA of femoro-popliteal occlusions provided that at least one infra-popliteal artery is patent.

Intra-arterial urokinase infusion in diabetic patients with rapidly progressive ischemic foot lesions.
Vannini P; Ciavarella A; Mustacchio A; Rossi C. Diabetes Care 1991; 14: 925–927.

OBJECTIVE: The effectiveness of local intra-arterial thrombolysis by urokinase was evaluated in eight non-insulin-dependent diabetic patients with angiographic evidence of infrapopliteal occlusive disease and rapidly progressive foot lesions. RESEARCH DESIGN AND METHODS: With an electric peristatic pump, urokinase was infused for 96 h by a 5–6 F catheter introduced into the femoral artery and placed immediately above the occluded infrapopliteal arteries. After baseline, angiography was repeated at 24- to 48-h intervals and at conclusion of the treatment. RESULTS: Six patients showed immediate improvement of clinical symptoms. Angiography revealed the reestablishment of blood flow in collateral vessels of the leg and foot in the dorsal pedal artery in three patients and in the plantar arch in two. Recanalization of the major arteries of the trifurcation was not achieved. After 12 mo of follow-up, all limbs were salvaged, although four patients required vascular reconstruction to further improve foot perfusion and complete healing. CONCLUSIONS: Intra-arterial urokinase, which opens collateral and smaller vessels of the leg and foot in patients with diabetes, may be effective in improving blood flow in lower extremities and in making the patient a better candidate for vascular surgery.

A protocol for the safe treatment of acute lower limb ischaemia with intra-arterial streptokinase and surgery.
Walker WJ; Giddings AE. Br J Surg 1988; 75: 1189–1192.

Over a 5-year period 70 patients, presenting with subacute ischaemia of the lowwr limb (more than 12 h), were treated with low-dose intra-arterial streptokinase. There were 72 infusions and effective lysis was achieved in 52 (72 per cent), with an average infusion time of 25 h. A total of 23 (32 per cent) also underwent percutaneous transluminal angioplasty when lysis showed an underlying stenosis, and a further 19 (26 per cent) required surgery to remove persistent stenosis, organized thrombus or atheromatous debris. Significant bleeding occurred in 4 patients (6 per cent) and 13 (18 per cent) underwent ampututution. There were five deaths (7 per cent), one of which was directly related to the infusion, while three were due to myocardial infarction. All of the major complications occurred in the early part of the study and both the selection of patients and the technique of infusion were modified to improve safety. Complementary treatment by percutaneous transluminal angioplasty and surgery was used more frequently in the later part of the study. The technique is not recommended for the white leg of acute ischaemia (less than 12 h), or for lysis of clot in a retroperitoneal Dacron great, but may be uniquely valuable to demonstrate the cause of subacute ischaemia.

Left ventricular thromboembolic occlusion of the popliteal artery treated nonoperatively with local urokinase infusion—a case report.
Weisman ID; Stanchfield WR Jr; Herzog CA; Ney AL; Blake DP. Angiology 1988; 39: 179–186.

Recently streptokinase and urokinase have been shown to be useful in the nonoperative treatment of thromboembolic disease. Urokinase is emerging as a safer and more effective thrombolytic agent when applied either to definitively lyse spontaneous thrombosis where no underlying structural lesion is present or to serve as an adjunct prior to surgical reconstruction or transluminal angioplasty. The authors report a case of a high-risk cardiac patient in whom an embolic occlusion of the distal popliteal artery was completely recanalized by using a localized catheter infusion of urokinase. The source of the embolus was a left ventricular thrombus. No serious bleeding or proximal or distal embolic complications occurred. The potential hazards of fragmentation of the embolic source in the presence of systemic thrombolysis, distal trifurcation embolization, and concomitant use of heparin are reviewed.

Fibrinolytic therapy for femoral arterial thrombosis after cardiac catheterization in infants and children.
Wessel DL; Keane JF; Fellows KE; Robichaud H; Lock JE. Am J Cardiol 1986; 58: 347–351.

The charts of 79 patients who required femoral arterial (FA) thrombectomy after cardiac catheterization were reviewed. Fifteen patients (19%) had poor pulses after thrombectomy and 2 had an extremity amputated. One thousand consecutive patients undergoing cardiac catheterization were also studied to prospectively determine the safety and efficacy of systemic fibrinolytic therapy for treatment of FA thrombosis. Among these, 771 patients underwent retrograde arterial catheterization, including 31 patients with left-sided obstructive lesions who had undergone transarterial balloon dilation procedures with large catheters. All patients were given heparin at the time of arterial cannulation. Patients who had a pulseless extremity 4 hours after catheterization continued to receive heparin therapy for 24 to 48 hours. If the extremity continued to have no palpable pulse and the systolic blood pressure was less than 50% of that in the contralateral leg, intravenous streptokinase infusion was begun. The overall incidence of FA thrombosis was 3.6% (28 of 771), including 39% (12 of 31) of all patients undergoing transarterial balloon dilation procedures; 97% (27 of 28) of patients weighed less than 14 kg and the majority weighed less than 10 kg. After an average treatment period of 33 hours, 16 patients continued to have a pulseless extremity and were treated with streptokinase for an average duration of 13 hours. Normal pulses and systolic blood pressure returned in 14 (88%) and were nearly normal in 1 other patient (6%). The incidence of bleeding at the arterial puncture site was 25% and was highest in the patients who had a transarterial balloon dilation procedure. No serious complications occurred.

Increased limb salvage with intraoperative and postoperative ankle level urokinase infusion in acute lower extremity ischemia.
Wyffels PL; DeBord JR; Marshall JS; Thors G; Marshall WH. J Vasc Surg 1992; 15(5): 771–778; discussion 778–779.

Over a 30-month period (May 1988 to November 1990) 143 acutely ischemic lower extremities (126 patients) were treated with an aggressive surgical approach that included ankle level tibial-peroneal artery thromboembolectomy. Twelve lower extremities in 10 patients that remained ischemic were further treated with adjuvant ankle level urokinase infusion. Sixteen ankle level arteries in 12 extremities were infused with an intraoperative bolus (1 to 2) of urokinase (50,000 to 100,000 units). Continuous postoperative urokinase (25,000 to 50,000 units per catheter per hour $\times$ 1 to 5 days) was infused through ankle level arteriotomies in 10 extremities (14 arteries) that did not improve with the initial intraoperative bolus. Concomitant bypass grafting was necessary in four extremities. With adequate inflow established, adjuvant ankle level urokinase salvaged all 12 extremities. The mean increase in ankle/brachial pressure index was 0.84. During continuous postoperative urokinase infusion, lower extremity bleeding requiring blood transfusion occurred in four patients (50%). No deaths occurred in the operative period. Although rhabdomyolysis occurred in 90% of patients, no patients had renal insufficiency. The addition of ankle level urokinase delivery increased the potential limb salvage from 90% of the entire 143 extremities treated during this period to an actual limb salvage of 98%. A mean follow up of 13 months (6 to 36 months) identified one late amputation. Despite the demanding postoperative management required in these patients and the frequent need for early reoperation, the limb salvage obtained justifies this aggressive adjuvant technique in the management of the acutely ischemic lower extremity.

II. Synopses of Pertinent Articles

B. Bypass Grafts: Aortic, Infrainguinal

Observations on the use of thrombolytic agents for thrombotic occlusion of infrainguinal vein grafts.
Belkin M; Donaldson MC; Whittemore AD; Polak JF; Grassi CJ; Harrington DP; Mannick JA. J Vasc Surg 1990; 11: 289–296.

Vein graft failure remains a major challenge for the vascular surgeon. Thrombolysis of occluded vein grafts has shown promising short-term results in restoring vein graft patency, however, the long-term results are not established. This study examines the long-term patency and limb salvage after successful thrombolysis and revision of 22 thrombosed vein grafts in 21 patients. There were 17 men and four women with an average age of 60 years (38 to 77 years). Failed vein grafts had an average primary patency of 19 months (1 to 84 months) and included eight in situ grafts and 14 non-in situ grafts. Twelve grafts were to the popliteal level, whereas 10 were infrapopliteal. Thrombolytic agents used included urokinase (15), tissue plasminogen activator (5), and streptokinase (2). After successful thrombolysis, 19 grafts underwent 26 additional procedures including percutaneous transluminal angioplasty (9), vein patch angioplasty (4), vein interposition or jump extension graft (9), or other procedures (4). Three patients had no additional procedure, but one was placed on sodium warfarin (Coumadin). After successful initial vein graft salvage, life-table analysis revealed a 36.6% +/- 11.9% patency at 1 year and a 22.9% +/- 11.6% patency at 3 years. After secondary failure six patients had further interventions contributing to an improved limb salvage of 66.9% +/- 11.6% at 1 year and 60.3% +/- 19.0% at 3 years. The results suggest that thrombosed vein grafts initially salvaged with thrombolysis and revision do not have a favorable long-term patency, and that a premium must be placed on the detection of the failing vein graft before thrombosis.

Successful thrombolytic therapy for acute and chronic occlusion of polytef vascular grafts.
Bisig CJ Jr; Kerstein MD. Arch Surg 1983; 118: 1218–1220.

Thrombolytic therapy for thrombosed arterial bypass grafts has received little attention in the medical literature. We carried out successful thrombolysis in occluded polytef arterial bypass grafts. A femoral-femoral artery crossover graft had been occluded 13 days, and a femoral-popliteal artery bypass graft had been occluded three months. No surgical intervention was required. Follow-up showed continued patency nine months following thrombolytic therapy. Long-term oral anticoagulation seems indicated. Also, data suggest thrombus in polytef grafts may be particularly susceptible to lyses. Thrombolytic therapy should play an increasing role in vascular surgery.

Two urokinase dose regimens in native arterial graft occlusions: initial results of a prospective, randomized clinical trial.
Cragg AH; Smith TP; Corson JD; Nakagawa N; Castaneda F; Kresowik TF; Sharp WJ; Shamma A; Berbaum KS. Radiology 1991; 178: 681–686.

The effects of two urokinase (UK) dose regimens on lysis time, lytic success, primary clinical success, and frequency of complications of peripheral thrombolysis were compared. Seventy-two intraarterial UK infusions were performed by means of standard catheter-directed infusion techniques in 63 patients with symptomatic peripheral arterial or bypass graft occlusions. Patients were prospectively randomized to high-dose (250,000 U/h for 4 hours and then 125,000 U/h) or low-dose (50,000 U/h) regimens. The mean time to complete lysis was 20.8, 26.0, 16.5, and 18.2 hours for the high-dose artery, low-dose artery, high-dose graft, and low-dose graft groups, respectively (P was not significant). Respective mean infusion durations were 27.1, 35.4, 22.2, and 25.3 hours. Clinical success was achieved in 65%–85% of cases. The frequency of complications was equivalent between groups, except for a higher frequency of minor bleeding complications in the high-dose group. The two urokinase dose regimens studied were equally effective in enabling peripheral thrombolysis.

High-dose thrombolytic therapy and angioplasty for thrombosis in a subacute femoropopliteal bypass graft.
Dieck JA; Benrey J. Tex Med 1991; 87: 80–82.

The rate of success in reoperation for thrombosed infrainguinal grafts is unimpressive, particularly in patients with disease of distal vessels. In certain cases, combining high-dose urokinase and angioplasty appears to offer a safe and effective alternative. We describe the successful use of this combined treatment in a patient with a recently occluded femoropopliteal bypass graft.

Regional infusion of urokinase into occluded lower-extremity bypass grafts: long-term clinical results.
Durham JD; Geller SC; Abbott WM; Shapiro H; Waltman AC; Walker TG; Brewster DC; Athanasoulis CA. Radiology 1989; 172: 83–87.

The initial outcome, long-term patency rate, and rate of limb salvage were studied in patients after regional urokinase infusion for treatment of thrombosed lower-extremity grafts. Seventy-one infusions were performed in 53 patients. Complete clot lysis occurred in 75% of grafts, with establishment of antegrade blood flow in 66%. Variables that favorably influenced clot lysis and the reestablishment of antegrade blood flow through the graft were a short duration of occlusion and a suprainguinal graft position. The median duration of patency after infusion and adjunctive therapy was 162 days, with 75% limb salvage at 301 days. No statistically significant variables that influenced the length of patency were identified. These long-term patency results are inferior to the reported results in suprainguinal grafts after reoperation. They appear similar to reported results for occluded infra-inguinal grafts treated with thrombectomy and patch grafting.

Salvage of occluded arterial bypass grafts by means of thrombolysis.
Gardiner GA Jr; Harrington DP; Koltun W; Whittemore A; Mannick JA; Levin DC. J Vasc Surg 1989; 9: 426–431.

Seventy-two thrombosed peripheral arterial bypass grafts in 62 patients were treated by local intraarterial thrombolytic infusion. The initial success rate was 69% (50 of 72 grafts). Graft material and location had no significant effect on the initial results. Urokinase was used in 43 cases with a 84% success rate, and streptokinase was used in 29 cases with a 48% success rate. After a follow-up period that ranged from 2 to 58 months, 27 grafts remained patent, with an average patency duration of 15 months (median 8 months). Overall graft patency at the end of 1 year was 60% applying life-table analysis. Factors that were evaluated to determine their effect on long-term patency included graft age and material, graft location, and the presence or absence of an underlying correctable lesion. The most significant factor in long-term patency was the presence of a lesion that was correctable by surgical revision or balloon angioplasty. In 25 grafts with underlying stenotic lesions, the 1-year patency was 86% after successful treatment. Twenty-five grafts without detectable lesions had 37% 1-year patency.

Thrombolysis of occluded femoropopliteal grafts.
Gardiner GA Jr; Koltun W; Kandarpa K; Whittemore A; Meyerovitz MF; Bettmann MA; Levin DC; Harrington DP. AJR 1986; 147: 621–626.

In a series of 44 occluded femoropopliteal grafts, streptokinase was used for thrombolytic therapy in 22 cases and urokinase in 22 cases. In most cases, thrombolytic agents were administered via an indwelling arterial catheter directly into the proximal thrombus. The catheter tip was advanced as thrombolysis occurred. Compared with streptokinase infusions, urokinase bolus injection followed by infusion had better results (77% vs 41%) and fewer complications (23% vs 50%). During thrombolytic infusion, concomitant heparin infusion was usually used to reduce the frequency of thrombus formation on the infusion catheter or recurrent thrombosis of the graft, once the tip of the infusion catheter was advanced distally. Follow-up in 23 of 26 successful cases showed that 11 of the grafts remained open at an average follow-up of 12 months or until the patient died. The 12 grafts that reoccluded remained open an average of 3 months. In none of the 18 failures was simple surgical thrombectomy or thrombectomy with graft revision effective in revascularizing the distal limb. The advantages of thrombolysis compared with thrombectomy are less trauma to the graft, which is especially important in vein grafts, and improved distal runoff due to lysis of infrapopliteal thrombus. Even among cases considered failures in this series, the surgical approach was often simplified because of partial thrombolysis. Thrombolysis requires a considerable amount of time, effort, and expense, but in certain patients where thrombectomy is indicated for the treatment of occluded femoropopliteal grafts this technique offers important advantages.

Local thrombolysis in the treatment of thrombosed arteries, bypass grafts, and arteriovenous fistulas.
Graor RA; Risius B; Denny KM; Young JR; Beven EG; Hertzer NR; Ruschhaupt WF 3d; O'Hara PJ; Geisinger MA; Zelch MG. J Vasc Surg 1985; 2: 406–414.

We reviewed the results, systemic effects, and complications associated with the selective infusion of low-dose streptokinase in 151 patients. Successful thrombus lysis was achieved in 78% of atherosclerotic thrombotic occlusions less than 30 days old, in 81% of post-procedural occlusions less than 14 days old, and in 87% of patients with thrombosed arteriovenous fistulas no more than 4 days old. During the first 12 hours of treatment 81% to 84% of patients had greater than 50% decrease in plasma fibrinogen levels and 100% showed the same decline after 24 hours of treatment. The thrombin time was prolonged to at least 1 ½ times the control thrombin time in 33% to 42% of patients measured at 4 hours of therapy and in 93% to 97% of patients measured at 24 hours of treatment. Fifteen patients (9.9%) had major ccmplications. Eleven of these had hemorrhagic complications, two had significant distal emboli, one had a thrombosed brachial artery, and one had a false aneurysm at the catheter entry site. We have found that selective low-dose streptokinase is effective in the treatment of acute and chronic thrombotic occlusions and is a useful adjuvant to vascular reconstruction or percutaneous transluminal angioplasty although the local infusion dose is substantially lower than the usual systemic dose, a systemic lytic effect was seen in all patients. Hemorrhagic complications occurred despite customary precautions.

Efficacy of low-dose streptokinase in acute arterial occluson and graft thrombosis.
Kakkasseril JS; Cranley JJ; Arbaugh JJ; Roedersheimer LR; Welling RE. Arch Surg 1985; 120: 427–429.

In a review of 35 patients undergoing local thrombolysis using selective infusion of low-dose streptokinase, the overall success rate was 43%. Streptokinase appears to be most effective in occlusion of native arteries, in high-flow segments, and in autogenous saphenous vein grafts. Local streptokinase was least effective in occluded prosthetic grafts in the femoropopliteal segment (19% success). Distal embolization and progression of thrombosis of the distal arterial tree may occur while the patient is undergoing local thrombolysis and may result in limb loss. Hence, local thrombolysis is not recommended when surgical treatment is an alternative. Despite the low dose, systemic fibrinolytic effects and hemorrhagic complications were common occurrences; hence, routine hematologic monitoring is mandatory in patients undergoing lytic therapy with local infusion of streptokinase.

Recombinant human tissue-type plasminogin activator is an effective agent for thrombolysis of peripheral arteries and bypass grafts: preliminary report.
Krupski WC; Feldman RK; Rapp JH. J Vasc Surg 1989; 10: 491–498; discussion 499–500.

The efficacy, safety, and effects on hemostasis and coagulation of two doses of human tissue-type plasminogen activator in patients with acute and subacute peripheral arterial occlusion were compared. Seven patients with lower extremity ischemia and one patient with upper extremity ischemia had peripheral arterial thromboses (five arteries, three grafts) confirmed by clinical history, physical examination, and angiography. The duration of occlusion ranged from 31 hours to 30 days (mean 11.9 days). Tissue-type plasminogen activator was infused via a catheter directly into the thrombus at a randomly assigned dose of 0.05 mg/kg/hr (n = 4) or 0.025 mg/kg/hr (n = 4). Thrombolysis was complete in seven patients and partial in one. Duration of infusion ranged from 1 hour to 21 hours (mean 7.4 hours). The low dose required a longer infusion than did the high dose, but they were both successful in achieving thrombolysis. The one patient with partial thrombolysis had abrupt discontinuation of infusion when extravasation through a recently endarterectomized femoral artery developed. Otherwise there were no significant complications from tissue-type plasminogen activator therapy. Secondary procedures to correct underlying arterial disease were performed in five of the seven patients (71%) who had complete thrombolysis. Even at low dosages, infusion of tissue-type plasminogen activator into arteries or bypass graft thrombus produced complete thrombolysis, and no major complications occurred. This allowed more systematic effects to diagnose and treat underlying arterial disease.

Treatment of peripheral arterial obstruction with streptokinase: results in arterial vs graft occlusions.
LeBolt SA; Tisnado J; Cho SR. AJR 1988: 151: 589–592.

A retrospective study of the efficacy of local low-dose intraarterial streptokinase for the treatment of peripheral arterial occlusion was performed in 60 cases. The results of treatment of occlusion of native arterial and arterial graft occlusions were compared. Twenty-two (73%) of 30 cases of arterial occlusion showed complete or partial angiographic resolution, compared with 16 (53%) of 30 cases of arterial graft occlusion. Ten (71%) of 14 patients with venous arterial grafts were successfully treated vs only six (38%) of 16 patients with prosthetic arterial grafts. These results suggest that streptokinase is an effective fibrinolytic agent for the treatment of arterial occlusion and arterial graft occlusion. Its effectiveness in arterial graft obstruction is comparatively low, although patients with venous grafts respond much more favorably than those with synthetic conduits.

The use of lytic therapy with endovascular "repair" for the failed infrainguinal graft
McNamara TO. Semin Vasc Surg 1990; 3: 59–65.

In summary, thrombolysis of occluded infrainguinal grafts is associated with a high incidence of initial success, a low incidence of significant complications, and a long-term patency rate that is competitive with thrombectomy and markedly improved if flow-limiting lesions can be identified and corrected by either PTA or surgery. The long-term secondary patency of vein grafts following thrombolysis is expected to be higher than that of synthetic grafts, but this has not been substantiated. Currently, PTA of stenosis is the mainstay of endovascular therapy following successful thrombolysis. However, all too often it is the presence of chronic occlusions of the trifurcation vessels that are the major source of outflow restriction. An endovascular method of restoring flow through chronically occluded trifurcation vessels would be expected to improve the long-term patency rates of the salvaged infrainguinal grafts, but such a method has proven elusive. Despite current shortcomings in long-term patency, thrombolysis continues to play an important role in the treatment of the failed infrainguinal graft. It can promptly restore flow to ischemic tissues and obviate the need for emergency surgery in most instances; lyse all of the clot, thereby reducing outflow resistance to a minimum; minimize intimal damage; and provide for excellent angiographic assessment for optimal treatment planning. In the patient who is not a candidate for secondary surgical reconstruction with a vein graft, thrombolysis followed by PTA or patch grafting may be the most attractive option for postponing further disability or for avoiding amputation in cases of failed infrainguinal grafts.

Thrombolysis of peripheral arterial and graft occlusions: improved results using high-dose urokinase.
McNamara TO; Fischer JR. AJR 1985; 144: 769–775.

Ninety-three thromboembolic occlusiona of peripheral arteries or grafts in 85 patients were treated with high-dose urokinase by direct intraarterial infusion. Urokinase was infused at 4000 IU/min until antegrade blood flow was reestablished and then at 1000 or 2000 IU/min until clot lysis was completed. Of the 93 infusions, 75 (81%) resulted in clinical improvement. The infusion therapy was incomplete in nine patients. The mean duration of the 84 completed infusions was 18 ± 20 hr, the incidence of complete clot lysis was 83%, and the incidence of clinical improvement was 89%. Significant bleeding, requiring transfusion, occurred during or after four of the urokinase infusions (4%). Other complications included distad clot migration, thrombus formation on the catheter, revascularization phenomena, oliguria, skin rash, pseudoaneurysm, balloon rupture during angioplasty, and vascular spasm. There were no instances of drug resistance or adverse drug reactions. These results indicate that an initially high-dose urokinase regimen accomplishes more rapid recanalization, a higher incidence of total clot lysis, and produces fweer complications than the standard low-dose streptokinase regimen.

Recombinant tissue-type plasminogen activator versus urokinase in peripheral arterial and graft occlusions: a randomized trial [see comments].
Meyerovitz MF; Goldhaber SZ; Reagan K; Polak JF; Kandarpa K; Grassi CJ; Donovan BC; Bettmann MA; Harrington DP. Radiology 1990; 175: 75–78; 34–36.

A randomized prospective trial was undertaken to compare intraarterial administration of recombinant human tissue-type plasminogen activator (rt-PA) with urokinase (UK) in 32 patients with peripheral arterial or bypass graft occlusions. Sixteen patients were randomized to receive rt-PA and 16 to receive UK. The rt-PA dose was administered as a 10-mg bolus into the thrombus, followed by 5 mg/h for up to 24 hours. The UK dose was administered as a 60,000 IU bolus into the thrombus, followed by 240,000

IU/h for 2 hours, 120,000 IU/h for 2 hours, and 60,000 IU/h for up to 20 hours. Serial arteriograms were obtained at baseline and at 4, 8 or 16, and 24 hours. The endpoint was defined as 95% of greater clot lysis. The cumulative numbers of patients with successful thrombolysis (rt-PA vs UK) were four vs none at 4 hours, seven vs one at 8 hours, seven vs three at 16 hours, and eight vs six at 24 hours. Lysis occurred more rapidly in the rt-PA group (P = .04). Major bleeding complications occurred in five rt-PA patients and two UK patients (P = .39). At 24 hours, fibrinogen levels were significantly lower in the rt-PA group than in the UK group (P = .01). There was no apparent difference in 30-day clinical success.

Outcome of intraarterial urokinase for acute vascular occlusion.
Parent FN 3d; Piotrowski J; Bernhard VM; Pond GD; Pabst TS 3d; Bull DA; Hunter GC; McIntyre KE. J Cardiovasc Surg (Torino) 1991; 32: 680–689.

Intraarterial urokinase (IAUK) was administered to 33 patients on 40 occasions for the treatment of acute extremity ischemia and long-term patency was assessed. Lysis was successful in 39 of the 40 cases (95%). Occlusive thrombus was cleared in 12 of 13 patients with native artery occlusion (7 complete, 5 partial), 8 of 9 with autologous vein grafts (5 complete, 3 partial), and in all 18 patients with synthetic grafts (17 complete, 1 partial). The primary cumulative patency following successful IAUK was 100% for native arteries and 47% for synthetic grafts at 12 months, and 23% for autologous grafts at 9 months. The difference in rethrombosis rate between autologous vein (67%) and native artery (0%) was significant (p = 0.02) as was the difference betwen infrainguinal prosthetic grafts (63%) and native artery (p = 0.025). IAUK is most effective for the treatment of native artery occlusion, but is significantly less effective for thrombosed infrainguinal autologous vein or synthetic grafts due to the likelihood of reocclusion, despite the high immediate success rate. For autologous vein grafts, lysis is frequently incomplete and patency rapidly deteriorates regardless of adjunctive therapy to relieve the underlying obstruction.

Transgraft hemorrhage: a serious complication of low-dose thrombolytic therapy.
Perler BA; Kinnison M; Halden WJ J Vasc Surg 1986; 3: 936–938.

A 71-year-old woman came to the hospital with a 24-hour-old occlusion of the left limb of an aortoiliac knitted Dacron graft and was treated with an intra-arterial infusion of urokinase, 40,000 U/hr. Although the graft limb was successfully recanalized in 16 hours, the patient suffered a massive retroperitoneal hemorrhage through the wall of the graft. Clinicians must be aware of this potentially serious complication of thrombolytic therapy in patients with thrombosed, knitted Dacron grafts.

Low dose thrombolytic therapy for infrainguinal graft occlusions: an idea whose time has passed?
Perler BA; White RI Jr; Ernst CB; Williams GM. J Vasc Surg 1985; 2: 799–805.

Despite the growing enthusiasm for low-dose intra-arterial thrombolytic therapy, the efficacy and risks in specific clinical situations have not been defined. During the past 13 months, 10 infrainguinal bypass graft occlusions occurred in nine patients 2 to 48 months postoperatively and were treated with local infusions of either streptokinase or urokinase. The grafts treated included two saphenous vein femoropopliteal grafts, two expanded polytetrafluoroethylene (PTFE) femoropopliteal grafts, four saphenous vein femoro-anterior tibial grafts, one saphenous vein-PTFE composite femoro-anterior tibial graft, and one saphenous vein-PTFE composite femoroperoneal graft. The graft occlusions occurred 2 to 14 days prior to initiation of treatment. The infusion failed to restore flow completely in seven grafts; and of the three successes, two patients required surgical treatment of complications. All successful recanalizations occurred within 48 hours of the initiation of thrombolytic therapy. Of the seven failures, two patients had viable limbs and were discharged, whereas two required amputation (one above and one below knee). Three patients underwent surgical thrombectomy and revisions that were successful in two and resulted in a below-knee amputation on the other. Despite all precautions, complications occurred in five patients. Low-dose intra-arterial thrombolytic therapy is a poorly efficacious, risky method of infrainguinal graft occlusion management.

Local thrombolysis in peripheral arteries and bypass grafts.
Pernes JM; De Almeida Augusto M; Vitoux JF; Raynaud A; Fiessinger JN; Brenot P; Fabiani JN; Murday A; Gaux JC. J Vasc Surg 1987; 6: 372–378.

Sixty-two patients hospitalized for recent angiographically documented arterial occlusion in the legs (46 femoropopliteal arteries and i6 grafts) benefited from local fibrinolytic therapy delivered at the site of the occlusion with a No. 4F or No. 5F catheter. This therapy combined a continuous urokinase (UK) infusion of 1000 U/kg/hr and a lysyl plasminogen (LYS-PLG) infusion of 15 mukat every 30 minutes. Angiographically confirmed lysis was obtained in 77% of the cases. Five percent of the patients had major and 8% had minor groin hematomas. Only two patients had concentrations of fibrinogen as low as 100 mg/dl. Intravascular infusion of UK and LYS-PLG is as effective as streptokinase but produces lower systemic fibrinolysis. However, local fibrinolysis remains a potentially hazardous procedure (10% suffered major complications) and must only be applied to patients with severe ischemia and little or no possibility of surgical intervention.

Acute peripheral arterial and graft occlusion: treatment with selective infusion of urokinase and lysyl plasminogen.
Pernes JM; Vitoux JF; Brenoit P; Raynaud A; Parola JL; Roth JP; Angel CY; Fiessinger JN; Roncato M; Gaux JC. Radiology 1986; 158: 481–485.

Thirty-five patients hospitalized for recent angiographically documented arterial occlusion in the legs (27 femoropopliteal arteries and eight grafts) benefited from local fibrinolytic therapy delivered at the site of the occlusion with a 4- or 5-F catheter. This therapy combined a continuous urokinase (UK) infusion of 1,000 U/kg/hour and a lysyl plasminogen (LYS-PLG) infusion pf 15 microkatals every 30 minutes. Angiographically confirmed lysis was obtained in 85% of the cases. Only 3% of the patients had major and 6% had minor groin hematomas. Only two patients had concentrations of fibrinogen as low as 100 mg/dl. Intravascular infusion of UK-LYS-PLG is as effective as streptokinase. Its excellent tolerance makes it a good alternative in the treatment of acute ischemia in the lower limbs.

Recombinant human tissue-type plasminogin activator for thrombolysis in peripheral arteries and bypass grafts.

Risius B; Graor RA; Geisinger MA; Zelch MG; Lucas FV; Young JR; Grossbard EB. Radiology 1986; 160: 183–188.

Recombinant human tissue-type plasminogen activator (rt-PA) was infused intraarterially at 0.1 mg/kg/h for 1–6 ½ hours in 25 patients with lower extremity thromboembolic occlusions (13 thrombosed arteries, 12 thrombosed bypass grafts). Occlusion duration ranged from 1 hour to 21 days. Thrombolysis occurred in 23 of 25 patients (92%). Time to lysis varied from 1 to 6.5 hours, with an average time of 3.6 hours. Twenty of 23 patients (87%) in whom thrombolysis was successful benefited clinically from thrombolytic therapy. Twelve of 23 patients (52%) required secondary procedures to maintain arterial segment patency. In 15 of 25 patients (60%) fibrinogen levels were maintained above 50% of baseline values. No major complications directly attributable to rt-PA infusions occurred. rt-PA is a potent, relatively fibrin-specific thrombolytic agent that can achieve rapid thrombolysis while usually avoiding the profound systemic fibrinogenolysis associated with currently available thrombolytic agents.

Combined thrombolytic therapy and percutaneous transluminal angioplasty for treatment of complex arterial graft thrombosis—a case report.

Rubin JR; Pond GD; Bernhard VM. Angiology 1988; 39: 169–173.

Combined catheter-directed thrombolytic therapy followed by percutaneous transluminal angioplasty (PTA) was successfully performed for the treatment of a thrombosed complex mesenteric artery bypass graft resulting from an anastomotic stenosis. Restenosis of the graft due to neointimal hyperplasia was subsequently treated by PTA, with resultant long-term patency. This approach is an attractive alternative to surgical thrombectomy and graft revision, especially in patients who are poor surgical risks owing to concurrent medical problems.

Percutaneous intraarterial thrombolysis in the treatment of thrombosis of lower extremity arterial reconstructions.

Seabrook GR; Mewissen MW; Schmitt DD; Reifsnyder T; Bandyk DF; Lipchik EO; Towne JB. J Vasc Surg 1991; 13: 646–651.

Vascular grafts may be salvaged with thrombolytic therapy after acute occlusion as an alternative to balloon catheter thrombectomy. From October 1987 to May 1990, 15 arterial bypasses to the lower extremity (infrainguinal saphenous vein [n = 7] or expanded polytetrafluoroethylene [n = 6], and Dacron aortofemoral bifurcation graft limbs [n = 2]) were treated for 30 occlusions with intraarterial urokinase (390,000 IU to 5,808,000 IU) infused from 3 to 40 hours. The origins of 15 graft occlusions were morphologic defects (intimal hyperplasia with anastomotic or conduit stricture), pseudoaneurysm, or progression of disease distal to the graft. Two occlusions were attributed to coagulation disorders. A cause could not be identified for 13 occlusions. Patency was initially restored to all grafts with use of thrombolytic therapy, however, adjunctive surgical thrombectomy to remove persistent thrombus from the graft or outflow vessels was required after six thrombolytic infusions. One graft in the series could not be salvaged leading to below-knee amputation. Graft defects were corrected by balloon angioplasty (n = 7) or surgical revision of the conduit (n = 8). Five significant hemorrhagic complications occurred from the catheter insertion site requiring four emergent surgical procedures and resulting in the death of a fifth patient from a myocardial infarction. This technique allows chemical thrombectomy of branch arteries distal to the graft and inaccessible to a balloon embolectomy catheter, and permits diagnosis of abnormal graft morphology that may be the cause of the graft occlusion. Graft reocclusion can be expected if technical defects in the arterial reconstruction are not revised or hypercoagulable states are not treated.

Lower-extremity in situ saphenous vein grafts: angiographic interventions.

Sniderman KW; Kalman PG; Shewchun J; Goldberg RE. Radiology 1989; 179: 1023–1027.

In 16 consecutive patients, thrombosis, anastomotic and intragraft stenoses, and residual venous communications (arteriovenous fistulas [AVFs]), after in situ saphenous vein bypass of femoropopliteal and infrapopliteal arteries, were treated with interventional angiographic techniques. Streptokinase infusion for graft thrombosis was performed in four patients with long-term clinical improvement in two; in the other two, early rethrombosis was treated with surgical thrombectomy. Delayed rethrombosis occurred at 13 months in another patient. Anastomotic (six occasions) and intragraft (four occasions) stenoses in six patients were dilated with percutaneous transluminal angioplasty (PTA). Two grafts subsequently occluded, one 3 weeks and one 3 months after PTA. Residual AVFs were occluded in ten patients. Ten of 16 patients remained clinically improved without further therapy. One complication occurred: A graft stenosis developed at the site where a coil, protruding from the AVF into the graft lumen, was successfully removed and replaced.

[Local thrombolysis in acute occlusion of a femoropopliteal Gore-Tex bypass] Lokale Thrombolyse bei akut verschlossenem femoropoplitealem Gore-Tex-Bypass.

Stiegler H; Lander T; Standl E; Steckmeier B. Dtsch Med Wochenschr 1986; 111: 99–101.

Occlusion of a femoro-popliteal Gore-Tex-bypass in two patients could be reopened using local low-dose thrombolytic therapy. Apart from the peripheral outflow effective anticoagulation treatment appears to have a deciding influence on long-term results. Application of the thrombolytic selectively to single vessels of the lower leg as well as a post-lysis effect offer the chance for an improvement in outflow. Combination of local lysis with vessel surgery may be an additional alternative for conservation of the extremities.

Efficacy of thrombolysis in infrainguinal bypass grafts.
Sullivan KL; Gardiner GA Jr; Kandarpa K; Bonn J; Shapiro MJ; Carabasi RA; Smullens S; Levin DC. Circulation 1991; 83(2 Suppl): I99–105.

The initial outcome of a consecutive series of 43 intra-arterial urokinase infusions for thrombosed infrainguinal grafts in 37 patients was analyzed. There was an 88% (38/43) technical success rate (complete clot lysis) and a (74%) (32/43) clinical success rate. Complications occurred in 10 patients (23%) and were related to bleeding in four patients (9%). Patient age, graft age, location, material, and the duration of occlusion did not significantly influence the initial outcome, although there was a trend toward a higher bleeding complication rate among grafts less than or equal to 1 month of age at the time of thrombolysis. A second group of 43 infrainguinal grafts successfully recanalized using regional infusions of thrombolytic agents were followed for long-term patency. This group included 32 grafts successfully treated with urokinase and 11 grafts recanalized with streptokinase. By life-table analysis there was a 55.6% 1-year patency, which fell to 42.4% at 4 years. Vein grafts had significantly (p = 0.01) better long-term patency than prosthetic grafts (69.3% versus 28.6% at 30 months). Grafts with flow-limiting lesions identified and corrected by angioplasty or surgery also had significantly (p = 0.01) better long-term patency than those without such lesions (79.0% versus 9.8% at 2 years). Based on the results of our study compared with a survey of long-term results following secondary surgical procedures for thrombosed infrainguinal grafts, thrombolysis can be recommended in several circumstances. Thrombolysis is indicated for thrombosed vein grafts or when thrombus is present in distal runoff vessels. Thrombosed prosthetic grafts should be replaced by autogenous vein grafts whenever possible (ABSTRACT TRUNCATED AT 250 WORDS)

Improved patient selection for enzymatic lysis of peripheral arterial and graft occlusion.
Sussman B; Dardik H; Ibrahim IM; Fox R; Mendes D; Kahn M. Am J Surg 1984; 148: 244–248.

Intraarterial thrombolysis by remote intravenous or direct intraarterial infusion of streptokinase is possible. The latter may be more effective with a lesser potential for systemic hemorrhagic complications because of the smaller dose administered directly in the area. Fifty patients with prosthetic graft, embolic, and renal artery occlusions were evaluated. Embolic occlusion responded dramatically, particularly since lytic therapy was initiated at an early stage. Patients with severe ischemia or those with simple localized occlusion were best treated by surgical means. Successful thrombolysis was also obtained with renal artery occlusions combined with percutaneous transluminal angioplasty. The management of patients with prosthetic graft occlusion by lytic therapy is complex. Optimal results can be obtained in patients presenting with occluded grafts after the immediate postoperative period and in those in whom previous satisfactory runoff has been demonstrated. Failure of lysis in this group is associated with a high incidence of limb loss due to unreconstructable obliterative disease. Successful lysis of occluded prosthetic grafts will often require corrective angioplasty or surgical revision.

II. Synopses of Pertinent Articles

C. Overview

Thrombolysis: the logical approach for the treatment of vascular occlusions (editorial).
Abel H. Acta Cardiol 1992; 47(4): 287–295.

Thrombotic and thromboembolic occlusions of arteries and veins represent acute and often life threatening complications requiring immediate therapeutic intervention. The most important clinical manifestations of vascular occlusions are myocardial infarction, peripheral arterial occlusion, pulmonary embolism, deep vein thrombosis and ischemic stroke. The logical approach for the treatment in these indications is the early restoration of blood circulation in order to preserve the organ deprived from oxygen supply and to prevent chronic sequelae. Recanalization by surgical intervention is only possible in some indications and is restricted to special clinics. Thrombolysis induced by agents activating plasminogen imitates the physiologic way of dissolving an occlusive clot by shifting the balance of the hemostatic and fibrinolytic system towards fibrinolysis. Streptokinase was the first effective thrombolytic drug used in patients. In the first years of its usage the identification of the appropriate indication and the dosage and application regimens used were based on little pharmacological knowledge and lack of appropriate dose finding. This resulted in suboptimal therapeutic efficacy and severe bleeding. Development of advanced diagnostic methods, more appropriate dose and application regimens and the development of more specific fibrinolytic drugs like rt-PA led to a remarkable improvement of its benefit-risk ratio and made thrombolysis to a widely accepted form of therapy in thrombotic and thromboembolic diseases. Early restoration of blood flow however is only the starting point of a therapeutic strategy, aiming at minimizing the risk of recurrence. (ABSTRACT TRUNCATED AT 250 WORDS)

Heparin-induced thrombocytopenia with thrombotic complications.
AbuRhama AF; Malik FS; Boland JP. W V Med J 1992; 88(3): 95–100.

Heparin-induced thrombocytopenia with thrombotic complications is a serious clinical problem. The diagnosis is confirmed by a positive heparin-induced platelet aggregation text and/or detection of white clots upon pathological exam after a presumptive diagnosis based on these criteria: (1) Development of thrombocytopenia of less than 100,000 mm3 while receiving heparin therapy; (2) Normalization of the platelet count after an interruption in heparin therapy; (3) The presence of thrombotic complications; and (4) Exclusion of other causes of thrombocytopenia. Eight patients with heparin-induced thrombocytopenia were encountered at the Charleston Area Medical Center, Memorial Division, in a recent 20-month period. Various types of heparin, routes of administration, and indications were implicated. The mean platelet nadir was 25,750 mm3 and the mean time to onset of heparin-induced thrombocytopenia was 4.9 days. Thrombotic complications included seven patients with artrial occlusions of the legs, six with deep-vein thrombosis of the legs (three had pulmonary embolism), and five with combined arterial and venous thrombosis. Treatment strategies included discontinuation of heparin in all patients; intravenous infusion of dextran in five patients, followed by arterial thrombectomy in three patients; urokinase therapy in two patients for arterial thrombotic complications; and insertion of Greenfield filters in four patients for venous thrombotic complications. All surviving patients were given warfarin. The mortality rate was 25 percent and the morbidity rate was 38 percent. In conclusion, an initial platelet count should be obtained on all patients prior to receiving heparin, followed by repeat platelet counts every two to three days. Once thrombocytopenia or thrombosis is diagnosed, heparin should be discontinued and other therapeutic modalities considered.

Intra-arterial fibrinolytic therapy: efficacy of streptokinase vs urokinase.
Belkin M; Belkin B; Bucknam CA; Straub JJ; Lowe R. Arch Surg 1986; 121: 769–773.

This study is a retrospective comparison of the results in 25 low-dose, intra-arterial streptokinase and 12 low-dose intra-arterial urokinase infusions for thromboembolic disease. Intra-arterial streptokinase was successful in 50% of infusions and was marked by significant abnormalities in the coagulation criteria. There was a high incidence of major and minor bleeding (48% overall), which could be attributed to systemic effects of the drug. Urokinase was successful in 100% of infusions, and showed no significant effects on systemic coagulation criteria. There were also fewer complications during urokinase infusion. The average pharmacy cost for a course of intra-arterial streptokinase was $165, while urokinase cost $1142. Despite the significant difference in expense, the increased efficacy and safety of urokinase make it the preferred agent for intra-arterial infusion. Theoretical reasons for the increased effectiveness of urokinase are discussed.

Pulsed-spray pharmacomechanical thrombolysis: preliminary clinical results.
Bookstein JJ; Fellmeth B; Roberts A; Valji K; Davis G; Machado T. AJR 1989; 152: 1097–1100.

Pulsed-spray pharmacomechanical thrombolysis was used to treat 41 patients with 47 complete thrombotic occlusions of hemodialysis grafts (n = 29), arterial bypass grafts (n = 10), or peripheral native arteries (n = 8). The procedure involves the use of small pulses of highly concentrated urokinase, which are forcefully sprayed throughout the thrombus during systemic heparinization. Virtually complete lysis was achieved in 46 of 47 occlusions. In the 46 thrombi that lysed, mean time for completion of lysis was 63 ± 35 min and initial partial return of flow required 26 ± 18 min. Complications included small peripheral emboli in one treated bypass graft (which cleared promptly after further pulse-spray therapy) and bleeding in three cases (one case of hematoma in the infused field at the site of recent surgery, one case of bilateral hematomas at the femoral puncture site, and one minor delayed self-limited gastrointestinal hemorrhage). Results to date suggest that the pulsed-spray pharmacomechanical method augments the speed, consistency, safety, and cost efficacy of clinical thrombolysis. Further study is warranted.

[Value of intraoperative lysis therapy as an adjuvant measure after late surgical embolectomy] Stellenwert der intraoperativen Lysetherapie als adjuvante Massnahme nach chirurgischer Spatembolektomie.
Boos C; Hohlbach G; Reusche E; Richter P. Langenbecks Arch Chir 1990; 435–436.

The effect of intraoperative local fibrinolysis after delayed catheterembolectomy (CE) of occluded arteries was examined in a model in the dogs hind limb; the superficial femoral artery was occluded by a rapid injection of an autologeous blood clot and ligation. Embolectomy was performed 24 h after occlusion with or without additional local fibrinolysis (urocinase, r-tPA). The success of revascularisation was estimated by measurement of the total periphereal resistance. There happened a total re-occlusion in all vessels within 48 h if only CE was performed; in contrast after additional fibrinolysis a complete revascularization could be achieved.

Local long-time lysis in combination with percutaneous transluminal angioplasty (TPA).
Brock FE; Nobbe F. Int Angiol 1986; 5: 155–160.

In order to produce an endogenous lysis in case of local longtime lysis Urokinase is infused directly into the occlusion in a maximum dosage of 40,000 U/h via an arterial catheter. Remaining stenoses are extended by means of a dilatation catheter. The so far obtained results concerning 72 patients with very long and/or very old arterial occlusions show a primary successrate of 96% and a 2 years' patency rate of 85% for all patients with a primary success of treatment. Complications and side-effects are scarce with this method. Therefore it can be applied with patients for whom other recanalising catheter methods are not indicated and with whom vascular surgery is not possible. However, a lasting success of treatment is only to be expected on the basis of the precise planning and careful performance of a long-term after treatment.

Accelerated thrombolysis using pulsed intra-thrombus recombinant human tissue type plasminogen activator (rt-PA).
Buckenham TM; George CD; Chester JF; Taylor RS; Dormandy JA. Eur J Vasc Surg 1992; 6(3): 237–240.

The efficacy of regional thrombolysis for treating leg ischaemia is well established, but the duration of infusion and the frequent complications remain major disadvantages. By delivering recombinant human tissue type plasminogen activatory (rt-PA) as pulsed intra-thrombus 5-mg aliquots combined with catheter manipulation to maintain an intra-thrombus location, the average time taken to achieve thrombolysis in 20 consecutive patients with infra-aortic occlusions was 109 min. Immediate thrombolysis was achieved in every case. Pulsed delivery of high dose rt-PA significantly accelerates thrombolysis, decreases dose and reduces costs.

In vivo effects of defibrotide on platelet c-AMP and blood prostanoid levels.
Cizmeci G. Haemostasis 1986; 16(Suppl 1): 31–35.

Patients were treated with defibrotide (3 X 200 mg/day) for 7 days. Plasma PG12 and TXB2 levels were measured by RIA using EDTA-aspisol as anticoagulant and cyclooxygenase inhibitor. Isolated platelet c-AMP levels were also determined by RIA, using EDTA-dipyridamole as anticoagulant and phosphodiesterase inhibitor. Blood PG12 levels were found to increase significantly upon treatment while the increase in TXB2 levels was not significant. Blood PG12/TXB2 ratio increased 51%, 30 min after intravenous injection and it remained 28% higher during therapy than the predrug blood level. Significantly higher platelet c-AMP levels were also obtained after the injection of drug (0.02 less than p less than 0.05).

Intra-arterial thrombolytic therapy in peripheral vascular disease.
Comerota AJ; Rubin RN; Tyson RR; White JV; Williams FF; Soulen RL; Sherry S. Surg Gynecol Obstet 1987; 165: 1–8.

This is a prospective analysis of patients undergoing 34 treatments for arterial thromboses and emboli with intra-arterial thrombolytic therapy. These included acute arterial thromboses, graft thromboses, arterial emboli and pulmonary emboli. Twenty-seven of 34 patients treated had evidence of lysis, 14 had complete lysis, 13 had partial lysis and seven had no lysis. Both patients with occlusions for longer than three weeks failed to respond to treatment. Thirty-two patients presented with ischemia of the extremity. Twenty-four of 32 patients had limb salvage with eight subsequently undergoing amputation. No patient who was treated for claudication or who had a patent popliteal artery distal to the acute thrombosis failed to respond. Extensive tibioperoneal occlusion generally responded poorly compared with femoropopliteal or more proximal thrombi. Complications are divided into direct (drug related) and indirect (technique related). Four of 34 patients had an extensive hemorrhagic event with two suffering intracranial bleeding who ultimately died. All of the patients with extensive hemorrhagic episodes had serum fibrinogen levels of less than 50 milligrams per cent. During infusion, extensive distal emboli occurred in three with two of these patients requiring thrombectomy; one instance resolved with infusion. Minor distal emboli occurred in three and all resolved with continued infusion. We believe that intra-arterial thrombolytic therapy is a valuable adjunct in the treatment of acute arterial occlusion. The local infusion of lytic agents appears to be more efficient than systemic therapy. The tip of the infusion catheter should be placed into the thrombus for optimal lysis, but not advanced too far. The fibrinogen level is a sensitive indicator of systemic lysis and should be maintained above 50 milligrams per cent. Systemic lysis is obtained even with low dose infusion when therapy exceeds six hours. Intra-arterial infusion of thrombolytic agents can be performed safely in the immediate postoperative period as well as intraoperatively if specific guidelines are followed. Patients with massive unilateral pulmonary embolism can be efficiently treated with intra-arterial lytic therapy.

[rt–PA in extracardiac thromboembolic vascular occlusions]. L'rt-PA nelle occlusioni vascolari trombo-emboliche extra-cardiache.

Cortellaro M; Cofrancesco E; Polli EE. Ann Ital Med Int 1990; 5: 61–69.

Recombinant tissue plasminogen activator (rt-PA) is a thrombolytic agent characterized by elevated but not absolute fibrin specificity. However, its therapeutic dose is high and associated with a variable degree of systemic activation of the fibrinolytic system. Thrombolytic drugs are widely used in acute myocardial infarction and have now begun to be considered for deep vein thrombosis (DVT), pulmonary embolism (PE), and peripheral artery thrombosis (PAT) as well. Although anticoagulant therapy is effective in reducing the immediate complications of venous thromboembolism, thrombolytic therapy has various advantages over anticoagulant therapy, including lysis of thrombi with recanalization of venous circulation, reduction of venous valve damage and prevention of post-phlebitic syndrome. The different dosage regimens of rt-PA recently evaluated (0.71 to 1.76 mg/kg/24 h for 2–4 days) in DVT have caused consistent thrombolysis but also excessive bleeding. The optimal therapeutic range for rt-PA in DVT remains to be determined. Thrombolytic therapy is superior to heparin treatment only in hemodynamically compromised patients with massive PE. The minor systemic fibrinolytic effect and the faster action on thrombi of rt-PA compared with the first generation thrombolytic agents, streptokinase (SK) and urokinase (UK), are very interesting and explain the positive results recently obtained in PE with this drug (50 mg over 2 h, followed, if necessary, by 40–50 mg over 4–5 h) by Goldhaber and Verstraete. (ABSTRACT TRUNCATED AT 250 WORDS)

Tissue plasminogen activator: a new thrombolytic agent (published erratum appears in Clin Pharm 1987 Dec; 6 (12):925).

Crabbe SJ; Cloninger CC. Clin Pharm 1987; 6: 373–386.

The chemistry, pharmacology, pharmacokinetics, clinical efficacy, adverse effects, contraindications, and dosage and administration of tissue plasminogen activator are reviewed. Tissue plasminogen activator (t-PA) is a serine protease that binds to fibrin-plasminogen complex, catalyzing the conversion of plasminogen to plasmin. Unlike streptokinase or urokinase, t-PA binds slowly, if at all, to free circulating plasminogen. This clot specificity suggests t-PA will not produce a systemic lytic effect; however, clot specificity appears to be dose-related, and concentrations similar to those achieved in recent clinical trials have been associated with hemostatic defects. Most clinical trials have used a recombinant DNA product (rt-PA). In the treatment of acute myocardial infarction, intravenous infusions of rt-PA appear to be more effective than intravenous streptokinase. Similar rates of hemorrhage, reperfusion arrhythmias, and reocclusion have been reported. Contraindications to rt-PA use are similar to those for other thrombolytic agents. Preliminary studies of rt-PA in various thromboembolic disorders are encouraging. Marketing approval of a t-PA product (rt-PA, Activase, Genetech, Inc.) is expected in the United States by mid-1987. Clinical trials suggest that rt-PA is more effective and as safe as intravenous streptokinase in lysing occlusive coronary-artery thrombi; however, safety and efficacy appear to be dose-related, and further study is needed to determine the optimal dose.

Cost-effectiveness of intra-arterial thrombolytic therapy.
Dacey LJ; Dow RW; McDaniel MD; Walsh DB; Zwolak RM; Cronenwett JL. Arch Surg 1988; 123: 1218–1223.

We reviewed the clinical course of 23 patients who received intra-arterial infusions of either streptokinase or urokinase to treat 14 arteries and ten arterial grafts that were occluded due to primary thrombosis (22) or artery-artery embolism (two). Time from symptom onset to treatment was one to 28 days (mean, 11 days). Five infusions (21%) were completely successful since symptoms were eliminated without subsequent operation. Seven infusions (29%) were partially successful since thrombolysis aided, limited, or postponed subsequent surgery. Six infusions (25%) were failures since thrombolysis or clinical improvement did not occur and surgery was required. Six infusions (25%) were associated with thrombolytic complications that required urgent operation (less severe complications occurred in an additional 17% of cases [4/24]). Of the 19 patients without complete success after thrombolytic therapy, 16 underwent surgery during the same admission, two were not operable due to distal disease, and one declined operation. Of the 16 operations, 15 (94%) were successful in restoring graft or artery patency and achieving limb salvage, whereas one failed. In the 12 patients with failure or major complications of thrombolytic treatment, all had successful surgical outcome without morbidity. The actual mean cost of thrombolytic treatment was $8,200 per patient and was comparable with the actual mean cost of subsequent surgical treatment in the 16 patients who required operation ($8,900 per patient). The effective cost of thrombolytic and surgical treatment was calculated by dividing the actual costs by the proportion of successful cases. The effective cost of thrombolytic therapy per complete success was $39,200 and per complete or partial success was $16,500. This was significantly more than the effective cost of $9,400 per complete success of surgical therapy.

[Treatment of massive arterial thrombosis caused by thrombocytopenia induced by heparin with local thrombolysis] Traitement par thrombolyse locale d'une thrombose arterielle massive par thrombopenie induite par l'heparine.
Delagardelle C; Harf C; Dondelinger RF; Goffette P; Beissel J; Pesch C; Welter R. Arch Mal Coeur 1990; 83: 113–115.

The authors report the case of a patient treated by subcutaneous injection of calcium heparin after deep vein thrombosis with floating thrombus and pulmonary embolism. She was readmitted to hospital after 16 days' treatment because of a massive aorto-iliac thrombosis due to heparin-induced thrombocytopenia (platelet count = 29.000). This thrombosis was treated by local injection of Urokinase (total dose = 7.425.000 U) over 93 hours without any major complications. The aorto-iliac circulation was completely restored to normal after treatment. Thrombotic complications secondary to immuno-allergic heparin-induced thrombocytopenia are relatively common because of the widespread use of heparin. From the therapeutic point of view, it is imperative to stop the heparin, which makes surgery very difficult, and the platelet-fibrin composition of these thrombi suggests that local thrombolysis with Urokinase is the treatment of choice in this syndrome.

Treatment modalities in peripheral vascular disease.
Doyle JE. Nurs Clin North Am 1986; 21: 241–253.

This section deals with two commonly encountered clinical problems lower extremity arterial occlusive disease and venous dysfunction. Medical and surgical treatment approaches are discussed, providing an overview of management options. Patients with peripheral arterial and venous disease present nursing with many challenges. Their problems are often chronic, enforcing the need for astute recognition and management as well as patient teaching. (29 Refs.)

Hypercoagulable states in arterial thromboembolism.
Eason JD; Mills JL; Beckett WC. Surg Gynecol Obstet 1992; 174(3): 211–215.

Hypercoagulable states are disorders of blood coagulation, which include deficiencies of natural antigoagulants, disorders of the fibrinolytic system, presence of antiphospholipid antibody and abnormalities of platelet function. These disorders are well known causes of venous thrombembolic disease and are being recognized in association with arterial thromboembolic occurrences with increasing frequency. The performance of standard prosthetic vascular reconstructions may result in disastrous outcomes in patients with unrecognized and untreated hypercoagulable states. From 1986 to 1990, we identified 12 patients with hypercoagulable states, six of whom presented with evidence of arterial thromboembolism. All of the patients were men who smoked and were somewhat younger than the usual patient with atherosclerosis. Their ages ranged from 41 to 62 years. Four patients presented with ischemic rest pain, one patient with blue toe syndrome and one with rapidly progressive claudication. Four patients had undergone prior vascular reconstruction and two had previous pulmonary emboli. Evaluation of these patients to identify hypercoagulability included determinations of prothrombin time (PT) and partial thromboplastin time (PTT), platelet count, antithrombin III, protein C, free protein S and total protein S levels, along with platelet aggregometry. Two patients had protein S deficiency, one had protein C deficiency, one patient had protein C and S deficiency and two patients had hyperaggregable platelets. Four patients had prosthetic reconstructions and two had autogenous reconstructions. Three of the four patients undergoing prosthetic reconstructions had subsequent loss of limb and one patient died. Only one patient with prosthetic reconstruction had a patent graft on long term anticoagulation. Both patients undergoing autogenous procedures had successful revascularization with limb salvage.

Complications of intraarterial urokinase-lys-plasminogen infusion therapy in arterial ischemia of lower limbs.
Fiessinger JN; Vitoux JF; Pernes JM; Roncato M; Aiach M; Gaux JG. AJR 1986; 146: 157–159.

Thirty-five patients with peripheral arterial occlusions were treated by intraarterial infusion of low-dose urokinase associated with bolus of lys-plasminogen. Thrombolysis was achieved in 26 cases (74%), but only 10 patients (28.5%) experienced sustained improvement. Complications of thrombolysis occurred in 11 patients: five patients developed groin hematoma, five had distal emboli. and one experienced macroscopic hematuria. Catheter-related thrombosis was observed in 14 patients (40%) despite intravenous heparin. Nine patients suffered from recurrent thrombosis and three from proximal emboli. A patient died from catheter-related infection. Limited fibrinolysis could increase pericatheter thrombosis, and further work will be necessary to assess the local risk of intraarterial thrombolysis.

Peripheral artery thrombolysis with urokinase-lys-plasminogen. A disappointing experience.
Fiessinger JN; Vitoux JF; Pernes JM; Roncato M; Aiach M; Gaux JG. Int Angiol 1987; 6: 183–186.

Thirty-five patients with peripheral arterial occlusion were treated by intraarterial infusion of low dose urokinase associated with bolus of lys-plasminogen. Systemic fibrinolysis was moderate, thrombolysis was achieved in 26 patients (74%). Only one patient required blood transfusion, five patients (14%) had distal emboli. Infection at the catheter entry site occurred in 2 patients, 3 patients experienced proximal embolism. Six patients required leg amputation, 4 died, in 2 of them deaths were related to arterial catheterization. Local thrombolysis with limited systemic fibrinolysis is associated to a high rate of catheter-related complications.

The role of intravenous streptokinase in acute arterial occlusions after cardiac catheterization.
Gagnon RM; Goudreau E; Joyal F; Morissette M; Roussin A. Cathet Cardiovasc Diagn 1985; 11: 409–412.

Arterial occlusions after cardiac catheterization are usually treated surgically. We report four patients with femoral thrombosis or distal emboli that developed after cardiac catheterization. Each patient was treated successfully with intravenous streptokinase. Therapy was initiated 6–60 hr after the procedure. The duration of infusion lasted 4–42 hr (mean 27 hr). Pulses were restored 4–19 hr after the beginning of infusion. There was no major hemorrhagic complication, even in patients with very early streptokinase infusion. Thus intravenous streptokinase may be an alternate choice to surgery for arterial occlusions after invasive procedures.

The use of antithrombotic drugs in artery disease.
Gallus AS. Clin Haematol 1986; 15: 509–559.

Evaluating the use of antithrombotic drugs in artery disease has been a long and difficult process, which is a far from complete. The aims of treatment have ranged from the primary prevention of myocardial infarction or stroke, through the restoration of blood flow to ischaemic organs in order to salvage threatened tissue, to the prevention of recurrent vascular occlusion. Drugs studied in depth by clinical trial include the oral anticoagulants, antiplatelet drugs (especially aspirin), and thrombolytic agents. Their results are considered under the headings of coronary artery disease, cerebral ischaemia, and peripheral vascular disease. Aspirin, with or without dipyridamole, prevents progression of unstable angina to myocardial infarction or death, probably reduces long-term mortality after myocardial infarction, and prevents aortocoronary bypass graft occlusion. It decreases the risks of stroke or death in patients with transient cerebral ischaemia, diminishes cardiovascular morbidity after a thrombotic stroke, and may improve the outcome after some kinds of surgery for peripheral vascular disease. The benefits of oral anticoagulant treatment to prevent artery occlusion remain poorly defined. Oral anticoagulants prevent systemic embolism in many groups of high-risk patients, and probably reduce the risk of recurrence after embolism has occurred whether their long-term use to prevent reinfarction in patients with a previous myocardial infarct can be justified remains uncertain. They are of little or no proven value in patients with transient cerebral ischaemia or thrombotic stroke. On the other hand, there is increasing support for early thrombolytic treatment after myocardial infarction, especially since two multicentre trials have now shown reduced mortality in patients treated with intracoronary streptokinase within 4–6 hours of infarction and a further large multicentre study also demonstrated reduced mortality in patients treated with early intravenous streptok. (278 Refs.)

Intraoperative intra-arterial urokinase infusion as an adjunct to Fogarty catheter embolectomy in acute arterial occlusion.
Garcia R; Saroyan RM; Senkowsky J; Smith F; Kerstein M. Surg Gynecol Obstet 1990; 171: 201–205.

Sixteen patients, seven men and nine women (mean age of 66 years), with acute arterial ischemia were treated with operative thromboembolectomy by Fogarty catheterization and urokinase. Seven patients were diabetic, ten were hypertensive and six had prior vascular surgical treatment. The operative arteriograms confirmed vascular occlusive phenomenon. The ankle to brachial ratio was a mean of 0.02. Perioperatively, patients had anticoagulation with heparin systemically. All patients underwent transfemoral embolectomy using a Fogarty catheter. An initial retrieval of clots was accomplished, with documentation by arteriography, instillation of urokinase (50,000 units) and clamping of vessel for 15 minutes. Subsequent passage of the Fogarty catheter and repeat urokinase infusion resulted in further retrieval of clots and improvement by repeat intraoperative arteriography. All interventions resulted in clinical restoration of perfusion to the affected limb. Six patients had amputations of the lower extremities (one transmetatarsal and one below the knee) during the 30 day postoperative period. Improvement in distal run-off was demonstrated by intraoperative arteriography and increases in the ankle to brachial ratio from 0.1 to 1.04, with a mean of 0.54, were noted. No complications from bleeding occurred. One patient died postoperatively because of myocardial infarction.

Salvage of the limb may increase with combined embolectomy and thrombolytic therapy.

Increased fibrinolytic potential induced by gliclazide in type I and type II diabetic patients.

Gram J; Jespersen J. Metabolism 1992; 41(5 Suppl 1): 25–29.

Despite the fact that the relationship between impaired diabetic control and the development of vascular complications now seems less controversial than before, we are still in a situation where interventions or strategies aimed at decreasing the complications of late diabetes have high priorities. It is believed that accelerated vascular disease in the diabetic population is caused by repeated intimal injury of the arteries, and there is also evidence that the accelerated vascular disease states cannot be attributed only to the hyperglycemic state. One factor of importance for delayed tissue repair and arteriosclerotic disease in diabetic patients might be a disordered endothelian cell-dependent fibrinolytic system. Here, we review the evidence of the relationship between increased fibrin deposition and defective fibrinolysis in diabetic patients, and, furthermore, we discuss the possible beneficial effects of an enhancement of endogenous endothelial cell-related fibrinolysis by sulphonylurea drugs. (43 Refs.)

Iliac artery stenting—clinical experience with the Palmaz stent, Wallstent, and Strecker stent.

Hausegger KA; Lammer J; Hagen B; Fluckiger F; Lafer M; Klein GE; Pilger E. Acta Radiol 1992; 33(4): 292–296.

A total of 82 iliac artery lesions (62 stenoses and 20 occlusions) were treated with 3 different types of endovascular metallic stents (12 lesions with the Palmaz stent, 36 with the Wallstent, and 34 with the Strecker stent). The complication rate was 12%. Occlusion of 2 Wallstents occurred 4 and 12 weeks after stent placement, respectively. Both stents were recanalized by local fibrinolysis. One Strecker stent occluded after 8 months. The observation period was 3 to 26 months (mean 9.7 months). The patency rate with secondary intervention (fibrinolysis) was 100% after 3 and 6 months, and 98% after 9 months. All 3 stent designs turned out to be effective in the treatment of complicated iliac artery occlusive disease.

Antithrombotic efficacy of low-molecular-weight heparin in deep arterial injury.

Heras M; Chesebro JH; Webster MW; Mruk JS; Grill DE; Fuster V. Arterioscler Thromb 1992; 12(2): 250–255.

Low-molecular-weight heparin subfractions more specifically inhibit factor Xa than thrombin, and they may have advantages over unfractionated heparin in arterial thrombosis. The antithrombotic efficacy of four dosages of a low-molecular-weight heparin (CY216 at 100, 200, 400, or 500 Institute Choay units/kg) was compared with unfractionated calcium heparin (100 US Pharmacopeia units/kg) and placebo during deep arterial injury produced by balloon dilatation of the carotid artery in the pig. The acute thrombotic end points were 111In-labeled platelet and 125I-labeled fibrinogen/fibrin deposition and macroscopic mural thrombosis; these were related to the anti-factor Xa and antithrombin effects of the heparin preparations. Platelet deposition in segments with deep arterial injury was 42 ± 28, 22 ± 5, 29 ± 12, 9 ± 2, and 11 ± 3 × 10(6)/cm2 (mean ± SEM) for pigs treated with placebo, with 100, 200, 400, and 500 units/kg CY216, and with 100 units/kg unfractionated heparin, respectively. Fibrinogen/fibrin deposition was 35 ± 8, 19 ± 2, 19 ± 4, 21 ± 3, 14 ± 4, and 12 ± 3 molecules × 10(12)/cm2, respectively; deposition was significantly reduced in pigs given 100 units/kg unfractionated heparin compared with placebo (p less than 0.05). Mural thrombosis was present in 74%, 45%, 30%, 14%, 5%, and 9% of deeply injured arterial segments, respectively (p = 0.02). Plasma anti-factor Xa activity and prolongation of the activated partial thromboplastin time (aPTT) with 100 units/kg unfractionated heparin were similar to that produced by 200 units/kg and 500 units/kg CY216, respectively. Thus, low-molecular-weight heparin, which predominantly inhibits factor Xa activity, was only moderately effective at reducing platelet thrombus deposition. It was less effective than 100 units/kg unfractionated heparin, except at high dosages, producing similar prolongation of the aPTT and the thrombin time. (ABSTRACT TRUNCATED AT 250 WORDS)

Errors and pitfalls in intraarterial thrombolytic therapy.
Hirshberg A; Schneiderman J; Garniek A; Walden R; Morag B; Thomson SR; Adar R. J Vasc Surg 1989; 10: 612–616.

Sixty complications occurred during 138 courses of intraarterial thrombolytic therapy in 122 patients during a 5-year period. These complications were recorded and analyzed prospectively to identify underlying errors in management. There were 31 bleeding episodes, 15 vascular complications, and 14 other complications. Twelve of the bleeding episodes occurred at the puncture site, and 19 occurred at remote sites, accounting for six of the eight deaths in the series. Management errors were clearly identified in 27 of the 60 complications. The three following patterns of errors were recognized: (1) mismanagement of bleeding (12 instances), (2) wrong patient selection (nine instances), and (3) breach of the administration protocol (six instances). The group of 27 complications with underlying management errors included seven of the eight deaths in the present series. Efforts to prevent complications from thrombolytic therapy should concentrate on the specific patterns of management errors identified. This study indicates that low-dose intraarterial thrombolytic therapy is not a low-risk alternative to surgical intervention but should be viewed as a prelude or possible alternative to surgery in selected patients despite the risks involved.

Surgical implications of fibrinolytic therapy.
Hurley JJ; Burrell MJ; Auer AI; Woods JJ Jr; Binnington HB; Hershey FB. Am J Surg 1984; 148: 830–835.

Intraarterial fibrinolytic therapy was used in 37 cases (34 patients) of severe peripheral ischemia. Nineteen patients (56 percent) required surgical intervention (5 amputations and 14 successful reconstructive procedures). Twenty-four patients (71 percent) were significantly improved (average ankle-to-arm index 0.84), whereas only 5 patients (15 percent) lost their limbs.

Five patients wwre angiographically unchanged with no or slight improvement in the ankle-to-arm index (0.22 to 0.32) and were discharged on anticoagulant therapy. One death and two cerebrovascular accidents occurred. The usefulness of intraarterial fibrinolytic therapy needs to be evaluated within the total realm of vascular surgery. It offers options for therapy where previously none existed. Some situations might be treated equally well with either intraarterial fibrinolytic therapy or surgery. Finally, surgery might be required to maintain initial successful results with intraarterial fibrinolytic therapy or to rescue intraarterial fibrinolytic therapy failures in striving to achieve superior results in limb salvage.

Thrombolytic therapy for femoral artery thrombosis after pediatric cardiac catheterization.
Ino T; Benson LN; Freedom RM; Barker GA; Aipursky A; Rowe RD. Am Heart J 1988; 115: 633–639.

Femoral artery thrombosis remains a well-known complication after cardiac catheterization. A study was undertaken to assess the efficacy of thrombolytic therapy for this complication. A total of 526 consecutive infants and children were prospectively evaluated after cardiac catheterization, and the medical charts of 42 patients who required femoral artery thrombectomy between 1975 and 1985 were reviewed. In the prospective study, patients were given a bolus injection of heparin, 150 U/kg, at the time the artery was entered. Patients with persistently absent or diminished pulse 2 hours after catheterization received a second bolus injection of 50 U/kg followed by an infusion of 20 U/kg/hr heparin for a maximum of 48 hours. If the affected leg pulse was absent or reduced and the systolic Doppler blood pressure was less than two thirds that of the unaffected leg, thrombolytic therapy was begun. In the 42 patients with surgical thrombectomy, there were no serious complications of surgery. Forty-five of the 526 patients (8.6%) had a decreased or absent pulse after catheterization. Of these 45 patients,32 (71.1%) improved with systemic heparinization only. Thirteen patients (28.9%) had a persistently absent pedal pulse suggesting femoral artery thrombosis, despite continuous heparinization. Eleven patients were successfully treated with thrombolytic therapy and two required surgical thrombectomy. Intraarterial balloon dilatation procedures were performed in 8 of these 13 patients. Prothrombin time was prolonged (11.5 ± 1.06 to 52.3 ± 40.4 seconds; p less than 0.025) and fibrinogen levels were significantly reduced (2.25 ± − .79 to 1.52 ± 0.52 gm/dl; p less than 0.01) during therapy. There were no serious complications, although four patients bled from the groin entry site.

Streptokinase in the treatment of acute arterial occlusion of the hand.
Jelalian C; Mehrhof A; Cohen IK; Richdrdson J; Merritt WH. J Hand Surg 1985; 10: 534–538.

Continuous, low-dose, intra-arterial streptokinase was used to treat six patients with ischemia of the hand secondary to distal arterial occlusion. A bolus dose of 100,000 U of streptokinase was administered, followed by a maintenance dose of 5000 U/hr, which was titrated against the patients' coagulation profile. The duration of infusion ranged from 16 to 96 hours. Recanalization was achieved in four patients who were treated within 36 hours of the onset of occlusion.

Intra-arterial thrombin activity produced by percutaneous transluminal angioplasty eliminated by segmentally enclosed thrombolysis.
Jorgensen B; Nielsen JD. Eur J Vas Surg 1992; 6(2): 153–157.

We determined the specific marker of thrombin activity, fibrinopeptide a (FPA), in the vicinity of dilated sites during percutaneous transluminal angioplasty (PTA) for femoro-popliteal obstructions in 24 patients. Blood samples were drawn proximal to dilated segments from a 4F catheter inserted retrogradely in the common femoral artery and distal to dilated segments from the balloon catheter tip. Median ± S.E. FPA concentration was 21.5 ± 4.4ng ml-1 before PTA. Immediately after dilatation, FPA concentrations were increased to 970.0 ± 836.9 ng ml-1 distal to dilated segments (p less than 0.00005) and to 48.5 ± 11.4 ng ml-1 proximally (p less than 0.003). Segmentally enclosed thrombolysis (SET) was undertaken immediately after PTA, when a double balloon catheter was positioned with a balloon at each end of dilated segments. Both balloons were inflated and 5 mg recombinant tissue plasminogen activator (rt-PA) and 1000 IU heparin were enclosed in the segments for 30 min. Immediately after SET, FPA concentration distal to dilated segments was 34.0 ± 14.2 ng ml-1 and not different from proximal concentrations found after PTA (p = 0.57). Intense fibrinolysis was indicated by significantly increased levels of cross-linked fibrin degradation products (D-dimer) for hours after SET, but FPA concentrations in peripheral blood remained near baseline values. This finding differed from increased thrombin activity found by others during systemic thrombolytic therapy. Early rethrombosis did not occur after PTA in this study. (ABSTRACT TRUNCATED AT 250 WORDS)

Urokinase thrombolysis using a multiple side hole multilumen infusion catheter.
Kaufman SL; Martin LG; Gilarsky BP; Finnegan MF Jr; Casarella WJ. Cardiovasc Intervent Radiol 1991; 14: 334–337.

A multilumen, multiple side hole infusion catheter was used for urokinase thrombolysis in 13 patients with thromboembolic occlusions of peripheral arteries and grafts. Balloon angioplasty was performed following urokinase infusion in 6 patients and atherectomy in 1 patient. There was one hemorrhagic complication. The major advantage of the multiple sidehole infusion catheter was the elimination of the need to reposition the catheter during the infusion and the reduction of the time burden on the angiographic facility. The success rate for the thrombolysis (77%) was comparable to results recorded in the literature. The total duration of infusion was not reduced compared to other series.

Streptokinase in the management of arterial thrombosis in infancy.
Kirk CR; Qureshi SA. Int J Cardiol 1989; 25: 15–20.

Fourteen children with a mean age of 9.7 months (range 0.1–34.0 months) and a mean weight of 5.4 kg (range 2.5–10.0 kg) received intravenous streptokinase following arterial thrombosis. A median loading dose of 1000 U/ kg (range 750–4000 U/kg) was given followed by an initial median infusion rate of 1000 U/kg/hr (range 750–1000 U/kg/hr). If thrombolysis did not occur and the fibrinogen level remained within the normal range (1.5–4.5 g/l) the infusion rate was increased to a maximum of 3000 U/kg/hr. Thrombolysis was achieved in all cases a mean of 16.7 hours (range 2–44 hours) after the start of treatment. The mean fibrinogen level at thrombolysis was 1.11 g/l (range 0.28–2.25 g/l) compared with pretreatment levels of 2.12 g/l (range 1.4–3.05 g/l). Minor bleeding from arterial puncture sites occurred in 6 children (43%). Streptokinase is a safe and effective treatment for arterial thrombosis in children.

Fibrinolytic therapy.
Klatte EC; Becker GJ; Holden RE; Yune HY. Radiology 1986; 159: 619–624.

The state of the art of fibrinolytic therapy is constantly changing; perhaps no other area of medicine is developing as rapidly. This paper presents the status of fibrinolytic therapy from the authors' viewpoint. Many statements are controversial. It is possible to find divergent opinions expressed by experts on almost any aspect of fibrinolysis. Objective data are rapidly accumulating, but because new substances continue to be ddveloped, the present and future statuses of fibrinolysis remain unclear. The current results of fibrinolytic therapy are excellent but will be dwarfed by the effects of new compounds and techniques in the near future. Continued developments in this field will have a major impact on improved health care delivery.

Local intra-arterial streptokinase therapy for acute peripheral arterial occlusions. Should thrombolytic therapy replace embolectomy?
Kolts RL; Kuehner ME; Swanson MK; Carlson RD; Myers WO; Friedenberg WR. Am Surg 1985; 51: 381–387.

Locally administered low-dose streptokinase was used in 13 patients with acute arterial occlusions. Systemic fibrinolytic effects were noted in each of 11 patients in whom some effective thrombolysis was demonstrated. In the two patients with no angiographically demonstrable thrombolysis, a systemic lytic effect was absent. Bleeding complications were frequent (31%). Three patients required amputations and one patient died. The systemic lytic effects of streptokinase appear to be necessary for complete clot lysis. Locally administered streptokinase appears to have no significant benefit compared to high-dose systemic administration. Occlusions accessible to balloon embolectomy should probably be treated surgically, reserving fibrinolytic therapy for inaccessible lesions. More research is needed to clarify the specific indications, as well as to determine optimal methods of administration and dosage.

Hemorheology in systemic ultrahigh-dose thrombolytic therapy with streptokinase and urokinase.
Koppensteiner R; Jung M; Minar E; Ehringer H. Thromb Res 1989; 56: 277–287.

The course of fibrinogen (Fgen), red cell aggregation (RCA), plasma viscosity (PV), platelet aggregation (PA) and hematocrit (Hc) was studied in patients with ultrahigh-dose thrombolytic therapy (1.5 × 10(6) units/hour for 6 hours = 1 cycle) with streptokinase (SK) or urokinase (UK) over a period of 3 cycles. Both ultrahigh-dose SK and UK produced significant changes in the course of Fgen, RCA and PV, whereas PA (spontaneous and ADP-induced) and Hc remained unchanged. After termination of each cycle Fgen progressively increased while RCA and PV further decreased. The extent of alteration in cycle 1—concerning the baseline values—was more pronounced with SK than with UK, but the overall effect of SK decreased through the consecutive cycles because of more rapid increase during the SK-free period. In UK-therapy hemorheological alterations were initially moderate but increased from cycle to cycle.

Catheter-lysis: indications and primary results.
Krings W; Roth FJ; Cappius G; Schmidtke I. Int Angiol 1985; 4: 117–123.

Catheter-lysis—local low-dose fibrinolytic therapy—extends the indication to catheter-treatment. Occlusions longer than 10 cm younger than 3 months may be treated by this method. This treatment is primarily indicated for Fontaine stage III/IV occlusions. The complication of acute embolism or acute reocclusion during routine angioplasty can be treated satisfactorily by catheter-lysis. The primary result of low-dose fibrinolysis depends on the clinical stage, peripheral outflow, age and length of the occlusion.

Intraarterial fibrinolysis: long-term results.
Lammer J; Pilger E; Neumayer K; Schreyer H. Radiology 1986; 161: 159–163.

Intraarterial fibrinolytic therapy was performed in 136 patients suffering from arteriosclerotic thrombosis of the iliac and femoropopliteal arteries. The initial success rate was 78%. Despite anticoagulation therapy, early recurrent thrombosis was observed in 10% of the patients. The 2-year cumulative patency rate after recanalization was 81%. These results are competitive with those of reconstructive vascular surgery. Therefore, intraarterial fibrinolysis has become a viable alternative to surgery in treating segmental peripheral occlusions more than 4 cm in length that are less than 6–9 months in duration.

[Systemic thrombolysis of arterial occlusions of the lower extremities. Comparison of various treatment schedules.]
Systemische Thrombolyse arterieller Verschlusse der unteren Extremitaten Vergleich verschiedener Behandlungsschemata.
Lammle B; Noll G; Christe M; Fritschi J; Czendlik C; Marbet GA; Biland L; Da Silva A; Huber P; Widmer LK; et al. Schweiz Med Wochenschr 1983; 113: 1570–1576.

From 1971–1982 121 patients with arterial occlusions of the lower limbs underwent systemic thrombolysis treatment at the Kantonsspital Basel. During 4 time-periods, 3 different treatment schedules were evaluated consecutively: a) individually titrated high dose streptokinase (SK), b) individuilly titrated low dose SK and c) p-plasmin, followed by low dose SK infusion. Thrombolytic success rates did not differ significantly with the 3 treatment schedules. Nevertheless, the p-plasmin-SK scheme tended to the thrombolytically more effective (68%) than high-dose (58%) or low-dose (50%) SK. The most frequent side effects were bleeding complications. In 6 out of the 121 patients, intracranial bleeding occurred and was lethal in 1 of the patients. The incidence of this most serious complication of 4/47 during the sequential p-plasmin-SK schedule led the authors to abandon this scheme for the treatment of arterial occlusions. The intracranial bleeding complications are much less frequent in patients with deep venous thrombosis undergoing systemic thrombolysis, and hence seem to be due in part to the generalized arteriopathy often present in patients with arterial occlusions. The p-plasmin-SK schedule induced the strongest systemic proteolysis in the light of thromboplastin time and factor V values. Comparison of these data with those of other authors is very difficult because of differences in patient selection, treatment schedules and observance of contraindications. The serious prognosis for patients with acute arterial occlusions, with an overall hospital mortality of 26% (experience at the Kantonsspital Basel, 1978–1982) relativizes the importance of the side effects due to systemic thrombolysis. (ABSTRACT TRUNCATED AT 250 WORDS)

Accelerated thrombolysis and angioplasty for hand ischemia in Buerger's disease.
Lang EV; Bookstein JJ. Cardiovasc Intervent Radiol 1989; 12: 95–97.

A patient with severe hand ischemia due to Buerger's disease was treated by a rapidly effective modification of percutaneous catheterization. Accelerated mechanical and pharmacologic thrombolysis of an occluded palmar arch with 200,000 U urokinase and subsequent small vessel angioplasty abolished pain and restored digital perfusion within 40 min.

Recombinant tissue-type plasminogen activator is superior to streptokinase for local intra-arterial thrombolysis.
Lonsdale RJ; Berridge DC; Earnshaw JJ; Harrison JD; Gregson RH; Wenham PW; Hopkinson BR; Makin GS. Br J Surg 1992; 79(3): 272–275.

The results of local intra-arterial thrombolysis in 98 patients treated with streptokinase and 69 patients treated with recombinant tissue plasminogen activator (rtPA) have been compared. The two gropus of patients were well matched and their treatment protocols were identical except with regard to the thrombolytic agent used. Strict criteria for defining successful thrombolysis were used. Successful lysis was achieved in 40 of 98 patients (41 percent) receiving streptokinase and 40 of 69 patients (58 percent) receiving rtPA (P less than 0.05). The time to lysis was significantly shorter with rtPA, median time 22 h, than with streptokinase, median time 40 h (P less than 0.002). There was no difference in the incidence of haemorrhagic complications. These results suggest that rtPA is superior to streptokinase for local intra-arterial thrombolysis.

Thrombolytic treatment with i.v. brinase of advanced arterial obliterative disease of the limbs.
Lund F; Ekestrom S; Frisch EP; Magaard F. Angiology 1975; 26: 534–556.

The material includes 17 patients suffering from different degrees of chronic peripheral arterial disease (11 chronic patients stage III and IV, two patients with acute arterial occlusion, and four patients stage II). Presence and extent of arterial occlusion was ascertained by initial arteriography. In twelve of the patients amputation had been considered. The patients were treated by a series of i.v. infusions of brinase, a proteolytic enzyme from Aspergillus oryzae. The brinase inhibitor capacity in plasma was determined by the azocollagen technique. Dosage of brinase was calculated to retain a rest-inhibitor capacity in order to avoid free proteolytic activity. In five patients the enzyme was also given preoperatively by intra-arterial instillation prior to a series of i v. brinase infusions. Thirteen patients showed clinical improvement after brinase treatment. The condition of two patients remained unchanged, and in two patients amputation could not be avoided. In fourteen patients the treatment results were followed by measurement of peripheral systolic blood pressure. In ten patients obvious increase of the peripheral systolic blood pressure was observed. Cutaneous microcirculation was studied in seven patients by i.v. sequential fluorescein angiography and signs of improved microcirculation (appearance time, intensity and/or extent of fluorescence) were found in all examined patients. One patient with acute arterial occlusion of the right leg with obstruction of blood flow from the external iliac artery showed complete disobliteration after a series of i.v. brinase infusions. Bleeding complications associated with brinase treatment were not observed in the material. In three patients brinase treatment was discontinued because of complications (2 brinase, 1 heparin).

Results of thrombolysis in the treatment of arterial ischemia of the limbs according to mode of administration.
Marzelle J; Combe S; Gigou F; Samama M. Int Angiol 1989; 8: 179–187.

After reviewing the principles, results and complications of thrombolytic therapy with "classical" agents (Streptokinase and Urokinase) used via intravenous, intraarterial route, or intraoperatively, and with more "modern" agents (APSAC, scuPA, tPA), we discuss the future of thrombolysis in the treatment of arterial ischemia of the limbs. Several items need to be clarified: —indication of thrombolysis among other treatments, mainly surgery, of arterial ischemia depends on the clinical staging of ischemia, its causes and the site of arterial obstruction; —method of delivery of the thrombolytic agent must provide the highest local concentration and the lowest systemic side effects; —efficacy of each thrombolytic agent must be analyzed when used in peripheral arterial ischemia, but also in other diseases such as myocardial infarction. (65 Refs.)

Discrepancy in the thrombolytic effect of UK between angiography and circulatory evaluations.
Matsuo O; Mihara H; Motomatsu K. Angiology 1984; 35: 523–527.

A clinical case in which angiographic and circulatory evaluations of the thrombolytic effect of urokinase (UK) were not correlated, is described. Circulatory improvement distal to the thrombosis was recognized on the basis of a rise in skin temperature and increased palpability of the pulse at the distal artery. However, angiography revealed the development of thrombosis. This discrepancy may have arisen from the hypotensive action of UK preparations due to increased flow in the collateral circulation. The significance of angiography in providing direct evidence for assessing the thrombolytic effect of UK as emphasized.

Management of thrombotic complications of invasive arterial monitoring of the upper extremity.
McFadden PM; Ochsner JL; Mills N. J Cardiovasc Surg (Torino) 1983; 24: 35–39.

Invasive arterial monitoring is essential intraoperative and perioperative management of vascular and cardiac patients. Complications resulting from arterial monitoring, although rare, can result in severe functional sequelae and loss of an extremity. Severe extremity ischemia and repeated thromboses in a 10-year-old male resulted from brachial arterial monitoring line, Multiple operative thrombectomies and systemic anticoagulation were unsuccessful. Limb salvage and arterial patency were achieved by saphenous vein patch angioplasty at site of arterial injury and intermittent intra-arterial streptokinase infusion placed into a natural side branch of the saphenous vein segment. Although many complications may result from arterial monitoring, the most serious is arterial thrombosis with impending degital or extremity gangrene. This constitutes a surgical emergency. When aggressive conventional surgical techniques alone fail to control catheter induced thrombosis, an innovative technique in combination with regional intra-arterial streptokinase therapy has been successful adjunctive measure in reestablishing microvascular patency resulting in limb salvage.

Technique and results of "higher-dose" infusion.
McNamara T. Cardiovasc Intervent Radiol 1988; 11 (Suppl): 48–57.

We experimented with thrombolytic technique in an attempt to maximize therapeutic outcome, selecting urokinase because of its proven safety and efficacy in clinical investigation. An initially "high-dose" regimen, starting at 4,000 U/min and decreasing to 1,000 U/min after restoration of antegrade blood flow, generally establishes lysis within 3–4 h—even after acute embolic or thrombolytic occlusion. It can also be used effectively and safely as a therapeutic trial. "High-doses" urokinase compares favorably with "low-dose" streptokinase and shows a lower incidence of bleeding and allergic complications.

Role of thrombolysis in peripheral arterial occlusion.
McNamara TO. Am J Med 1987; 83: 6–10.

In an initial study, 85 patients with 93 thromboembolic occlusions of peripheral arteries or grafts were treated with urokinase by direct intra-arterial infusion. Urokinase was infused directly into the proximal portion of the clot at 4,000 IU/minute for two hours. Arteriography was then repeated. If a channel had been lysed in the proximal part of the clot, but the distal part remained occluded, the catheter was gently advanced into the still occluded portion of the clot and the infusion was resumed at 4,000 IU/minute until antegrade blood flow was reestablished. Then the catheter was repositioned to be proximal to all of the remaining clot. The urokinase dosage was reduced to 1,000 IU/minute and the infusion continued with reexaminations at eight-hour intervals. The infusion was continued until complete clot lysis was accomplished. A search for a flow-limiting lesion on which to perform a percutaneous transluminal angioplasty was then performed. The lack of at least a 10 percent reduction in clot length after a 500,000-IC cumulative infusion dose of urokinase was an indication for termination of the regimen. Seventy-five percent of the 93 infusions resulted in complete clot lysis, even though in nine patients (10 percent) the infusion could not be completed. Eighty-one percent of the 84 completed infusions resulted in complete clot lysis, and the incidence of clinical improvement was 89 percent. The average duration of infusion was 18 hours. Major bleeding (requiring transfusion) occurred in only 4 percent of the patients. This regimen has now been applied to 150 occlusions, and the results are approximately the same. Review of our experience demonstrated that the ability to easily advance an angiographic guide wire through an occlusion has been the best predictor that a given clot would lyse irrespective of the clot's location or the duration of symptoms. Easy guide wire traversal appears to rule out the presence of either advanced changes of clot organization throughout the occlusion or a rare completely obstructing atherosclerotic lesion. A review of the published experience of 155 direct intra-thrombus infusions of 5,000 IU/hour of streptokinase demonstrated only a 45 percent incidence of complete clot lysis. Also, infusion times were quite prolonged (41 hours), and major bleeding complications were surprisingly common (13 percent). The results with urokinase thus indicate that it is preferable to streptokinase since it produces fewer complications and accomplishes more rapid recanalization and a higher incidence of total clot lysis.

The role of thrombolytic therapy in surgical practice.
Moran KT; Jewell ER; Persson AV. Br J Surg 1989; 76: 298–304.

The ability of streptokinase and urokinase to lyse intravascular fibrin-based clots is firmly established. However, there is a lack of enthusiasm for these agents because of serious haemorrhagic complications and a lack of controlled randomized studies indicating their efficacy. Thrombolytic therapy is suitable in only 15 percent of patients with acute deep venous thrombosis. It restores the venous circulation to normal in up to 95 percent of these patients if therapy is instituted within 5 days of the onset of symptoms. These patients have significantly fewer symptoms on follow-up than patients treated with heparin although the ability of thrombolytic therapy to preserve venous valvular function and to prevent the post-phlebitic syndrome is now in question. Thrombolytic therapy is as effective as heparin in preventing pulmonary embolism and may be superior in its treatment. Pulmonary haemodynamics are rapidly improved, diffusion capacity is restored and, although the evidence is inconclusive, long-term pulmonary hypertension may be prevented. Although the mortality rate is not decreased, controlled studies show that thrombolytic therapy may be beneficial in massive pulmonary embolism with clinical shock. Thrombolytic therapy is indicated for acute arterial and acute bypass graft occlusion when the surgical alternative is associated with a higher morbidity and mortality. Partial thrombolysis is achieved in up to 90 percent of cases and the need for further therapeutic intervention is eliminated in one-third of the patients treated.

New thrombolytic agents with greater specificity and potentially greater efficacy and fewer complications are being developed. Tissue plasminogen activator has been successfully used. Prourokinase, fibrin-seeking urokinase and acetylated streptokinase-plasmin ogen complex may expand the role of thrombolytic therapy in surgical practice. (99 Refs.)

Review: Stratton Lecture. Thrombosis and atherogenesis: molecular connections.
Nachman RL. Blood 1992; 79(8): 1897–1906.

Treatment with stanozolol before thrombolysis in patients with arterial occlusions.
Noll G; Lammle B; Duckert F. Thromb Res 1985; 37: 529–532.

The administration of the anabolic steroid stanozolol during 7, 8 days as pretreatment before thrombolytic therapy of acute or subacute arterial occlusions enhances the fibrinolytic potential significantly. On average the plasminogen increased from 101% to 133%, the euglobulin lysis time after venous stasis was shortened and the alpha 2-antiplasmin remained constant. This effect could be favourable to prepare patients undergoing thrombolytic treatment.

Reduced synthesis of tissue plasminogen activator by vascular endothelium during acute myocardial infarction.
Norris RM; Ockelford PA; Cross DB; Rivers JT; Smith JM; Takayama M; White HD. Aust N Z J Med 1992; 22(3): 261–264.

We measured levels of tissue plasminogen activator (t-PA) antigen in 100 patients within six hours of the onset of acute myocardial infarction, in 34 patients with chronic angina but no recent infarction, and in 36 normal subjects. We also assayed von Willebrand factor in the acute patients and in the normal subjects. Measurements were repeated in 40 acute patients at three weeks after myocardial infarction. Although resting levels of t-PA antigen were not significantly different from normal during myocardial infarction, the capacity of the vascular endothelium to release t-PA after five minutes of venous occlusion was impaired (p less than 0.01). The acute phase vessel wall release of von Willebrand factor was increased during acute infarction (p less than 0.01). We conclude that impairment of t-PA production is associated with acute coronary thrombosis, although it is not possible to differentiate between a causative role or a secondary response due to exhaustion of the t-PA producing mechanism.

Thermographic evaluation of the hemodynamic effect of the antithrombotic drug cilostazol in peripheral arterial occlusion.
Ohashi S; Iwatoni M; Hyakuna Y; Morioka Y. Arzneimittelforschung 1985; 35: 1203–1208.

Cilostazol (6-[4-(1-cyclohexyl-1H-tetrazol-5-yl) butoxy]-3,4-dihydro-2(1H0)-quinolinone, OPC-13013) was evaluated experimentally to be effective in increasing blood flow in arterial occlusive disease. The hemodynamic effect of the drug on peripheral arterial occlusion was examined using a noninvasive thermographic technique over a certain period of time. The study included 10 patients with peripheral arterial occlusion, 7 with thromboangiitis obliterans and 3 with arteriosclerosis obliterans. Cilostazol was administered at 200 mg/day for 6 successive weeks to 7 patients (10 lower limbs and 1 upper limb) and at 100 mg/day for 6 weeks to 2 patients (3 lower limbs) and 4 weeks to 1 (1 lower limb), and the skin temperature and skin blood flow were measured in the limbs of these patients. The 200-mg/day dose brought about elevation of the two parameters at 4 and 6 weeks. The increase in skin temperature in the leg and foot at 6 weeks was statistically significant (p less than 0.05, t-test), and the increase in skin blood flow was also signaficant in the leg (p less than 0/05) and foot (p less than 0.1). Such increase was obtained at the lower dose of 100 mg/day, but the number of cases was too small to statistically analyze patient response.

Inhibitor of plasminogen activator in human arterial wall. I. Histochemical study.

Okamura T; Nanno S; Sueishi K; Tanaka K. Acta Pathol Jpn 1984; 34: 743–747.

An inhibitor of urokinase, human urinary plasminogen activator, was found in the media of human arteries using a histochemical method (fibrin slide sandwich technique). Arteriosclerotic lesions, especially atherosclerosis, apparently contained the urokinase inhibitor. The inhibator did not alter plasmin activity. This inhibitor of urokinase may be involved in regulation of fibrinolysis in arterial wall and thus a significant role in atherogenesis.

Inhibitor of plasminogen activator in human arterial wall. II. Biochemical characterization.

Okamura T; Nanno S; Sueishi K; Tanaka K. Acta Pathol Jpn 1984; 34: 749–757.

Fibrinolytic inhibitor was prepared from human aortas and some of its biochemical properties were investigated. The fibrinolytic inhibitor suppressed urokinase activity, but did not inhibit plasmin activity when assayed by fibrin plate method and synthetic fluorogenic substrate method. The urokinase inhibitor was a glycoprotein and migrated similar to alpha-globulin upon fibrin-ager electrophoresis. The molecular weight determined by gel filtration was approximately 98,000. The urokinase inhibitor was immunologically different from other known plasma protease inhibitors, such as alpha 2-plasmin inhibitor, alpha 2-macroglobulin, and alpha 2-antitrypsin. The interaction of urokinase with the inhibitor was dose-dependent. Progressive inactivation of urokinase occurred by increasing time of incubation with the inhibitor at 37 degrees C, and over 90% inhibition of urokinase required 30 min of incubation. The inhibitor of plasminogen activator in human aorta may be noteworthy in relation to thrombogenesis and atherogenesis.

Thrombolytic therapy in the treatment of peripheral arterial occlusions.

Olin JW; Graor RA. Ann Emerg Med 1988; 17: 1210–1215.

Intra-arterial infusions of thrombolytic agents are useful adjuncts to surgery and percutaneous transluminal angioplasty. The best results occur when the thrombus is lysed within 30 days; however, successful thrombolysis has occurred up to four months after an arterial occlusion. Thrombolysis allows dissolution of thrombus in the small distal runoff vessels, decreasing outflow resistance and enabling the native artery or bypass graft to remain open longer. When native arteries are lysed successfully, underlying area of stenosis is usually identified and thus able to be corrected with either surgery or percutaneous transluminal angioplasty. When bypass grafts thrombose, thrombolytic agents are usually successful in lysing the thrombus and identifying the cause for the thrombosis. With local intra-arterial infusions, side effects and complications may be kept to a minimum. (34 Refs.)

Fibrinolytic treatment of residual thrombus after catheter embolectomy for severe lower limb ischemia.
Parent FN 3d; Bernhard VM; Pabst TS 3d; McIntyre KE; Hunter GC; Malone JM. J Vasc Surg 1989; 9: 153–160.

Intraoperative intraarterial fibrinolytic therapy (IIFT) was employed in 28 patients with acute limb ischemia. In 17 patients, significant residual calf thrombus was demonstrated by completion arteriography after standard balloon catheter thromboembolectomy, whereas in 11, pretreatment arteriography was not obtained. With the patient systemically heparinized, a bolus of fibrinolytic agent was instilled into the distal vessels below an inflow occlusion clamp. Among the 17 patients under angiographic control, arteriography was repeated after 30 minutes and a second bolus was injected if significant residual thrombus was still present. Successful lysis was achieved in 88% of these 17 limbs and streptokinase (SK) and urokinase (UK) were equally effective. The dosage of SK varied between 50,000 and 150,000 units (seven patients) and of UK between 35,000 and 150,000 units (21 patients). Serum fibrinogen levels declined significantly after IIFT (t test; p less than 0.05), but the average level remained within the normal range. Major bleeding developed in two patients, both of whom received SK and underwent a concomitant major abdominal vascular procedure, with a severe fall in fibrinogen values to 10 and 17 mg/dl. A minor groin hematoma occurred in one patient treated with UK. There was a significant difference in the incidence of bleeding between SK (2/7) and UK (1/21) (chi 2; p less than 0.05). Compartment syndrome developed in six limbs (21%). Amputation was required in two patients (7%). There was no correlation between prolongation of ischemia time as a result of IIFT and the incience of compartment syndrome. (ABSTRACT TRUNCATED AT 250 WORDS)

Outcome of intraarterial urokinase for acute vascular occlusion.
Parent FN 3d; Piotrowski J; Bernhard VM; Pond GD; Pabst TS 3d; Bull DA; Hunter GC; McIntyre KE. J Cardiovasc Surg (Torino) 1991; 32: 680–689.

Intraarterial urokinase (IAUK) was administered to 33 patients on 40 occasions for the treatment of acute extremity ischemia and long-term patency was assessed. Lysis was successful in 39 of the 40 cases (95%). Occlusive thrombus was cleared in 12 of 13 patients with native artery occlusion (7 complete, 5 partial), 8 of 9 with autologous vein grafts (5 complete, 3 partial), and in all 18 patients with synthetic grafts (17 complete, 1 partial). The primary cumulative patency following successful IAUK was 100% for native arteries and 47% for synthetic grafts at 12 months, and 23% for autologous grafts at 9 months. The difference in rethrombosis rate between autologous vein (67%) and native artery (0%) was significant (p = 0.02) as was the difference betwen infrainguinal prosthetic grafts (63%) and native artery (p = 0.025). IAUK is most effective for the treatment of native artery occlusion, but is significantly less effective for thrombosed infrainguinal autologous vein or synthetic grafts due to the likelihood of reocclusion, despite the high immediate success rate. For autologous vein grafts, lysis is frequently incomplete and patency rapidly deteriorates regardless of adjunctive therapy to relieve the underlying obstruction.

Immediate post-operative urokinase infusion: extending the limits of limb salvage surgery.
Perler BA; Osterman FA. J Cardiovasc Surg (Torino) 1990; 31: 184–188.

We report the case of a 74-year-old woman with multi-level arterial occlusive disease and severe ischemia of the right lower extremity who underwent a re-operative femoro-femoral and a right femoro-popliteal bypass graft. Her right foot remained non-viable post-operatively despite patent grafts. She then underwent a 12-hour infusion of urokinase through a percutaneously placed popliteal artery catheter during that first post-operative day, with salvage of the right leg.

Intraarterial fibrinolysis: in vitro and prospective clinical evaluation of three thrombolytic agents.
Pilger E; Lammer J; Bertuch H; Steiner H. Radiology 1986; 161: 597–599.

In order to investigate and compare the fibrinolytic activity of streptokinase, streptokinase-Glutamine-plasminogen, and urokinise for intraarterial fibrinolysis, as in vitro test and a prospective trial were performed. For the in vitro demonstration of lytic activity, fibrin plates with plasminogen and fibrin plates without plasminogen were incubated with streptokinase; with streptokinase-plasminogen in molar proportions of 1:1, 1:2, and 2:1, and with urokinase. In order to examine the in vivo activity of the different lytic solutions, 98 patients suffering from peripheral arterial occlusions were divided into three homogeneous groups for treatment with streptokinase, streptokinase-plasminogen, and urokinase. Although urokinase was superior to streptokinase on the fibrin plate with plasminogen, no difference was demonstrated in vivo between the two lytic agents. Streptokinase-plasminogen in a molar proportion of 1:2 showed significantly higher fibrinolytic activity than any other solution. Therefore, the fibrinolytic agent of choice for intrathrombotic infections seems to be a 1:2 solution of streptokinase with plasminogen or with the lytic enzyme plasmin itself.

Blood and plasma viscosity in experimentally induced hyper- and hypo-fibrinogenaemia.
Pola P; Flore R; Tondi P. Int J Tissue React 1986; 8: 333–336.

For some time now fibrinogen has been attributed considerable importance in influencing blood and plasma viscosity. This paper attempts to experimentally confirm this statement in vivo: two groups of arteriopathic patients were selected for investigating viscosity in hyper- and hypo-fibrinogenaemia induced by PTA and a cycle of fibrinolytic treatment with urokinase respectively. Although fibrinogenaemia exhibited highly significant changes under such conditions, there was no important change in viscosity. Probably the role of fibrinogen in influencing viscosity has been overestimated in the past and it is likely that there are other more important factors.

Antiplatelet drugs or dicoumarol: what is the most effective prophylaxis in occlusive arterial disease?
Poliwoda H; Avenarius HJ. Int Angiol 1986; 5: 169–180.

Arterial thromboses lead to disturbances of vital function: myocardial infarction, ischemic cerebral infarction, disorders of peripheral blood flow, nephrosclerosis. Prophylaxis of thrombosis is still an unsolved problem, since diseases caused by thrombosis remain the first cause of death, at least in Western countries. After describing the pathomorphological and pathobiochemical findings, a survey of the literature on prophylaxis of occlusive arterial diseases is presented and the difference between anticoagulants and aggregation inhibitors is pointed out.

Late results of local thrombolytic treatment of peripheral arterial occlusions.
Poredos P; Keber D; Videcnik V. Angiology 1989; 40: 941–947.

One hundred thirty-four patients, in whom acute and subacute arterial occlusions of lower limbs were treated with low dose intraarterial streptokinase, were observed for periods of up to five years. Primary recanalization of occluded vessels was achieved in 66 patients, but in the remaining 68 patients recanalization was not observed. In 45% of the patients with successful thrombolytic treatment, percutaneous dilatation (PTA) of remnant stenosis was performed. In patients with successful recanalization the reocclusion rate was greatest in the first year (17.4%); the first two weeks after therapy were most critical in this respect. The reocclusion rate during the succeeding years ranged from 4% to 9% per year. The cumulative patency rate after five years was 63.4%. Late results were better in patients in whom more proximal vascular segments were affected. The preservation of vessel patency was highly dependent on the severity and extent of the previous atherosclerotic process and especially on the state of peripheral (runoff) arteries. Presence of diabetes mellitus increased the reocclusion rate of recanalized vessels. Of the patients with unsuccessful recanalization, only 5 reported some symptomatic improvement during the observation period, 39 (57%) needed immediate amputation, and an additional 8 (4.7%) were amputated later on. Considering the fact that all patients were previously refused for bypass surgery owing to unsuitable runoff vessels or bad general condition, the long-term results were surprisingly good, suggesting that thrombolytic treatment, combined in remnant stenosis with PTA, was an efficient method in patients with acute or subacute arterial occlusions.

Intraoperative infusion of lytic drugs for thrombotic complications of revascularization.
Quinones-Baldrich WJ; Baker JD; Busuttil RW; Machleder HI; Moore WS. J Vasc Surg 1989; 10: 408–417.

Between August 1983 and December 1987, 23 patients received a 30-minute intraoperative, intraarterial infusion of streptokinase (seven patients) or urokinase (16 patients) because of residual thrombus or persistent ischemia or both after thromboembolectomy. Ages ranged from 21 to 77 years (mean, 58 years). In 15 patients intraoperative lytic therapy was part of the initial operation, whereas in eight patients intraoperative lytic therapy was performed during a secondary operation to treat thrombosis of a recently placed graft. Seven patients in the latter group had hypercoagulable conditions (five had heparin-induced thrombosis; one had protein C deficiency; one had polycythemia with thrombocytosis). Improvement after intraoperative lytic therapy was seen on angiography performed after infusion in 13 of 17 (76%) patients in whom angiography was performed both before and after intraoperative lytic therapy. Grafts in 12 of these patients remained patent without additional intervention, and in one graft thrombus formed again. In contrast, among four patients without angiographic evidence of improvement, thrombus formed again in four grafts (p less than 0.004). Intraoperative lytic therapy was considered successful in 74% of instances (17/23), including four of seven patients with hypercoagulable states. Three of six patients whose grafts failed had major amputations, whereas there were no amputations after successful infusions. Twelve patients were heparinized after intraoperative lytic therapy. Ten patients in this group were considered treatment successes, and two were considered treatment failures. Three of 11 patients not heparinized after intraoperative lytic therapy were considered treatment failures. Four hematomas occurred in the former group and none in the latter (p less than 0.03). No hematomas occurred in the heparin-induced thrombosis group in spite of anticoagulation with sodium warfarin (Coumadin). Only one hematoma occurred within 6 hours of intraoperative lytic therapy, and thus it was attributable to the infusion. We conclude that intraoperative lytic therapy is an effective adjunct to manage residual thrombus or persistent ischemia or both after lower extremity revascularization. Postinfusion angiography is of prognostic value. Heparinization after intraoperative lytic therapy seems beneficial but significantly increases the risk of bleeding complications.

Intraoperative fibrinolytic therapy: an adjunct to catheter thromboembolectomy.
Quinones-Baldrich WJ; Zierler RE; Hiatt JC. J Vasc Surg 1985; 2: 319–326.

This article describes our initial experience with intraoperative infusion of the fibrinolytic agent streptokinase. Five patients with various complications of atherosclerosis manifested by limb-threatening ischemia were treated by balloon-catheter thromboembolectomy followed by intra-arterial streptokinase infusion. In each patient viability of the involved extremity was questionable after removal of all thrombus accessible to the balloon catheter. Fibrinolytic therapy was used when operative arteriography showed residual thrombus distal to the popliteal artery. All patients were systemically heparinized during the operation, and three patients were maintained on anticoagulants during the initial postoperative period. A streptokinase solution containing 7S0 U/ml was infused intra-arterially proximal to the residual thrombus. The total dosage ranged from 20,000 to 100,000 units per patient. This treatment was considered successful in all five patiints, as documented by return of palpable pulses, audible Doppler flow signals where none was present prior to infusion, and operative arteriography. There were no complications related to intraoperative streptokinase infusion. We conclude that intraoperative fibrinolytic therapy is a safe adjunct to catheter thromboembolectomy. The observed improvement in limb perfusion can be attributed to lysis of thrombus in the distal arteries that could not be retrieved with the balloon catheter. Laboratory studies are in progress to establish precise indications for intraoperative streptokinase and to determine the most effective dosage and rate of administration.

Use and limitations of thrombolytic therapy in the treatment of peripheral arterial ischemia: results of a multi-institutional questionnaire.
Ricotta JJ; Green RM; DeWeese JA. J Vasc Surg 1987; 6: 45–50.

In an attempt to assess the efficacy of thrombolytic infusions for arterial ischemia, a questionnaire was distributed to 142 vascular surgeons. Data from 45 respondents who had experience with thrombolytic infusion in 623 patients were reviewed. A successful outcome was obtained in 313 of 623 patients (50.2%). Morbidity was significant. with hemorrhage requiring transfusion or operation in 125 cases (20.1%) and major amputation in 103 cases (16.5%). There were nine strokes associated with thrombolytic infusion (1.4%), six of which were fatal. Sixteen deaths were associated with thrombolytic therapy, for a mortality rate of 2.5% (16 of 623 patients). Analysis of results by grouping centers according to numbers of lytic infusions failed to show significant correlation with center experience. Furthermore, morbidity and mortality were seen in centers with both limited and extensive experience with thrombolytic infusion. The initial enthusiasm for thrombolytic infusion to treat arterial ischemia is not substantiated by our data. Carefully controlled prospective trials are needed before this method can be offered as an alternative to arterial reconstruction.

Axillary artery compression and thrombosis in throwing athletes.
Rohrer MJ; Cardullo PA; Pappas AM; Phillips DA; Wheeler HB. J Vasc Surg 1990; 11: 761–769.

A 28-year-old major league baseball pitcher sustained an axillary artery thrombosis which was successfully treated with intraarterial urokinase. Subsequent angiography and duplex scanning with the arm elevated in the pitching position demonstrated inducible compression of the axillary artery by the humeral head as well as compression at the thoracic outlet. To determine the incidence of axillary and subclavian artery compression and to investigate the mechanism of injury, brachial artery blood pressures and duplex scans of the subclavian and axillary arteries were performed in both the neutral position and the throwing position in the 92 extremities of 19 major league baseball pitchers, 16 non-pitching major league players, and 11 nonathlete controls. A drop in blood pressure of greater than 20 mm Hg was noted in the position in 56% of extremities tested, with a loss of a detectable blood pressure in 13%. Compression of the axillary artery by the humeral head was documented in 83% of extremities, but in only 7.6% was a greater than 50% stenosis inducible. No statistical difference was found in the incidence of arterial compression between the three groups tested or between their dominant and nondominant extremities. Dissection of the axillary artery in two cadavers documented that abduction and external rotation of the arm causes compression of the axillary artery by the humeral head, which acts as a fulcrum. We conclude that the repetitive mechanical trauma of the throwing motion can cause intermittent compression and contusion of the axillary artery by the humeral head and predisposes the athlete who throws to thrombosis of the axillary artery.

The treatment of venous thrombosis of the upper and lower limbs with "APSAC" (p-anisoylated striptokinase-plasminogen complex).
Ruckley CV; Boulton FE; Redhead D. Eur J Vasc Surg 1987 1: 107–112.

APSAC, administered by bolus injection, has been used to treat 28 patients: 14 with ilio-femoral venous thrombosis, 6 with "spontaneous" axillary-sub-clavian thrombosis and eight with superior vena-caval thrombosis associated with perenteral nutrition catheter. Four of the patients with lower limb deep vein thrombosis (DVT) showed partial lysis whereas the remaining 10 showed no change. Of the patients with upper limb and/or superior caval DVT seven showed complete lysis three showed partial lysis and four showed no benefit. APSAC is an effective treatment of venous thrombosis of the upper limbs.

Increased type 1 plasminogen activator inhibitor gene expression in atherosclerotic human arteries.
Schneiderman J; Sawdey MS; Keeton MR; Bordin GM; Bernstein EF; Dilley RB; Loskutoff DJ. Proc Natl Acad Sci USA 1992; 89(15): 6998–7002.

Decreased fibrinolytic capacity has been suggested to accelerate the process of arterial atherogenesis by facilitating thrombosis and fibrin deposition within developing atherosclerotic lesions. Type 1 plasminogen activator inhibitor (PAI-1) is the primary inhibitor of tissue-type plasminogen activator and has been found to be increased in a number of clinical conditions generally defined as prothrombotic. To investigate the potential role of this inhibitor in atherosclerosis, we examined the expression of PAI-1 mRNA in segments of 11 severely diseased and 5 relatively normal human arteries obtained from 16 different patients undergoing reconstructive surgery for aortic occlusive or aneurysmal disease. Densitometric scanning of RNA (Northern) blot autoradiograms revealed significantly increased levels of PAI-1 mRNA in severely atherosclerotic vessels (mean densitometric value, 1.7 ± 0.28 SEM) compared with normal or mildly affected arteries (mean densitometric value, 0.63 ± 0.09 SEM; P less than 0.05). In most instances, the level of PAI-1 mRNA was correlated with the degree of atherosclerosis. Analysis of adjacent tissue sections from the same patients by in situ hybridization demonstrated an abundance of PAI-1 mRNA-positive cells within the thickened intima of atherosclerotic arteries, mainly around the base of the plaque. PAI-1 mRNA could also be detected in cells scattered within the necrotic material and in endothelial cells of adventitial vessels. In contrast to these results, PAI-1 mRNA was visualized primarily within luminal endothelial cells of normal-appearing aortic tissue. Our data provide initial evidence for the increased expression of PAI-1 mRNA in severely artherosclerotic human arteries and suggest a role for PAI-1 in the progression of human atherosclerotic disease.

Cholesterol embolization syndrome. Occurrence after intravenous streptokinase therapy for myocardial infarction.
Schwartz MW; McDonald GB. JAMA 1987; 258(14): 1934–1935.

Two patients developed the cholesterol embolization syndrome after coronary angiography and intravenous streptokinase therapy for acute myocardial infarction. Clinical manifestations included cyanosis, ulcers, gangrene of the hands and feet, myalgias, intestinal infarction, eosinophilia, and renal failure. One patient dies; one has survived with chronic renal failure. Streptokinase therapy may expose atheromatous plaques to the circulation by lysing platelet-fibrin thrombi.

Fibrinogen/fibrin in atherogenesis.
Smith EB; Thompson WD; Crosbie L; Stirk CM. Eur J Epidemiol 1992; 8(Suppl 1): 83–87.

Fibrin is a major component of many atherosclerotic plaques. Within the intima there is continuous formation of fibrin, and continuous fibrinolysis. In aortic lesions, a lipoprotein bound to fibrin can be released by incubation with plasmin. Most of this lipoprotein is accounted for by Lp(a). The atherogenicity of Lp(a) may be more associated with lipid deposition than with inhibition of fibrinolysis. Fibrin degradation products may be chemotactic to monocyte-macrophages and stimulate smooth muscle cell proliferation. (15 Refs.)

Percutaneous aspiration thromboembolectomy.
Starck EE; McDermott JC; Crummy AB; Turnipseed WD; Acher CW; Burgess JH. Radiology 1985; 156: 61–66.

Percutaneous aspiration thromboembolectomy (PAT) was used as an angioplastic tool to remove from arteries of the lower limbs thromboembolitic material originating from any source. PAT was performed with a custom-designed catheter/sheath system, alone or in combination with balloon dilatation and/or local lytic infusion therapy with streptokinase or urokinase. PAT completed the restoration of blood flow, thus improving the results of the preceding angioplastic interventions. Clinical improvement was high, with 93% success (42 of 45 procedures). Only one below-the-knee amputation occurred, and could not be prevented. No patient became worse because of PAT intervention. The Fogarty catheter technique remains the method of choice for removing emboli within the aorto-iliac region, but in the smaller vessels below the inguinal ligament-especially in the distal superficial femoral, popliteal, and tibial regions—in our experience PAT is superior. This has been substantiated also in studies of laboratory animals, using barium-impregnated emboli.

[Rotation aspiration thromboembolectomy] Rotations-Aspirations-Thromboembolektomie.
Starck EE; Wagner HJ. Dtsch Med Wochenschr 1991; 116: 1–6.

Rotating aspiration thromboembolectomy (RAT) was performed in 32 patients (11 women and 21 men; mean age 68 [41–92] years with infrainguinal arterial occlusion, various conventional angioplasty techniques having been unsuccessful. Mean length of occlusion was 19.7 cm (2–47 cm). 17 patients were in stage IIb, 8 in stage III and 7 in stage IV (Fontaine classification). RAT consists of mechanical fragmentation of thrombotic or embolic occlusion material during simultaneous infusion of urokinase, followed by aspiration of the material. Primary success (residual stenosis less than or equal to 50%) was demonstrated by angiography in 31 of 32 patients, while primary clinical success (reduction by at least one Fontaine stage) occurred in 29 patients. These results demonstrate that RAT is a suitable method for the percutaneous intraluminal treatment of long thrombotic or embolic occlusions in which conventional angioplasty techniques have previously failed.

Arterial occlusions in neonates: use of fibrinolytic therapy.
Strife JL; Ball WS Jr; Towbin R; Keller MS; Dillon T. Radiology 1988; 166: 395–400.

For neonates with ischemia of an extremity or extensive thrombosis of the aorta after umbilical artery catheterization, prompt recognition and management decisions are necessary. The cases of eight infants with symptomatic thrombosis who were treated with fibrinolytic agents were retrospectively reviewed to study means of diagnosis and response to therapy. Peripheral thrombosis was seen in two otherwise healthy infants; fibrinolytic therapy produced complete lysis in one and partial lysis in the other. The six infants with central thrombosis presented with low Apgar scores and multiple clinical problems; umbilical catheters were already in place. To assess the clot, real-time sonography was performed in all six patients, and umbilical arteriograms were obtained in five. Fibrinolytic therapy produced complete lysis of clot in five of the six infants. The one death occurred in a premature infant in whom a large intracranial hemorrhage developed 6 hours after institution of therapy.

Acceleration of thrombolysis with a high-dose transthrombus bolus technique.
Sullivan KL; Gardiner GA Jr; Shapiro MJ; Bonn J; Levin DC. Radiology 1989; 173: 805–808.

The rate of complication and the time necessary to achieve thrombolysis remain major disadvantages of regional thrombolytic therapy. By lacing the entire length of arterial or arterial bypass graft occlusions in the lower extremities of 49 patients with one of two different bolus doses of urokinase (mean, 52,000 International U in 35 infusions = low-dose group [28 patients]; mean, 230,000 U in 23 infusions = high-dose group [21 patients]) prior to identical continuous infusions, it was possible to demonstrate a decrease in the time needed to complete thrombolysis from 33.6 hours in the low-dose group to 10.4 hours in the high-dose group (P less than .001). The total urokinase dose necessary for successful thrombolysis was also significantly less in the high-dose group (P less than .001). The major complication rate was 22.9% in the low-dose group and 3.7% in the high-dose group, although the difference was not statistically significant. The use of urokinase and a high-dose transthrombus bolus injection technique significantly accelerates thrombolysis, decreases the total urokinase dose needed, and may lower the major complication rate.

Application of thrombolytic therapy in vascular occlusive disease. A surgical view.
Towne JB; Bandyk DF. Am J Surg 1987; 154: 548–559.

The use of fibrinolytic agents to control the fibrinolytic enzyme system and lyse pathologic fibrin deposits or thrombus has now assumed a position with anticoagulants and vascular surgery in the physician's therapeutic armamentarium. The principal exogenous activators that are used clinically are streptokinase, urokinase, and tissue plasminogen activator. Acute arterial occlusions are more likely than chronic occlusions to respond to thrombolytic therapy, especially if treatment is instituted within a few hours of onset of symptoms and if the disease is due to embolic material rather than in situ thrombosis. Since the duration of drug infusion necessary to lyse arterial thrombus cannot be predicted, patients in whom tissue viability cannot be determined or in whom ischemia cannot be tolerated during the drug infusion interval are not candidates for intraarterial fibrinolytic drug infusion. In treating patients with venous occlusion, thrombolytic therapy is more effective against proximal clots than in calf thrombosis. No protective effect from pulmonary embolism has been noted in trials comparing heparin with streptokinase. Fifty percent of patients with an initial episode of deep venous thrombosis treated within 72 hours of onset will have complete resolution of thrombus with preservation of valve function.

Intraarterial fibrinolytic therapy for popliteal and tibial artery obstruction: comparison of streptokinase and urokinase.
Traughber PD; Cook PS; Micklos TJ; Miller FJ. AJR 1987; 149: 453–456.

Experience with using intraarterial fibrinolysis in the treatment of occlusive disease of the popliteal artery and runoff vessels is limited. We describe the techniques and results in 25 patients with 30 fibrinolytic infusions of the popliteal and tibial arteries and compare them with the initial and long-term results of treatment using streptokinase and urokinase. The roles of catheter delivery systems and systemic heparin in the prevention of pericatheter thrombus were also studied. Urokinase was initially successful in 18 (90%) of 20 intraarterial infusions, whereas streptokinase was effective in 8 (80%) of 10 intraarterial infusions. Urokinase had the advantages of a shorter effective infusion time and fewer complications. Long-term follow-up was available in 20 of the successfully treeted patients. Sixteen of these patients were doing well with an average follow-up of 27 months. The duration of the initial occlusion may be useful in identifying patients at risk for early reocclusion. No limbs were lost because of complications of therapy. The coaxial catheter system with a divided fibrinolytic dose provided protection against pericatheter thrombus, while systemic heparin was ineffective. Our results suggest that urokinase is more effective than streptokinase for intraarterial infusion in the treatment of occlusion of the popliteal and tibial arteries; this procedure is an important alternative to surgery or an adjuvant to surgery in selected patients.

Percutaneous aspiration thromboembolectomy (PAT): an alternative to surgical balloon techniques for clot retrieval.
Turnipseed WD; Starck EE; McDermott JC; Crummy AB; Acher CW; Jensen SR; Voegeli DR. J Vasc Surg 1986; 3: 437–441.

Percutaneous aspiration thromboembolectomy (PAT) is an angiographic technique that can be used to remove thromboembolic debris from the distal lower extremity circulation. This procedure employs a specially designed catheter-sheath system, which can be used alone or in combination with balloon angioplasty or thrombolytic drugs (streptokinase 10,000 U/hr or urokinase 100,000 U/hr for 6 hours) to remove thromboembolic material. PAT is best suited for treating iatrogenic emboli resulting from intra-arterial catheterization or balloon angioplasty but can be used as a supplement to Fogarty embolectomy when retained distal clot cannot be retrieved by surgical means and for removal of primary distal emboli of peripheral vascular or cardiac origin. PAT was used in 42 patients with acute threatening limb ischemia. Successful clot retrieval and limb salvage were achieved in 40 of the 42 patients (95%). The major complication was groin hematoma (7 of 42 patients, 17%) and one death occurred as a result of myocardial infarction (2.4%). PAT enhances the therapeutic role of angiography and can be used as an alternative to surgical embolectomy in selected patients.

Pulsed–spray thrombolysis of arterial and bypass graft occlusions.
Valji K; Roberts AC; Davis GB; Bookstein JJ. AJR 1991; 156: 617–621.

Pulsed-spray thrombolysis is accomplished through forceful injection of a spray of highly concentrated urokinase into clot by using catheters with multiple side holes. We previously reported the immediate technical efficacy of the method in eight arterial and 10 bypass graft occlusions. We now describe the clinical efficacy of the method in a second, larger series of 23 native artery occlusions and 25 bypass graft occlusions. Transluminal angioplasty was performed after thrombolysis in 21 of the arteries and 24 of the bypass grafts. Initial thrombolysis was observed in all artery occlusions and all but one bypass graft occlusion with an average time for pulsed-spray lysis of 65 +/− 28 min in native arteries and 93 +/− 38 min in bypass grafts. Recanalization with improvement in symptoms or distal pulses after thrombolysis and angioplasty was achieved in 74% of treated arterial occlusions and 92% of treated graft occlusions. Of the 15 arteries that were recanalized and did not require adjunctive surgery, seven remained patent at 3–28 months follow-up. Nine of 23 recanalized bypass grafts required early adjunctive surgery. Of the nine synthetic and five saphenous vein grafts successfully recanalized and not requiring surgical revision, the mean patency was 4.3 +/− 3.1 months and 3.0 +/− 2.2 months, respectively. Minor complications were seen in 23% of cases. The two major complications (4%) involved one groin hematoma requiring surgery and one episode of gastrointestinal hemorrhage. We conclude that combined pulsed-spray thrombolysis and angioplasty achieve rapid and consistent arterial and graft recanalization with minimal risk. The method offers a favorable alternative to standard thrombolytic therapy of arterial occlusions. (Abstract truncated)

Urokinase versus streptokinase in local thrombolysis.
Van Breda A; Katzen BT; Deutsch AS. Radiology 1987; 165: 109–111.

In a retrospective analysis, the efficacy of lysis, the degree of systemic thrombolytic effect, and the rate of complications during local thrombolytic therapy with either streptokinase (SK) or urokinase (UK) were compared in 47 patients. There were 24 infusions of each agent; one patient in the UK group received two infusions. The overall efficacy of lysis was better in the UK-treated group (8o% vs. 63%). The UK group had a lower frequency of systemic thrombolytic effect and of bleeding complications SK antibody titers were measured in all patients who received infusions. Patients with high titers who were treated with SK responded poorly (20% lysis); patients with low titers responded at a rate equal to that of UK-treated patients. Three patients with high titers of SK antibodies did not respond to SK, but subsequent successful lysis did occur with UK. In conclusion, UK is believed to be preferable to SK for local thrombolytic therapy due to increased efficacy of lysis and decreased rate of systemic fibrinolytic effect and bleeding complications.

Use of thrombolytic drugs in non-coronary disorders.
Verstraete M. Drugs 1989; 38: 801–821.

Clinical experience with thrombolytics in non-coronary disorders is limited to the plasminogen activators streptokinase, urokinase and alteplase; therapeutic trials with anistreplase (APSAC) are almost, and with saruplase completely, limited to acute myocardial infarction. In terms of thrombus clearance, thrombolytic drugs are superior to heparin in patients with recent deep vein thrombosis in the pelvis or lower limbs. In aggregate, thrombi younger than 8 days are lysed in approximately 60% of patients treated with streptokinase, urokinase or alteplase. The results of studies assessing the subsequent development of the postphlebitic syndrome are conflicting, but most suggest that thrombolytic therapy can reduce symptoms of chronic venous insufficiency. Currently, the combination of systemic thrombolytic drugs followed by heparin is recommended for patients with acute major pulmonary embolism who are haemodynamically unstable. Streptokinase, urokinase and alteplase have all been shown to accelerate the lysis of pulmonary emboli and to decrease pulmonary vascular obstruction and pulmonary hypertension. Systemic venous or intrapulmonary infusions of alteplase offers the same benefit in terms of angiographic and haemodynamic improvement. A short infusion of 100 mg alteplase over 2 hours seems to be superior to a 24-hour infusion of urokinase. None of the thrombolytic trials in pulmonary embolism have been large enough to demonstrate a reduction in mortality. It is now generally accepted that, unless contraindicated, thrombolytic therapy is the front-line treatment for patients with massive pulmonary embolism and major haemodynamic disturbance. The local treatment of acute arterial occlusion in limb arteries results in rapid clearing of the artery in 67% of patients treated with streptokinase; the corresponding success rates for urokinase and alteplase are 81% and 88 to 94%, respectively. The main question appears to be the identification of patients in whom local thrombolysis is the treatment of choice, as opposed to established therapeutic modalities. Thrombolytic treatment following a major ischaemic stroke is hazardous, although clinical improvement has been noted in a minority of patients with recanalised cerebral arteries. The safety and efficacy of thrombolytic treatment remains unproven for this indication, and its use must be restricted to experimental protocols. Thrombolytic treatment in retinal artery or vein occlusion has, in practice, been abandoned. (132 Refs.)

[Intra-arterial thrombolysis with the combination of urokinase and lysyl-plasminogen. 27 cases of acute arterial obliteration of the lower limbs] Thrombolyse intra-arterielle par l'association urokinase-lysyl-plasminoge ne.
Vitoux JF; Pernes JM; Roncato M; Aiach M; Fiessinger JN; Gaux JC; Housset E. Rev Med Interne 1984; 5: 255–261.

Twenty-five in situ thrombolysis using Lysyl Plasminogen and low doses of urokinase were performed on 25 acute, recent and severe arterial occlusion of lower limbs. Early success were 56% and 44% with a follow up of 5 months. Complications were very limited. Thus the thrombolytic treatment used in this study appears as effective as locally administered streptokinase but higher tolerated. It seems to be able to win one of the best places in the treatment of the arterial disease of the lower limbs.

[Treatment with the urokinase-lysyl plasminogen combination of developmental outbreaks of arteriopathies] Traitement par l'association urokinase-lysyl-plasminogene des poussees evolutives des arteriopathies.
Vitoux JF; Roncato M; Pernes JM; Fiessinger JN; Aiach M; Gaux JC. Ann Med Interne (Paris) 1986; 137: 105–107.

Thirty patients with acute severe lower limb arterial obstruction were treated with local administration of low dose Urokinase associated with Lysyl Plasminogen. Fifty-three percent primary and 40 p. 100 secondary successes were obtained with few complications but one death due to cerebral embolism related to the catheterisation procedure. This intra-arterial therapeutic association seems to be as effective as local streptokinase infusion, but it is much better tolerated than other forms of treatment. It could be the treatment of choice in acute occlusive arterial disease of the lower limbs providing the therapeutic indications are strictly respected.

II. Synopses of Pertinent Articles

D. Renal, Hepatic, Visceral Occlusions, Aortic

**Local thrombolytic therapy for hepatic artery thrombosis
following chemotherapy infusion catheter placement.**
*Andrews JC; Griggs TJ; Ensminger WD; Gyves JW; Cho KJ. Invest Radiol
1987; 22: 467–471.*

Nine patients with hepatic artery thrombosis subsequent to catheter placement (four surgical and five percutaneous) for hepatic arterial infusion
chemotherapy were treated with local thrombolytic therapy. The thromboses were located in the common hepatic, proper hepatic and hepatic arteries.
Thrombolytic therapy was instituted within seven days of catheter placement, at a rate of 5,000 to 20,000 units/hour (streptokinase) or 5,000 to
15,000 units/hour (urokinase) for 15 to 64 hours. All patients had repeat
angiography and 99mTc-MAA hepatic artery perfusion scintigraphy after
the infusion. In eight of the patients, thrombolytic therapy resulted in dissolution of the thrombus and recanalization of the hepatic artery. In three of
these patients, rethrombosis occurred within a few days, and was attributed
to underlying arterial abnormalities. The other five had documented continued hepatic arterial patency allowing completion of the chemotherapy
course. The patient who did not respond to the lytic therapy had developed
extensive collateral flow through the gastroduodenal artery to the liver.

**Portal thrombosis: percutaneous transhepatic treatment with
urokinase—a case report.**
*Bilbao JI; Rodriguez-Cabello J; Longo J; Zornoza G; Paramo J; Lecumberri
FJ. Gastrointest Radiol 1989; 14: 326–328.*

We present a case report of a patient suffering from portal and superior
mesenteric vein thrombosis secondary to splenectomy. No surgical procedure could be performed due to the extension of thrombus. Local fibrinolysis
treatment with urokinase through a percutaneous transhepatic approach
was decided upon, and this procedure had a successful patient outcome.

**Response of an abdominal aortic thrombotic occlusion to local
low-dose streptokinase therapy.**
*Cunningham MW; May S; Tucker WY; Gerlock AJ Jr. Surgery 1983; 93:
541–544.*

Local low-dose streptokinase infusion (5000 to 6000 IU/hr) as compared to
systemic streptokinase infusion (loading dose 250,000 IU/hr. maintenance
dose 100,000 IU/hr) successfully relieved a total thrombotic abdominal aortic occlusion complications of bleeding or distal embolization occurred during streptokinase therapy, which required only 8 days of hospitalization.

When seen at 4 months after streptokinase infusion, the patient was free of symptoms. When no immediate threat of ischemic limb exists, streptokinase may offer a promising therapeutic surgical intervention for patients who represent a poor operative risk.

Acute occlusion of the left renal artery manifested by hypertensive crisis.
Dell'Aria JC; Petrilli R; Schwartz E. J Emerg Med 1988; 6: 23–27.

Because the signs and symptoms of acute renal artery occlusion mimic those of many more common diseases, prompt diagnosis is aided by an awareness that an occlusive renovascular event may have occurred. No routine, noninvasive laboratory test can confirm the diagnosis. Renal arteriography is the procedure of choice after excretory urograms have ruled out an obstructive uropathy. Early assessment of kidney viability is important. The endpoints of emergency treatment are to decrease symptoms, decrease diastolic blood pressure to less than or equal to 105 mm Hg, and to maintain urine output at greater than 50 mL/h. Restoration of a lower blood pressure must not be so prompt that renal perfusion decreases too rapidly. Definitive surgical treatment versus medical management of the renal artery occlusion remains a controversial topic. Where surgery is not feasible, medical management consists of streptokinase acutely followed by heparin and then chronic coumarin therapy.

Failure of systemic thrombolytic and heparin therapy in the treatment of neonatal aortic thrombosis.
Emami A; Saldanha R; Knupp C; Kodroff M. Pediatrics 1987; 79: 773–777.

An unsuccessful attempt was made to lyse a large aortic thrombus in a newborn using systemic high-dose streptokinase and urokinase therapy and subsequently the use of heparin failed to prevent the propagation of thrombus. The patient was a seven-day old premature, sick neonate in whom an aortic thrombosis developed following umbilical artery catheterization. Surgical thrombectomy could not be performed in this patient, and local thrombolytic therapy was not technically feasible. Systemic thrombolytic therapy failed to induce any notable clinical or laboratory response, and the use of heparin failed to prevent thrombus extension. Experience with the use of fibrinolytic agents in neonates is limited. Local therapy has been variably effective, and systemic therapy has not been adequately investigated. The thrombotic phenomenon in neonates and the role of umbilical vessel catheterization as a cause are discussed in reference to this patient and suggestions are made regarding the management of similar cases.

Renal artery embolism treated with intra-arterial streptokinase infusion results in patent but small renal arteries.
Frey FJ; Stirnemann P; Fritschi P; Mahler F. Am J Nephrol 1986; 6: 214–216.

A low intra-arterial dose of streptokinase was used to dissolve a renal artery embolus in 2 patients. Angiography at the end of the streptokinase therapy disclosed patent renal arteries. Arteriograms performed 3 months and 2 years later demonstrated patent but small renal arteries. These cases confirm the limited experience reported in the literature that even though initial restoration of renal artery patency is possible, the ultimate renal function is poor after intra-arterial streptokinase therapy.

Local infusion of low-dose streptokinase for renal artery thromboembolism.

Gagnon RF; Horosko F; Herba MJ. Can Med Assoc J 1984; 131: 1089–1091.

Although local low-dose therapy with streptokinase has been found to be effective in patients with recent arterial occlusions, there have been few reports of its use in those with renal artery occlusion, perhaps because this condition is difficult to diagnose early. This paper describes a patient with acute renal artery thromboembolism and intermittent tachyarrhythmias in whom treatment with a local low-dose infusion of streptokinase resulted in complete recanalization of the main artery and good recovery of renal function.

Renal artery embolism: clinical features and therapeutic options.

Gasparini M; Hofmann R; Stoller M. J Urol 1992; 147(3): 567–572.

Local urokinase infusion for total occlusion of the lower abdominal aorta. Report of two cases and a review of the literature.

Goffette P; Kurdziel JC; Dondelinger RF. Eur J Radiol 1989; 9: 121–124.

Two patients with acute occlusion of the lower abdominal aorta have been successfully treated with total of 7,425,000 and 8,850,000 units of urokinase infused locally over 93 and 86 hours respectively, with restoration of flow. No complications occurred.

Neonatal aortic thrombosis treated with intra-arterial urokinase therapy.

Goldberg RE; Cohen AM; Bryan PJ; Olsen M; Martin RJ. Can Assoc Radiol J 1989; 40: 55–56.

We report a newborn infant with neonatal aortic thrombosis (a complication of umbilical artery catheterization) successfully treated by intra-arterial urokinase therapy.

Successful thrombolysis of an aortic-arch thrombus in a patient after mesenteric embolism (letter).

Hausmann D; Gulba D; Bargheer K; Niedermeyer J; Comess KA; Daniel WG. N Engl J Med 1992; 327(7): 500–501.

High-dose intra-arterial urokinase for the treatment of hepatic artery thrombosis in liver transplantation.

Hidalgo EG; Abad J; Cantarero JM; Fernandez R; Parga G; Jover JM; Manzanares J; Moreno E. Hepatogastroenterology 1989; 36: 529–532.

Two recipients of orthotopic liver transplants (OLT) underwent intra arterial thrombolytic treatment for hepatic artery thrombosis. Complete clot lysis was achieved in both using infusion of high-dose urokinase directly into the thrombus for 12 and 3 hours, respectively. Percutaneous transluminal angioplasty (PTA) was later carried out successfully on various strictures. Doppler ultrasonography confirmed arterial permeability one month after treatment. Liver transplantation is now an accepted therapeutic option in some patients with irreversible liver failure. Although the results of this procedure have improved radically since cyclosporine was introduced in 1978, life-threatening postoperative complications still occur. The one with the worst prognosis is hepatic artery thrombosis (HAT), with 64% mortality despite retransplantation. HAT was found in 7.4% of liver transplant recipients in a recent review of the most important group of these patients. Fibrinolytic treatment using an exogenous plasminogen activator, urokinase (UK), is effective and safe in the thrombotic obstruction of acute pulmonary embolism, acute myocardial infarction, and graft or peripheral arterial occlusion. We used intra-arterial thrombolysis in two patients with HAT of the liver graft, to avoid retransplantation and to treat a complication secondary to percutaneous transluminal angioplasty (PTA) of an anastomotic stricture, respectively. To our knowledge, this is the first report of treatment of HAT by direct infusion of urokinase in liver transplantation.

Brachial approach to management of an abdominal aortic occlusion with prolonged lysis and subsequent angioplasty.
Iyer SS; Hall P; Dorros G. Cathet Cardiovasc Diagn 1991; 23: 290–293.

The brachial approach for recanalizing an abdominal aortic occlusion utilizing a combination of thrombolysis and balloon angioplasty is described. The patient was deemed too ill to permit any surgical intervention. The unique aspects of the procedure are described including angioplasty of the unmasked (by lytic therapy) aortoiliac bifurcation stenoses utilizing double wires and double balloons through a single arteriotomy site. The advantages of the brachial approach in managing this unusual entity are outlined.

Percutaneous transcatheter recanalization in the management of acute renal failure due to sudden occlusion of the renal artery to a solitary kidney.
Kadir S; Watson A; Burrow C. Am J Nephrol 1987; 7: 445–449.

Percutaneous angioplasty was attempted in 5 patients with acute renal failure due to occlusion of the artery to a solitary functioning kidney. Angioplasty was technically successful in all patients. Renal function was completely restored in 3 and renal perfusion improved in 1 patient. In the fifth patient, renal function did not return despite ultrasound and radionuclide scan evidence of renal reperfusion. Transcatheter thrombolytic therapy was attempted in 2 patients, 1 of whom also underwent angioplasty. In this patient, perfusion was restored to most of the kidney. In the other patient an infrarenal aortic occlusion was present. During thrombolytic therapy, intrarenal microembolization occurred from lysis of the aortic thrombus, leading to irreversible renal damage.

**[Intra–arterial fibrinolysis of superior mesenteric artery embolism]
Fibrinolyse intra-arterielle d'une embolie de l'artere mesenterique
superieure.**
*Rodde A; Peiffert B; Bazin C; Amrein D; Regent D; Mathieu P. J Radiol
1991; 72: 239–242.*

Intra arterial fibrinolysis for acute mesenteric embolism. Acute mesenteric
ischemia has a poor prognosis because the diagnosis is often too late (greater
than 12 h), leading to a difficult surgery in old patients. The lesions of the
bowel don't always allow a single operative embolectomy but often need a
resection when there is a long time interval between onset of symptoms and
therapy. We report a case of acute embolism in the superior mesenteric
artery with the clot located in its terminal part. A rapid diagnosis was made
by arteriography and intra-arterial fibrinolysis was attempted with success
permitting the complete cure of the affection, without sequellae. This treatment is only likely to be successful if it is carried out within 10–12 hours
of the onset of clinical signs and symptoms.

**[Local fibrinolysis in renal artery occlusion] Die lokale Fibrinolyse
bei Nierenarterienverschlussen.**
*Schunk K; Schild H; Wandel E; Schinzel H; Weingartner K. ROFO 1990;
152: 147–150.*

The indications and technique of local fibrinolysis therapy of acute renal
artery occlusions are discussed in relation to four patients. Because of the
short period for which ischaemia is tolerated by the kidney, the result of
treatment depends largely on the time interval between occlusion and the
beginning of treatment. Partial perfusion of the renal artery was obtained
in three patients. Since the "ischaemia time" of the kidneys had been exceeded, it was not possible to obtain complete restitution of renal function
in any of these patients.

**Recovery of function in a solitary kidney after intra-arterial
thrombolytic therapy.**
*Skinner RE; Hefty T; Long TD; Rosch J; Forsyth M. J Urol 1989; 141:
108–110.*

Renal artery thromboembolism is a rare event that most often occurs in
patients with cardiac dysrhythmias. Surgical thromboembolectomy is risky
and medical therapy with intra-arterial thrombolytic agents has become
increasingly popular. Although successful clot dissolution has been well
documented, renal function often is not recovered. We describe a patient
with anuria from thromboembolism to a solitary kidney, treated with low
dose intra-arterial streptokinase infusion. There were no adverse effects
from therapy and renal function returned to a point where dialysis was no
longer required. A review of the literature is included with special attention
to various protocols for infusion. Early diagnosis and prompt initiation of
therapy may result in clinically significant recovery of renal function.

Acute renal vein thrombosis: successful treatment with intraarterial urokinase.
Vogelzang RL; Moel DI; Cohn RA; Donaldson JS; Langman CB; Nemcek AA Jr. Radiology 1988; 169: 681–682.

When acute renal vein thrombosis associated with renal failure, aggressive therapy to eliminate the venous obstruction is indicated. There are reports of successful treetment of this condition with thrombolytic agents adminis-tered systemically or directly into the renal vein. Renal arterial administra-tion of urokinase was used successfully to treat acute renal vein thrombosis associated with renal failure in a 9 ½-year-old child.

Intraarterial low-dose streptokinase infusion in the treatment of acute renal thromboembolism.
Wilms G; Vermylen J; Baert A. Eur J Radiol 1987; 7: 72–74.

A case of acute renal thromboembolism treated by intraarterial low dose streptokinase infusion is reported. The treatment appears effective, safe and less-invasive then surgery, with quick relief of pain and normalisation of blood pressure and renal function. It is concluded that intraarterial infusion of thrombolytic agents should be attempted first in the treatment of renal arterial thrombo-embolism.

II. Synopses of Pertinent Articles

E. Brachiocephalic: Subclavian, Carotid, Ultracranial

**[Thrombolysis in acute occlusion of cerebral blood vessels]
Thrombolyse beim akuten Verschluss zerebraler Gefasse.**
Adelwohrer C; Bohm-Jurkovic H; Brucker B; Deisenhammer E; Laich E; Loffler W; Markut H; Migl F; Nada E; Sommer R; et al. Wien Klin Wochenschr 1991; 103: 197–200.

Thrombolysis may achieve recanalization in cases of occlusion of the cerebral vessels. If therapy is initiated in good time, development of cerebral infarction may be at least partially prevented. Thrombolytic treatment was performed in 14 patients at the Wagner-Jauregg Hospital within a period of one year. Urokinase was given locally, while rtPA was applied locally and/or systemically. 4 patients had an occlusion of the internal carotid artery, 6 an occlusion of the middle cerebral artery, and 4 an occlusion of the basilar artery. Complete recanalization was achieved in 6 patients, partial recanalization in 4, and no recanalization in 4. The neurological outcome of the cases with complete recanalization was good with the exception of one patients who died. Partial recanalization resulted in a fair outcome in 2 patients, while the other 2 died. 3 out of the 4 patients in whom no recanalization was achieved died. Our findings show that this form of therapy may considerably improve the natural history of the disease, provided recanalization is achieved in good time. They encourage us to continue this form of therapy and to work at improving the therapeutic criteria.

Local thrombolytic therapy for thromboembolic occlusion o the middle cerebral artery.
Berg Dammer E; Mobius E; Nahser HC; Kuhne D. Neurol Res 1992; 14(2 Suppl): 164–166.

We report on 10 patients with thromboembolic occlusion of the middle cerebral artery (MCA) who underwent local thrombolytic therapy. Six patients developed a MCA occlusion during long-standing interventional neuroradiological procedures, while four had a proven or suspected cardio-embolic stroke. Streptokinase or urokinase was applied by a microcatheter placed into the thrombus within six hours of clinical onset. Complete or partial revascularization was achieved in all patients. Recovery was complete in seven and partial in three of the patients. In two patients, minor haemorrhagic transformation of the infarct occurred, which did not lead to neurological deterioration. It is concluded that in a selected group of patients with MCA occlusion, local thrombolytic therapy represents a safe and effective therapy.

Putaminal haemorrhage after recanalization of an embolic MCA occlusion treated with tissue plasminogen activator.
Bruckmann H; Ferbert A. Neuroradiology 1989; 31: 95–97.

We present the case of a 42-year-old female, who suffered an embolic occlusion of the right middle cerebral artery (MCA). Recanalization was achieved with tissue plasminogen activator (t-PA) within 7 h after onset of stroke. Post-TPA infusion angiographic and CT examinations revealed fragmentation of the thrombus and a small putaminal haemorrhage associated with early reperfusion of the MCA. No clinical deterioration was observed and complete recovery occurred within 10 days.

Vascular recanalizing techniques in the hind brain circulation.
Bruckmann HJ; Ringelstein EB; Buchner H; Zeumer H. Neurosurg Rev 1987; 10: 197–198, 200.

Percutaneous transluminal angioplasty (PTA) was performed in 45 patients with a manifest subclavian steal syndrome. Thirty-five of those patients were subjected to follow up examinations over a period of 6 to 18 months. Five patients suffered from severe restenosis and were treated again. Two thirds of the patients benefited from the treatment. PTA of the proximal vertebral artery was performed in 15 patients with bilateral occlusive lesions of the extracranial vertebral arteries. In 13 of these cases the neurological and the vascular states of the patients were regularly reexamined, 8 showed a marked improvement. During the 2 to 25 month observation period (average 15 months post-PTA) reocclusion was observed in only two cases. These showed no recurrent neurological sequelae. Forty-three consecutive patients with acute vertebro-basilar or basilar occlusion received intraarterial fibrinolytic therapy with streptokinase or urokinase. Twenty-three of these had presented severe deficits at the beginning of therapy (e g. complete tetraplegia, comatous state for more than 6 hours). None of this group survived. By contrast the 20 other patients in this group presented with incomplete fluctuating or progressive motor deficits. None was comatous for more than 6 hours. Fourteen patients (33% in this group) survived. Local intraarterial fibrinolytic therapy is the only therapy successful in the treatment of progressive stroke from vertebro-basilar thrombosis.

Intra-arteral thrombolytic therapy improves outcome in patients with acute vertebrobasilar occlusive disease.
Hacke W; Zeumer H; Ferbert A; Bruckmann H; Del Zoppo GJ. Stroke 1988; 19: 1216–1222.

In this retrospective analysis we report our treatment experience in 65 consecutive patients with clinical signs of severe brainstem ischemia with angiographically demonstrated thrombotic vertebrobasilar artery occlusions who received either local intra-arterial thrombolytic therapy (urokinase or streptokinase) (43 patients) or conventional therapy (antiplatelet agents or anticoagulants) (22 patients). We analyzed the data with respect to cerebral artery occlusion patterns, posttreatment arterial recanalization, and the clinical categories of favorable/unfavorable outcome and survival/death. In subgroup analyses, recanalization in patients who received thrombolytic therapy correlated significantly with clinical outcome; in 19 of 43 patients, recanalization was demonstrated angiographically, while in 24 patients the occlusion persisted. All patients without recanalization died, but 14 of the 19 patients displaying recanalization survived (p = 0.000007), 10 with a favorable clinical outcome. Only three of the 22 patients who received conventional therapy survived, all with a moderate clinical deficit. When we compared the treatment groups, highly significant differences in both outcome quality (p = 0.017) and survival (p = 0 0005) were found to depend on establishing recanalazation. Our data support the concept that technically successful thrombolysis of vertebrobasilar artery occlusions is associated with beneficial clinical outcome.

[Regional lysis of acute basilar artery occlusion—case report]
Regionale Lyse eines akuten Basilarisarterienverschlusses—ein Fallbericht.
Karnik R; Perneczky G; Ammerer HP; Brenner H; Slany J. Wien Klin Wochenschr 1984; 96: 26–30.

Thrombosis of the basilar artery is not a rare disease, and the mortality is reported to be 60 to 80%. Present standard therapy with heparin infusions yields poor results. The high risk of intracerebral haemorrhage prohibits systemic fibrinolytic therapy. Due to these facts and good experience in our department with the use of local intracoronary lysis in acute myocardial infarction, the method of local thrombolysis was applied in a case of acute basilar artery thrombosis. Fibrinolytic therapy was started via an angiography catheter placed in the vertebral artery in a 28 year-old woman with hemiplegia and severe brain stem symptoms. The patient received 200,000 IU streptokinase within 2 hours and subsequently 300,000 IU urokinase within 10 hours. The vessel re-opened completely. The neurological symptoms decreased during the following weeks. Based on this experience and according to rare reports in the literature we believe local low-dose thrombolysis to be a causal therapy promising success for acute thrombosis of the basilar artery. This therapy can be carried out in every medical centre able to perform selective angiography and experienced in the administration of fibrinolytic drugs.

Transcranial Doppler sonography monitoring of local intra-arterial thrombolysis in acute occlusion of the middle cerebral artery.
Karnik R; Stelzer P; Slany J. Stroke 1992; 23(2): 284–287.

BACKGROUND AND PURPOSE: The aim of this study is to report on the use of transcranial Doppler ultrasonography as a noninvasive diagnostic monitoring tool during local intra-arterial thrombolysis in a patient with acute embolic occlusion of the middle cerebral artery. CASE DESCRIPTION: We describe a 41-year-old woman with mitral valve stenosis suffering from embolism of the middle cerebral artery. Local thrombolysis was performed with tissue plasminogen activator at a dosage of 0.05 mg/kg/hr. Progress of the thrombolysis was monitored by transcranial Doppler. The steps of recanalization could be ascertained by transcranial ultrasound showing a hemodynamically relevant residual stenosis after the first 120 minutes and complete patency of the M1 segment of the middle cerebral artery 180 minutes later. One branch of the middle cerebral artery still showed a filling defect. CONCLUSIONS: Our report demonstrates the potential usefulness of transcranial Doppler monitoring during thrombolysis of a proximal occlusion of the middle cerebral artery for guiding the treatment by assessing the reperfusion of the obstructed artery.

Thrombolytic therapy and posterior circulation extracranial-intracranial bypass for acute basilar artery thrombosis. Case report.
Morgan JK; Sadasivan B; Ausman JI; Mehta B. Surg Neurol 1990; 33: 43–47.

Basilar artery thrombosis has a very poor prognosis. A 56-year-old comatose man with acute basilar artery occlusion was successfully treated with local urokinase infusion which reopened the basilar artery and revealed a mid-basilar stenotic plaque. This procedure was followed by a superficial temporal artery to superior cerebellar artery anastomosis for protection of the posterior circulation.

Carotid urokinase with thromboembolic occlusion of the middle cerebral artery.
Mori E; Tabuchi M; Yoshida T; Yamadori A. Stroke 1988; 19: 802–812.

Intracarotid urokinase infusion therapy was performed on 22 patients with evolving cerebral infarction due to acute thromboembolic occlusion of the middle cerebral artery. Mean time from onset of symptoms to start of infusion and mean dosage of urokinase were 4.5 hours and 927,000 units, respectively. Immediate recanalization was achieved in 10 patients (45%) after urokanase therapy. In patients with successful recanalization, rapid amelioration of symptoms followed the restoration of blood flow. Thrombolytic recanalization was associated with reduction of neurologic deficits and of computed tomography-demonstrable infarction volume. The reduction of infarction volume and functional outcome correlated highly with the degree of reflow. Hemorrhagic transformation of infarction occurred in four patients and controllable extracranial bleeding in three patients. These results support the safety and efficacy of urokinase therapy for acute thromboembolic occlusion of the middle cerebral artery.

Intraarterial thrombolytic therapy in acute stroke.
Poeck K. Acta Neurol Belg 1988; 88: 35–45.

Intraarterial thrombolytic therapy by means of urokinase has proved to be effective and safe in certain instances of acute thromboembolic occlusion of the vertabral and/or the basilar artery. Small hemorrhages have not led to deterioration on the patients, neurological state. In the territory of the carotid artery local thrombolytic therapy may be effective in very selected cases of acute thromboembolic occlusion. There is a high risk of intracerebral hemorrhage. Possibly intravenous administration of tPA will replace local intraarterial thrombolysis, provided a strict regimen is established for selection of patients, determination of dosage and time constraints for the application of this therapy.

Reproducibility of noninvasive ultrasonic measurement of carotid atherosclerosis. The Asymptomatic Carotid Artery Plaque Study.
Riley WA; Barnes RW; Applegate WB; Dempsey R; Hartwell T; Davis VG; Bond MG; Furberg CD. Stroke 1992; 23(8): 1062–1068.

BACKGROUND AND PURPOSE: To determine the effect of a lipid-lowering agent and/or a low-dose antithrombotic agent on the progression of early-stage carotid atherosclerosis, noninvasive B-mode ultrasound was used to measure intimal-medial thickness in asymptomatic individuals with moderately elevated lipids as part of the ongoing multicenter Asymptomatic Carotid Artery Plaque Study. METHODS: Uniform ultrasonic scanning and reading protocols were implemented to obtain maximum intimal-medial thickness measurements in 12 standard segments in patients having a small to moderate wall thickness (1.5–3.5 mm) in at least one of the carotid arteries. Paired B-mode image recordings on 858 patients, performed 1 month apart and read at a core laboratory (each pair by the same reader), determined both within-sonographer (W, n = 405) and between-sonographer (B, n = 453) reproducibility. RESULTS: The primary end point (mean ± SD), defined in each individual as the mean value of the 12 maximum intimal-medial thickness measurements, was 1.31 ± 0.21 mm (W) and 1.32 ± 0.22 (B) at the time of the second examination. The mean difference in the primary end point (exam 2-exam 1) was −0.01 ± 0.13 mm (W) and 0.00 ± 0.15 mm (B). The Pearson correlation coefficients were 0.79 (W) and 0.75 (B). In 90% of the patients, the absolute difference in the primary end point was less than 0.22 mm (W) and less than 0.24 mm (B). Variability of the secondary end point, defined as the single largest intimal-medial thickness measurement in a patient, was between three and four times larger than the variability for the primary end point. Differences in sonographer performance between clinical centers were very small. CONCLUSIONS: The results demonstrate that standardized noninvasive ultrasonic techniques yield highly reproducible measures of carotid intimal-medial thickness, which can serve as a measure of carotid atherosclerosis in clinical trials that monitor small rates of lesion progression.

[Intra-arterial fibrinolysis in central artery occlusion]
Intraarterielle Fibrinolyse bei Zentralarterienverschluss.
Schumacher M; Schmidt D; Wakhloo AK. Radiologe 1991; 31: 240–243.

Central retinal artery occlusion is known to have a poor natural outcome, and also conventional therapeutic procedures e.g. paracentesis, hemodilution or local massage show unfavorable results. As in intraarterial fibrinolytic therapy in cerebral vessels, we also applied this method to the territory of the ophthalmic artery in 6 patients with occlusion of the central retinal artery. The fibrinolysis was done with a microcatheter superselectively, placed in the proximal part of the opthalmic artery. The amount of urokinase varied from 200,000 to 900,000 IU, diluted in saline solution. In 5 patients, fluorescein angiography was carried out before and after fibrinolytic therapy, confirming the significant improvement of retinal and choroidal perfusion seen on the arterial ophthalmic angiogram. All patients showed an improvement of visual function after therapy, two patients even had a complete recovery of visual acuity.

Treatment of a case of thromboembolism resulting from thoracic outlet syndrome with intra-arterial urokinase infusion.
Sullivan KL; Minken SL; White RI Jr. J Vasc Surg 1988; 7: 568–571.

A 36-year-old man with thoracic outlet syndrome, admitted to the hospital with digital ischemia from subclavian artery thrombosis and distal embolization, was given intra-arterial urokinase. Thrombus in the subclavian artery was lysed successfully and peripheral emboli were partially cleared, resulting in relief of digital symptoms. Although surgical decompression and vascular reconstruction at the thoracic outlet may be necessary, this technique provides a means of recanalizing small distal vessels.

Local intraarterial fibrinolysis in the carotid territory.
Theron J; Courtheoux P; Casasco A; Alachkar F; Notari F; Ganem F; Maiza D. AJNR 1989; 10: 753–765.

A series comprising 12 patients who had intraarterial local fibrinolysis in the carotid territory is reported. A classification is proposed that divides the different types of occlusions into three groups on the basis of angiographic location. Group 1 (two cases) comprises occlusion of the extra- and/or intracranial carotid artery with patency of the circle of Willis and the lenticulostriate arteries. In this group, there is no brain infarction, the CT findings are normal, and the clinical signs are mainly hemodynamic and intermittent. Fibrinolysis may be performed late and rather safely and completed by surgery or angioplasty of the neck vessel stenosis responsible for the occlusion. Group 2 (five cases) comprises occlusions of the cortical arteries without involvement of the lenticulostriate arteries. The mechanism of the occlusion can be hemodynamic or embolic. Group 3 (five cases) comprises occlusions of intracerebral arteries involving the lenticulostriate arteries. In groups 2 and 3 with brain infarction, fibrinolysis will only be able to restore viability of the area of cerebral tissue surrounding the infarction (penumbra). The time factor is particularly critical in group 3 because lenticulostriate arteries are terminal vessels whose revascularization may induce hemorrhages with increasing frequency as the occlusion time is prolonged. The time factor is less critical in group 2 because collaterals make the ischemia less severe in the infarcted area and the vital and functional consequences of hemorrhage are not as serious as in group 3 because of the location. In this series, all the symptomatic complications of hemorrhage (two cases) occurred in group 3, in patients treated later than 6 hr after clinical onset. Given the time delay inherent in performing CT and angiography and in making the medical decision, it is considered dangerous to undertake fibrinolytic therapy in group 3, unless it can be started before 4 or 5 hr after clinical onset.

Fibrinolytic therapy for upper-extremity arterial occlusions.
Widlus DM; Venbrux AC; Benenati JF; Mitchell SE; Lynch-Nyhan A: Cassidy FP Jr; Osterman FA Jr. Radiology 1990; 175: 393–399.

Acute upper-extremity arterial occlusion may be due to embolic phenomena or de novo thrombosis. If the occlusion is left untreated, claudication or ischemia necessitating amputation can occur. Operative Fogarty-balloon embolectomy has been the treatment of choice for this entity. In a 6-year period the authors used fibrinolysis on nine occasions in eight patients to treat acute upper-extremity arterial occlusions. Concomitant balloon angioplasty was helpful in four cases. Success, defined as a normal hand with at least one artery that was continuously patent to the wrist, was achieved in all patients. A single significant groin hematoma was seen. Neither stroke nor death occurred in any case, and no amputations were necessary. Local transcatheter intraarterial administration of urokinase can be considered a first-line treatment for brachial artery embolus and other causes of acute upper-extremity arterial occlusion.

Vascular recanalizing techniques in interventional neuroradiology.
Zeumer H. J Neurol 1985; 231: 287–294.

Vascular recanalizing techniques only recently became methods of some clinical importance. Angioplasty of the subclavian artery in cases with subclavion steal syndrome has now been performed in so many instances that it can be judged safe. Angioplasty at the origin of the vertebral artery has not yet been performed in as many cases. However, even there this method is obviously less hazardous than surgery. Local intraarterial fibrinolytic therapy is the only therapy providing some success in progressive stroke from vertebrobasilar thrombosis. In contrast to the vertebrobasilar territory local fibrinolytic therapy within the carotid territory has to be strictly limited to some special indications.

Local intraarterial fibrinolytic therapy in inaccessible internal carotid occlusion.
Zeumer H; Hundgen R; Ferbert A; Ringelstein EB. Neuroradiology 1984; 26: 315–317.

Two exemplary cases of upper carotid occlusion and successful local intraarterial fibrinolytic therapy are described. To achieve a positive result one has to perform a balloon occlusion of the affected internal carotid artery while applying the fibrinolytic agent. Possible time limits instigating therapy are discussed especially if the lenticulostriatal arteries are additionally affected.

II. Synopses of Pertinent Articles

F. Venous

How to select patients with deep vein thrombosis for tPA therapy.
Brown WD; Goldhaber SZ. Chest 1989; 95 (5 Suppl): 276S–278S.

Despite enthusiasm for using thrombolytic therapy to treat proximal deep venous thrombosis (DVT), the proportion of patients eligible for this therapeutic strategy is unknown. Therefore, we screened all patients at Brigham and Women's Hospital who underwent leg venography in 1987. Of 240 patients with suspected DVT, 87 (36%) had positive venograms. Of those with positive venograms, 72 (83%) had proximal DVT, and 15 (17%) had DVT limited to calf veins. Overall, 22% of patients with proximal DVT were eligible for thrombolytic therapy. The major exclusion criteria were: (2) recent trauma or surgery, (2) recent GI bleeding, and (3) history of a bleeding disorder. Thus, thrombolytic therapy could be given to approximately one-fifth of our patients with proximal DVT.

[Acute arterial occlusive syndrome in streptokinase treatment of deep venous thrombosis: successful therapy with urokinase] Das acute arterielle Verschlussyyndrom unter der Streptokinasebehandlung einer teifen Venenthrombose: erfolgreiche Therapie mit Urokinase.
Franke D; Lutze G; Presser HJ; Grungreiff K. Z Gesamte Inn Med 1987; 42: 343–346.

Arterial embolism or thrombosis are very rare complications of the fibrinolytic therapy of deep venous thrombosis. The characteristics symptoms of these illness are the acute arterial failure of the concerned extremity during venous thrombolysis. The diagnosis take place by angiography, by ultrasonics, and in particular cases by the skin thermographic method. If the arterial occlusion is not operable, the thrombolysis by urokinase is discussed. This seems to be the last possible method to support the extremity.

Thrombosed iliac venous aneurysm: a rare cause of left lower extremity venous obstruction.
Hurwitz RL; Gelabert H. J Vasc Surg 1989; 9: 822–824.

A patient who had deep venous obstruction of the left lower limb was shown to have thrombosis of a venous aneurysm of the left common iliac vein that measured 8.8 cm at the largest diameter. The aneurysm was suspected on the basis of preoperative noninvasive testing. Findings at surgery suggested the left iliac vein was being compressed by the right iliac artery. The aneurysm was resected and prosthetic graft material was used to reconstruct the venous system. A 22-month follow-up is recorded. Literature pertaining to the case is discussed.

Haemodynamics of the postphlebitic syndrome.
Schmidt C; Schmitt J; Scheffmann M. Int Angiol 1987; 6: 187–192.

The venous function has been assessed after deep vein thrombosis (DVT) by Doppler, strain gauge plethysmography (55 patients) and exercise plethysmography (10 patients) for a mean period of 63 weeks. Venous volume and venous outflow remain significantly lower throughout the study, whatever the site of thrombosis and the initial therapy (Heparin, local or general Urokinase). There are no significant correlations between clinical and functional parameters except for patients with proximal obstruction and popliteal valvular incompetence. Exercise plethysmography evaluates the importance of the calf pump in the postphlebitic syndrome. Static plethysmographic measurements prove to be unreliable for the long term prognosis whereas associated dynamic tests should be a better way to assess the haemodynamic changes after DVT and to control the efficiency of the prevention of the post-phlebitic syndrome.

Thrombectomy for acute deep vein thrombosis: prevention of postthrombotic syndrome.
Shionoya S; Yamada I; Sakurai T; Ohta T; Matsubara J. J Cardiovasc Surg 1989; 30: 484–489.

Ninety-six limbs of 89 patients with acute deep vein thrombosis of the lower extremity were followed for 1 to 18 years. In the thrombectomy group (43 limbs), the cumulative incidence of pigmentation at the 15th year was 15%, but no stasis ulcers occurred throughout the follow-up period. In the conservative treatment group (53 limbs), the cumulative incidence of pigmentation at the 15th year was 41%, and that of stasis ulceration was 27%. Fogarty thrombectomy restricted below the pelvic vein spur and removal of thrombi in the leg veins by manual milking is sufficient to relieve early morbidity, preserve venous valve function, and promote intrapelvic collateral circulation. Preservation of venous valves in the femoropopliteal region is a key to the prevention of postthrombotic syndrome. Thrombectomy within 5 days of the onset of symptoms is recommended for patients with iliofemoropopliteal venous thrombosis.

Section 5

Author Index
(Primary Authors Only)